DRUG ACTION
AT THE MOLECULAR LEVEL

1969 Cuthbert: *Calcium and Cellular Function*
1970 Aldridge: *Mechanisms of Toxicity*
1971 Rabin and Freedman: *Effects of Drugs on Cellular Control Mechanisms*
1972 Rang: *Drug Receptors*
1973 Callingham: *Drugs and Transport Processes*
1974 Parsons: *Peptide Hormones*
1975 Grahame-Smith: *Drug Interactions*

BIOLOGICAL COUNCIL
The Co-ordinating Committee for Symposia
on Drug Action

DRUG ACTION AT THE MOLECULAR LEVEL

Edited by

G. C. K. ROBERTS

*National Institute for Medical Research,
Mill Hill London*

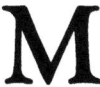

© Institute of Biology Endowment Trust Fund 1977

Softcover reprint of the hardcover 1st edition 1977

All rights reserved. No part of this publication may be reproduced or transmitted, in any form or by any means, without permission

First published 1977 by
THE MACMILLAN PRESS LTD
London and Basingstoke
Associated companies in New York   Dublin
Melbourne   Johannesburg   and   Madras

ISBN 978-1-349-03232-7   ISBN 978-1-349-03230-3 (eBook)
DOI 10.1007/978-1-349-03230-3

Typeset by Reproduction Drawings Ltd., Sutton, Surrey.

This book is sold subject to the standard conditions of the Net Book Agreement

Biological Council
Coordinating Committee for Symposia on Drug Action

Report of a symposium held on 12 and 13 April 1976 at the Middlesex Hospital Medical School, London, UK

Sponsored by:
International Union of Pharmacology
International Union of Pure and Applied Chemistry
Biochemical Society
British Biophysical Society
British Pharmacological Society
British Society for Antimicrobial Chemotherapy
British Society for Cell Biology
British Society for Immunology
Chemical Society
Pharmaceutical Society of Great Britain
Physiological Society
Royal Society of Medicine
Society of Chemical Industry (Fine Chemicals Group)
Society for Endocrinology

Organised by a committee consisting of:
G. C. K. Roberts (Chairman and Hon. Secretary)
Sir Arnold Burgen, FRS
T. J Franklin
C. R. Ganellin
D. W. Straughan

The symposium was made possible by generous donations from:
The Wellcome Trust
    and
Boehringer Ingelheim
Fisons
Imperial Chemical Industries
Eli Lilly & Co.
Parke-Davis & Co.
Roche Products
Sandoz Products
Smith Kline & French Laboratories
Syntex Pharmaceuticals

Foreword

Sir Arnold Burgen, FRS (National Institute for Medical Research,
Mill Hill, London, UK)

One of the delights of pharmacology is that its intellectual range spreads from the severely practical matters of therapeutics of human disease to inquiries at more and more penetrating levels into the way in which chemical substances can produce the biological responses which we call drug action. Inevitably the boundaries of such a subject will be ill-defined and will overlap into neighbouring disciplines. This is especially evident when one is considering the molecular aspects of drug action because here the basic molecular sciences, physics and chemistry, will provide the grammatical framework within which the investigator must proceed.

Herein lies a major problem, since pharmacologists in general are not conversant with such disciplines as chemical crystallography, molecular orbital theory or atomic magnetism, which are relevant to this level of explanation, and are therefore liable to turn over the pages hurriedly when such considerations intrude into a pharmacological explanation. Yet the necessity for penetrating to this level is very obvious if we are to have any real knowledge of the relationship of drug action to chemical structure. In the great majority of instances drugs act through the formation of non-covalent molecular complexes with a biological receptive molecule. Such interactions cannot be described at all comprehensively by a simple chemical equation (which suffices only for evaluation of net thermodynamic properties) since they are due to electrical forces between atoms in the drug and in the binding site arranged in three-dimensional space. Indeed it is this spatial ordering which is the essential feature in determining both potency and specificity.

It is also unfortunate that most investigations of pharmacological action at the molecular level are not necessarily applied to areas of pharmacology which are undergoing the most rapid advance at other levels of study. The reasons for this are obvious enough – the technical constraints of the molecular techniques available at present may restrict studies to molecules which have been sufficiently purified, are readily available and have favourable physical properties. Furthermore, the molecular approach is in such an early stage of its development that too few well studied examples are available to permit many wide generalisations.

The ideal method for molecular pharmacology is a topographical method that permits the definition of the position in space of all the atoms in a drug–receptor complex. X-ray crystallography comes near to meeting this requirement, and one such study is presented in this symposium. The limitations of X-ray studies are well known and include the restriction to well-crystallised complexes, the lack of dynamic information and some intrinsic uncertainties (~ 0.2 Å) in the precision of the coordinates of the atoms. Nevertheless the contributions that X-ray studies have made to our notions of complex formation have been revolutionary. What is not so clearly perceived is that even if we had quite ideal structural information, we would still be unable at present to translate this information into the energetic terms within which quantitative binding data need to be evaluated.

Interatomic potentials have mostly been derived from gas phase studies of simple molecules. Their application to condensed systems is hampered by uncertainties about the dielectric through which the electric forces operate, and the entropic and other problems of dealing with larger assemblies of atoms extended in space. The position is that, whereas the atomic arrangement may suggest, for instance, that an ionic interaction is involved in a particular complex, a much better estimate of the actual energetic contribution of such an interaction is likely to come from an experimental study of binding as a function of pH than from any theoretical calculation. The papers by Ganellin and Richards in this symposium deal with aspects of this problem, namely the difficulty of defining the formal ionisation state, and the delocalisation of the charge over a multiatomic molecule. The same kind of difficulty is seen with the sulphonamide - carbonic anhydrase complexes. There is no doubt that coordination of the sulphonamide group to the zinc atom in the enzyme contributes a major part of the binding energy but such binding has not been found in model systems and there is no way yet of understanding theoretically why such coordination should be so significant.

Indeed the assessment of positive contributions to binding is so unsatisfactory that at least one may take comfort in the clear results obtained where the inability to fit a group into the structure indicates a steric prohibition of binding. This is important because specificity is concerned as much with which molecules cannot bind as with what causes others to bind. However, where structural features are as well understood as in haemoglobin, the paper by Goodford reveals how this information can be used in the rational design of ligands.

While no other method can replace X-ray crystallography in its wealth of topographical detail, spectroscopic methods can provide much useful information that enriches simple binding data. NMR spectroscopy of both drug and binding molecule is capable of giving information about the involvement of groups in binding and also about conformation changes, as Roberts shows in his study of dihydrofolate reductase. This paper also deals with another of the perennial problems of structure - activity relationships, namely how far the binding energy of a molecule can be considered as a linear sum of the interaction energies of parts of the molecule.

Essentially the methods so far considered are limited to some systems that have been well characterised and purified. They are still restricted to rather simple systems, yet many important drug actions are exerted in complex multiunit systems, or in membrane-bound receptors. After all, the identification of a receptor is itself a landmark in understanding the action of a drug, and from this, further characterisation and useful molecular studies can proceed. The latter part of this symposium is concerned with these more complex sites of drug action and illustrates the remarkable progress that can be made in understanding them even if we cannot yet characterise them in terms of atomic structure.

Symposia such as the present one are only organised by dint of hard work and a good deal of money. The hard work was provided by Dr Gordon Roberts, who was Chairman and Secretary of the organising committee, and Miss Blunt, who supplied a long experience of organising these symposia to seeing that all went smoothly, as indeed it did.

This particular symposium is of particular interest in being the first in which the sponsorship of the International Union of Pharmacology and of the International Union of Pure and Applied Chemistry has met in this important interfacial area. It is likely to be only the first of such meetings, since a second symposium is already being planned to be held in Holland in 1977 and to concentrate on problems of structure-activity relationships.

The financial support of the symposium came from the interested societies but it was also most generously supplemented by the Wellcome Trust and by a number of pharmaceutical firms that are listed at the beginning of this volume.

Contents

Sponsoring Societies, Organising Committee and bodies from whom
financial support was received   v
Foreword   vi

1. Chemical constitution and prototropic equilibria in structure – activity analysis. C. R. Ganellin   1
2. Calculation of essential drug conformations and electron distributions. W. G. Richards   41
3. The conformation of hormonal peptides in solution. J. Feeney   55
4. Structure and function of carbonic anhydrase: comparative studies of sulphonamide binding to human erythrocyte carbonic anhydrases B and C. K. K. Kannan, I. Vaara, B. Nostrand, S. Lövgren, A. Borell, K. Fridborg and M. Petef   73
5. Kinetic aspects of structure – activity relationships in the carbonic anhydrase – sulphonamide system. R. W. King   93
6. The haemoglobin molecule as a model drug receptor. P. J. Goodford   109
7. Substrate and inhibitor binding to dihydrofolate reductase. G. C. K. Roberts   127
8. The molecular basis for the inhibitory action of 6-(arylhydrazino) pyrimidines on the replication-specific DNA polymerase III of Gram-positive bacteria. N. C. Brown and G. E. Wright   151
9. Structural and conformational studies on quinoxaline antibiotics in relation to the molecular basis of their interaction with DNA. M. J. Waring   167
10. The receptor site for chloramphenicol *in vitro* and *in vivo*. O. Pongs   190
11. The mechanism of cytochrome P450-catalysed drug oxidations. V. Ullrich   201
12. Interaction of ouabain and cassaine with $Na^+ + K^+$-ATPase and its relationship to their inotropic actions. T. Tobin and T. Akera   213
13. Adenylate cyclase: actions and interactions of regulatory ligands. C. Londos and M. Rodbell   235
14. Properties and function of the acetylcholine receptor of vertebrate skeletal muscle. E. A. Barnard   249

Index   275

1
Chemical constitution and prototropic equilibria in structure – activity analysis

C. R. Ganellin (The Research Institute, Smith Kline & French Laboratories Ltd, Welwyn Garden City, Hertfordshire, UK)

CHEMICAL CONSTITUTION AND STRUCTURE – ACTIVITY ANALYSIS

Chemical Characterisation of Drug Molecules
It seems to me appropriate that the first paper in a symposium on Drug Action at the Molecular Level should discuss the chemical characterisation of drug molecules. Attempts to establish why drug substances exert particular biological effects is a pursuit of long standing (for discussion of this see Sexton, 1963; Barlow, 1964; Albert, 1968; Burger, 1970). As our chemical understanding has advanced, we have become more sophisticated in the way we view the chemical constitution of drug molecules and in the way we attempt to relate this to biological action.

Drug molecules must exert their biological actions through their ability to interact at the molecular level – for example, with enzymes or receptor structures. These molecular interactions are determined, fundamentally, by the size and shape of molecules and by the electron density distribution and polarisabilities within molecules. The intermolecular forces at work are electrical in origin; there are short-range forces present when molecules are close enough for their electron clouds to overlap, as occurs with donor–acceptor bonding of lone electron pairs and charge-transfer complexation. When molecules are further apart, long-range forces act – for example, electrostatic (due to the interaction of the permanent charge distribution of the molecules), induction (due to the distortion of the charge distribution of one molecule by the permanent charge distribution of its neighbours) and dispersion (resulting from correlation of the fluctuations of the electron positions); induction and dispersion forces are related to the polarisability of molecules (Buckingham, 1975). Thus polar bonds, bond polarisabilities, lone pairs of electrons, π-electrons and charges, and their relative spatial orientation in drug molecules, can be crucial for drug action, and must be identified. Particular manifestations of these forces are the non-covalent interactions which have special importance in biology, such as hydrogen bonding and van der Waals attraction, these may be involved in the binding of drugs to biological macro-

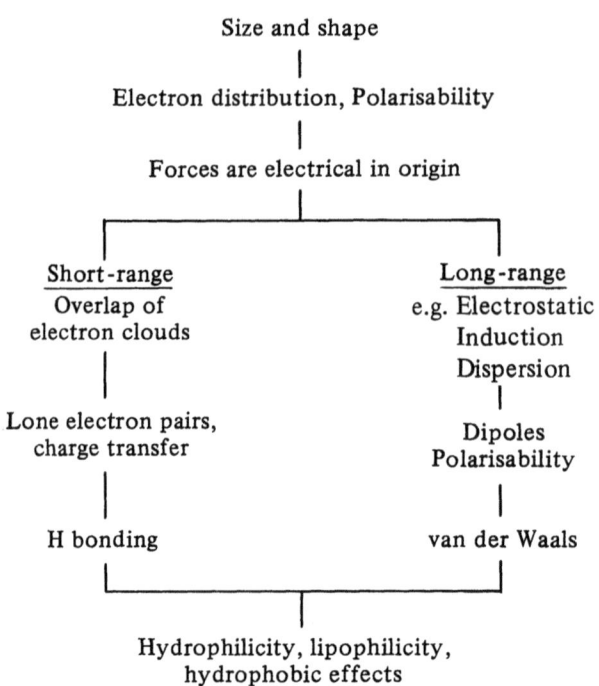

Scheme 1.1 Molecular characteristics and interactions

molecules and they also determine such properties as hydrophilicity, hydrophobic effects and lipophilicity (Gill, 1965; Nemethy, 1969; Frieden, 1975). Chemical reactivity involved in the making and breaking of covalent bonds is another manifestation of these forces but it will not be specifically considered in this chapter.

Relating Chemical Features to Biological Activity
From the above description of the fundamental characteristics of a molecule (summarised in Scheme 1.1) we have to identify those features that appear to determine the biological action of the drug. This is an analytical process and there is an established procedure for carrying it out (summarised in Scheme 1.2); however, it is often not explicitly recognised as such, since the methods are largely intuitive.

One selects particular chemical characteristics for investigation and modifies them by changing the drug structure. If this results in a corresponding alteration of the characteristic biological activity, the possibility of a direct association between these chemical aspects and drug action may be considered as a working hypothesis. One may then design further compounds with the aim of testing the hypothesis, or with the intention of deliberately modifying biological activity in a desired direction. Analogues may be made either to exaggerate the chemical

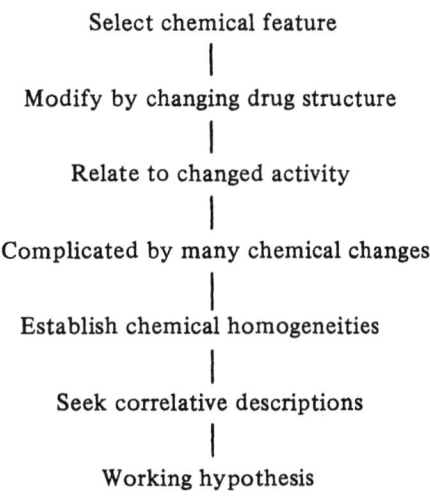

Scheme 1.2 Analytical procedure

characteristics or to minimise them or to leave them unaffected, depending upon the purpose. This statement is of course a gross oversimplification of the real procedure, because, in practice, it is not possible to introduce a change in drug structure that has a unique effect on drug chemistry. A simple structural change can alter many chemical aspects of a molecule. This gives the subject its complexity because we do not know, *a priori*, which of the chemical changes determine the biological outcome. Unravelling this complexity is fundamental to the discipline of medicinal chemistry, and it has a further aim of interpreting drug chemistry in terms of a chemical mechanism of drug action.

The working method consists of comparing compounds in which drug structure has been modified in ways that permit this analysis to be made. As the analysis proceeds, a short series of compounds may be constructed, which may be extended as required. One attempts to keep the series as chemically homogeneous as is possible and to identify for each compound the change in its chemistry; within the series there may run different threads of chemical homogeneity. Correlations are then sought between a particular chemical aspect or property, or set of properties (there are usually several properties contributing to different extents), and drug activity. This then allows the biological action of the drug to be described in terms of drug chemistry; rarely, however, does one find a unique description — that is, there are often several ways in which one can select combinations of various facets of drug chemistry and obtain a significant correlation. All such correlations have to be borne in mind and the implications of each correlation have to be examined separately. Sometimes this may lead one to make the same chemical change for apparently opposing reasons. Thus each correlation (or description) becomes a working hypothesis, to be refined, modified or discarded, depending upon the result obtained from the next compound tested. This procedure is well known to many medicinal chemists, but we need to keep reminding ourselves of its value.

It is of course implicit in any discussion of structure – activity analysis that in a series of compounds homogeneity of biological action is maintained. We cannot correlate chemical properties with a particular biological property if there has been a change in the biological mechanism. Ing (1964) very clearly pointed out that structure – activity studies really involve two separate biological inquiries: how changes in structure affect the mechanism of action and how they influence the intensity of action. It is no good the chemist trying to correlate changes in potency of compounds if they are acting by different mechanisms; furthermore, the determination of relative potency is based on the relative amounts of drug administered, whereas potency really depends on the concentration of drug at the active site. Therefore within a series of compounds changes in drug access, metabolism or elimination will have to be considered and allowed for in any correlation.

A further problem to be faced in the method of structure – activity analysis described above is the identification of particular chemical properties for consideration. The need to have some idea of the chemical properties likely to be of consequence in a given biological action is especially taxing to the imagination of medicinal chemists. The organic chemist's training gives a view of molecules which does not necessarily indicate the way drug molecules are perceived by a piece of guinea-pig tissue or by a cell membrane. The medicinal chemist has to acquire an appreciation of the molecular interactions that might occur between drug molecules and the biological milieu and to identify the chemical properties which reflect these interactions (Korolkovas, 1970). This part of the procedure depends, therefore, on the state of knowledge of the chemistry involved in maintenance of biological systems.

In attempting to relate drug chemistry to activity in a series of compounds, one may be faced with having to correlate changes in several chemical properties, unless a simple relationship is found between activity and a particular property. Use of the statistical techniques of multiple regression analysis may be helpful, but great care is required in the selection and number of parameters used in order to attain sufficient statistical significance and minimise chance correlations (Topliss and Costello, 1972).

Correlation Analysis of Substituent Effects

In principle, a similar procedure to the above is used in the technique pioneered by Hansch (summarised in Scheme 1.3), whereby drug molecules are considered as comprising a prototype structure plus substitutents. The description of a drug molecule is approached by using substituent constants to represent the substituent effect and, by use of linear free energy relationships (LFER), correlations are sought between the substituent contribution and activity. The effects of substituents may be characterised parametrically in terms of size (for example, E_s), electronic character (for example, σ), and contribution to lipophilicity (for exam-

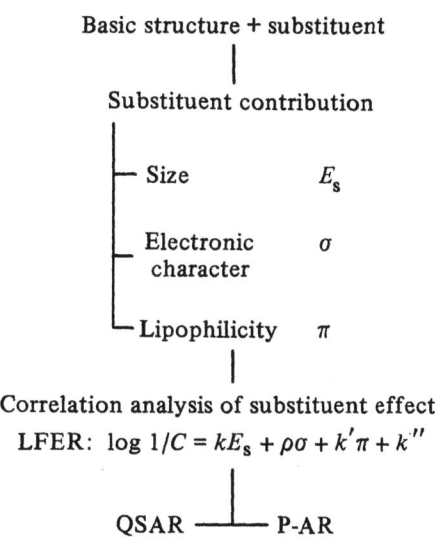

Scheme 1.3 Hansch analysis

ple, π) (Hansch, Deutsch and Smith, 1965; Hansch, 1969; Lien, 1969). Other parameters or substituent constants may be used as alternative manifestations of the substituent effect (Leo, Hansch and Church, 1969; Lien, 1969; Higuchi and Davis, 1970; Craig, 1971; Hansch et al., 1973a). Regression analysis is then used to distinguish between the roles of steric, electronic and hydrophobic parameters (Purcell, Bass and Clayton, 1973). By identifying particular dominant molecular characteristics this approach can suggest something about the mechanism of drug action (see, for example, Tute, 1970). This method draws particular attention to the role of lipophilic or hydrophobic properties in drug action, but it is less able to take account of the effect of molecular shape. The method can be a very powerful tool for directing attention to particular properties, but there is a danger that by relying too heavily on the statistical approach one may obscure what is really happening, chemically.

There is a burgeoning literature on the strategy of drug design in which methods for conducting Hansch analysis are debated and various alternative ways of approaching the problem are identified. The seeking of relationships between drug structure and biological activity has become correlation analysis of substituent effects (Silipo and Hansch, 1975) in which the selection of substituents has to be made with a view to conducting this type of analysis (Craig, 1971; Hansch, Unger and Forsythe, 1973b; Wootton et al., 1975). This is fine if substituent effects are the determining influence on activity. Undoubtedly, correlation analysis of substituent effects is a powerful technique, but its use must be carefully prescribed. In contrast to past situations of purely empirical molecular modification in the search for new drugs, we have entered a new phase in drug studies where we attempt to quantify drug chemistry by computation of selected properties with a view to obtaining quantitative structure - activity relationships (QSAR) (Purcell *et al.*, 1973; Hansch, 1976). If, however, the information is handled in a purely statistical manner, the procedure again becomes highly empirical. In directing attention to substituents there is a tendency to forget the rest of the molecule. Furthermore, this type of analysis may not contain sufficient information about drug structure, as has been pointed out by Goodford (1973), who suggests that we should really use the term 'physicochemical-activity relationships' (PAR). This approach is very helpful for studying the influence of physicochemical properties on drug activity, but it may not apply when activity is very sensitive to drug structure.

One of the properties most widely considered is that of octanol - water partition; it is especially useful when one tackles problems of drug penetration and access or hydrophobic effects. However, the partition of a molecule is largely determined by the sum of the component parts, although in certain situations it may also be sensitive to their arrangement (Hansch, Leo and Nikaitani, 1972; Nys and Rekker, 1973; Hine and Mookerjee, 1975). Although a given molecule may have a particular partition coefficient, this will be an inadequate descriptor of structure because there remain too many ways of altering drug structure without affecting the partition coefficient. There may be circumstances in which partition coefficients reflect changes in drug conformation, but, in general, partition coefficients do not adequately reflect molecular shape, so that their use often fails to provide correlations in structure - activity analysis where drug distribution or hydrophobic effects are not key issues (see discussion by Higuchi and Davis, 1970).

Physical chemists faced an analogous problem much earlier in this century and made a distinction between *additive* properties and *constitutive* properties (see Scheme 1.4). An additive property is one which is merely the sum of the various parts. The most obvious example is molecular weight: the mass of the molecule is

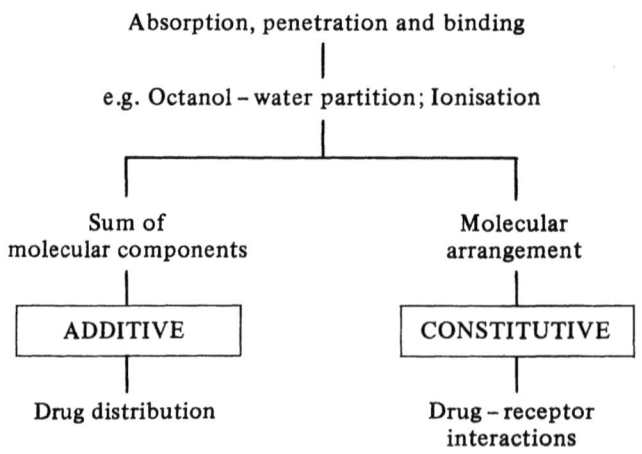

Scheme 1.4 Property – activity relationships

the sum of the masses of its atoms. A constitutive property depends primarily on the arrangement of the atoms in a molecule — that is, on the molecular constitution. Many molecular properties are partly additive and partly constitutive, but the balance between the two differs — for example, refractive index is largely additive and boiling point depends more on constitution (Kellie and Riddell, 1975). In this sense partition is more an additive property, although not entirely so (Hansch *et al.*, 1972). *Specific* biological activity is usually much more a constitutive property. Our chemical analysis of the problems should reflect these observations.

Dynamic Structure – Activity Analysis (DSAA)
To focus attention on the constitutive properties embodied in the chemical structures of drug molecules requires that we should know something about their shape and charge distribution. When we take this standpoint, we immediately perceive a new problem. We find that many drug molecules do not have unique shapes or single charge distributions. It is quite usual to find that drugs may exist in several charged species and assume several shapes. Furthermore these different forms are usually interconvertible; they exist in equilibrium. So not only do we have to identify the separate forms, we must also identify their probable importance. We must know something about their relative populations; how likely is it that a molecule adopts a particular conformation, or a particular charge distribution? The point is that changing a drug's structure may also change the relative impor-

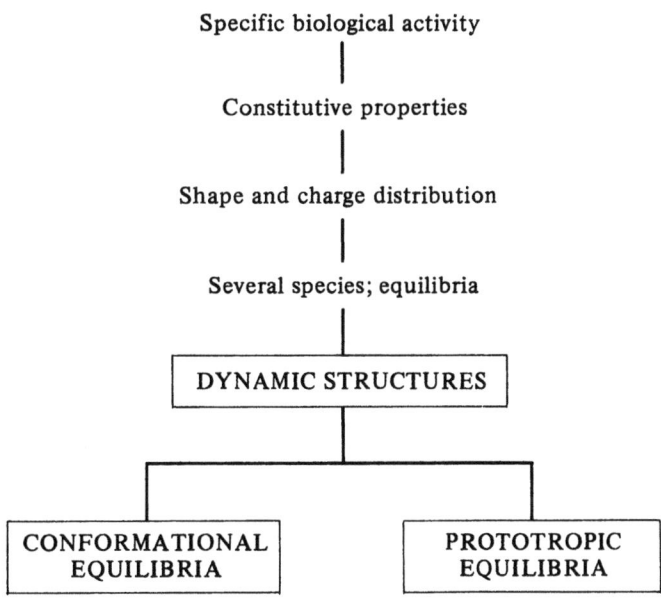

Scheme 1.5 Dynamic structure – activity analysis

tance of particular forms and this may affect activity. Perhaps we could identify this aspect as *dynamic structure-activity analysis* (DSAA) (Scheme 1.5); for example, if altering structure disfavours the biologically active form, then presumably this would reduce activity. Indeed, one may go further — it is conceivable that on occasions an equilibrium between two forms is mechanistically necessary. These notions are not universally applicable, but for molecules that participate in equilibria, we must try to understand these chemical aspects if we are to relate chemical structure to biological activity.

One may thus take as a starting point the chemical characterisation of the drug molecule in terms of its different species, i.e. conformations and protonated (or ionised) forms, and the quantitiative interrelationships between the species (e.g. equilibrium constants, free energy differences, energy barriers to interconversion). One may then modify structure to alter a particular equilibrium or favour (or disfavour) a particular species and investigate whether the changes correlate with altered biological activity. By this means it may be possible to infer something about the chemical mechanism of drug action, and it may also indicate the way to alter drug structure in order to deliberately modify drug activity — that is, provide a method for drug design.

Protropic equilibria

Investigation of conformation and conformational equilibria are the subjects of the two following papers by Drs Richards and Feeney. The present paper considers the complementary set of equilibria involving hydrogen atoms. Hydrogen atoms occupy a special position in chemistry. They are a constituent of most organic substances, and the covalent bonds linking hydrogen atoms in molecules are often of relatively low energy, so that some hydrogen atoms are relatively mobile. Thus many drugs are acids or bases, and charged species may well be involved in their pharmacological action. Changing a drug's structure may affect the equilibrium between protonated and non-protonated forms, and thereby affect activity. Since this involves the transfer of protons, we can call it *prototropic*.

There are several reasons for selecting prototropic equilibria for discussion.

(1) It appears to be of fundamental importance to the action of many drugs (Albert, 1968, Ch. 8; Tolstoouhov, 1955).

(2) Drug ionisation is widely considered as affecting drug solubility, drug absorption and membrane penetration, i.e. as a problem of drug access and the consequent effect on drug activity (see Albert, 1952), but it is often overlooked in relationship to the mechanism of drug action, e.g. in the specific molecular interactions that must occur at receptors. Some well-known cases where drug ionisation has been studied in relation to the mechanism of action are found in the work on sulphonamides (Bell and Roblin, 1942; Cammarata and Allen, 1967; Seydel, 1968) and amino-acridines (Albert, 1966).

(3) It is an area where the scientific literature abounds with mistakes: sometimes the site of proton mobility in the drug molecule is wrongly assigned;

sometimes it is not appreciated that the situation is complicated by the existence of multiple sites of proton mobility (the empirically determined ionisation constant is then a composite of microionisation constants; see below). Wrong interpretation of the sites of proton loss is a frequently occurring problem to be found in present-day publications.

(4) The ionisation state of a molecule may affect the fundamental properties of conformation and charge distribution in a drug, so that it is important to first identify the particular drug species for investigation.

(5) A drug's ionisation state may also affect such properties as hydrogen-bonding ability, hydrophilicity and lipid solubility, so that correlation analysis involving these physicochemical properties may be greatly affected.

(6) Finally, some examples are given of problems involving prototropic equilibria. These illustrate aspects which may be helpful in drug design and in thinking about the chemistry of drug action.

PROTOTROPIC EQUILIBRIA AND STRUCTURE – ACTIVITY ANALYSIS

Equilibrium Constants

The equilibria between protonated and unprotonated forms are represented by the equilibrium constant, K_a. For example,

(i) Dissociation of cations: $R\overset{+}{N}H_3 \rightleftharpoons RNH_2 + H^+$; $K_a = \dfrac{[RNH_2][H^+]}{[RNH_3^+]}$ (1.1)

(ii) Dissociation to anions: $RCO_2H \rightleftharpoons RCO_2^- + H^+$; $K_a = \dfrac{[RCO_2^-][H^+]}{[RCO_2H]}$ (1.2)

Thus pK_a is taken as a measure of proton acidity; the lower the pK_a, the greater is the tendency for an acid to dissociate into conjugate base and proton. In water, the relative concentration of species present is determined by K_a and the hydrogen ion concentration $[H^+]$; these are related by the formula

$$\text{percentage unprotonated} = \frac{[RNH_2] \times 100}{[RNH_2] + [R\overset{+}{N}H_3]} = \frac{100}{1 + \text{antilog}(pK_a - pH)} \quad (1.3)$$

likewise for anions; it should be noted that for the ammonium cation the unprotonated conjugate base is formally uncharged, whereas for the carboxylic acid the unprotonated conjugate base is a negatively charged ion. When $pH = pK_a$, it follows that there are equal amounts present of the conjugate acid and base.

(iii) sequential dissociation of two protons: $H\overset{+}{X}H \underset{}{\overset{K_{a_1}}{\rightleftharpoons}} HX + H^+ \underset{}{\overset{K_{a_2}}{\rightleftharpoons}} X^- + 2H^+$

In the general case where a cation [HXH$^+$] dissociates into an uncharged form [HX] which further dissociates to give an anion [X$^-$], the equilibrium constants for the first and second proton dissociations are represented, respectively, by K_{a_1} and K_{a_2}

(iv) Dissociation from two alternative sites: if the first proton can dissociate from two alternative sites (thus: H + H → HX + H$^+$ or H$^+$ + XH), the overall stoiechiometry is still such ahat each molecule of conjugate acid provides one proton, but there is a mixture of conjugate bases, viz. HX + XH; K_a is now a mixed constant (or *macroscopic* constant) and is a composite of the individual ionisations from the two sites, i.e. the *microscopic* constants k_1 and k_2. The three species are interrelated thus:

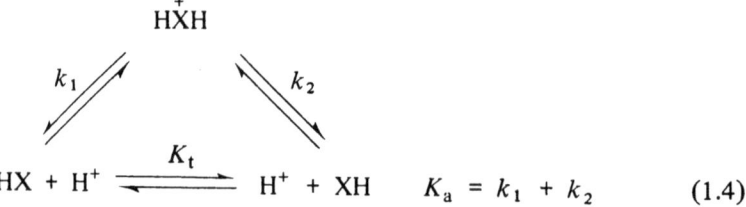

$$K_a = k_1 + k_2 \qquad (1.4)$$

HX and XH are tautomers and they differ in the siting of a proton; their respective concentrations are related by the tautomeric equilibrium constant, K_t, whence

$$K_t = \frac{[XH]}{[HX]} = \frac{k_2}{k_1} \qquad (1.5)$$

(v) Sequential dissociation of two protons involving alternative sites. Combining cases (iii) and (iv) above, we have

$$H\overset{+}{X}H \rightarrow [HX + H^+ \text{ or } H^+ + XH] \rightarrow X^- + 2H^+$$

The four species are interrelated thus:

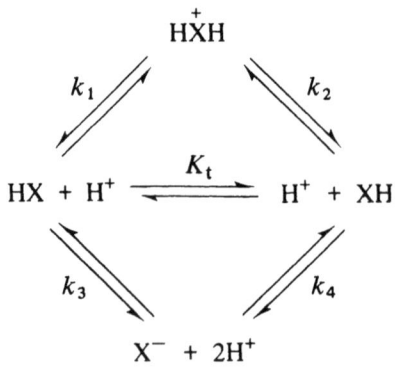

The macroscopic constants are given by

$$K_{a_1} = k_1 + k_2 \quad \text{(as before)}$$

$$\frac{1}{K_{a_2}} = \frac{1}{k_3} + \frac{1}{k_4} \tag{1.6}$$

whence

$$K_{a_1} K_{a_2} = k_1 k_3 = k_2 k_4 \tag{1.7}$$

The tautomeric equilibrium constant is given by

$$K_t = \frac{k_2}{k_1} = \frac{k_3}{k_4} \tag{1.8}$$

For discussions of the study of tautomeric equilibria and the treatment of overlapping ionisation constants see Katritzky and Lagowski (1963a), Jaffé and Jones (1964), Albert and Serjeant (1971) and Liler (1975).

Example 1: Site of Protonation in Thiamine

Most titration work on thiamine (vitamin B_1) has been concerned with the problem of estimating the pK_a of the CH acidity at relatively high pH. However, the titration curve, first described by Williams and Ruehle (1935), possesses two steps and the first titratable acid group (pK_a around 4.5) has since been assigned to NH dissociation from the aminopyrimidine moiety. The pK_a in water at 25°C has subsequently been reported to be 4.76 (Watanabe and Asahi, 1955) and, more

1A Proton on amino N   1B Proton assigned to ring N
(incorrect assignment)   Thiamine   (as in crystal)
structures

recently, 4.75 (Hopmann and Brugnoni, 1973). It is widely assumed that the site of protonation is the amino group giving $-NH_3^+$, structure 1A (e.g. Viscontini et al., 1951; Watanabe and Asahi, 1955; Breslow, 1958; Krampitz, 1969; Hopmann and Brugnoni, 1973; Risinger, Gore and Pulver, 1974; Rouvray, 1975).

In aminopyrimidines, however, protonation occurs on N in the pyrimidine ring (Albert, Goldacre and Phillips, 1948; Brown, Hoerger and Mason, 1955; Liler, 1975, p. 313) and this is in accord with other amino heterocycles (Osborn,

Table 1.1 pK_a values of some aminopyrimidines

Structure	pK_a
4-aminopyrimidine	2.50[a]
2-aminopyrimidine	3.54[a]
2-aminopyrimidine (isomer)	5.71[a]
4-amino-5-aminomethyl-2-methylpyrimidine	4.0[b]
cf. pyrimidine	1.30[a]

[a] Albert et al. (1948).
[b] Korte and Weitkamp (1959); pK_{a_2} = 7.1.

Schofield and Short, 1956); comparison with model compounds (Table 1.1) indicates that the main site of protonation in thiamine should be the N atom *para* to the amino group, i.e. structure 1B. This structure is also found in the crystalline state for thiamine hydrochloride, pyrophosphate (for examples see Kraut and Reed, 1962; Pletcher and Sax, 1972) and other salts (Richardson, Franklin and Thompson, 1975). The implication is that the NH_2 group is a very weak base and that the basic centre is the N atom in the *para* position of the pyrimidine ring.

The mechanisms of thiamine catalysis are well discussed by Bruice and Benkovic (1966) but the role of the aminopyrimidine moiety is poorly understood (Hopmann and Brugnoni, 1973). Breslow (1958) pointed out that the amino group of thiamine is quite unreactive, owing to resonance. This is in accord with its weak basicity. Thus interpretation of the pK_a data directs attention to these special features. The amino group is unlikely to act as an electron-pair donor; it might function as a proton donor in H bonding, or its main purpose may be to render the *para* N atom sufficiently basic for the latter to act as an electron-pair donor.

Example 2: Catecholamines and Zwitterion Formation

Knowledge of the chemistry of the catecholamines is fundamental to understanding the molecular mechanisms of their biological actions. The subject is complicated by the fact that the catecholamines exist as equilibrium mixtures of different ionic species and conformers, and there have been various studies to determine proton dissociation constants (Leffler, Spencer and Burger, 1951; Albert, 1952; Lewis, 1954; Tuckerman, Mayer and Nachod, 1959; Sinistri and Villa, 1962; Kappe and Armstrong, 1965; Jameson and Neillie, 1965; Rajan et al., 1972; Antikainen and Witikainen, 1973) and conformational preference (for reviews with leading references see Roberts, 1974; Green, Johnson and Kang, 1974). The studies have a twofold purpose, viz. to chemically characterise physiological amines and to try to account for the changed biological properties of synthetic analogues. Of prime interest in this area are the effects of N-alkyl substitution. The well-known classification of α and β adrenergic receptors by Ahlquist (1948) depended mainly on results obtained using α-methyladrenaline, and α-methylnoradrenaline, and the simple series 2 (Scheme 1.6), R = H, Me, ^{i}Pr (noradrenaline, adrenaline and isoprenaline). Isoprenaline is the least active at α receptors but the most active β receptor stimulant and the chemical basis for the selectivity imparted by the isopropyl substituent continues to be intriguing. The simplest explanation usually offered for the effect of the isopropyl substituent is that it sterically hinders interaction at the α receptor but contributes additional binding at the β receptor; various molecular models for the receptor site interaction have been reviewed by Brittain, Jack and Ritchie (1970). However, there is no proven mechanism and it is important, therefore, to continue to examine catecholamine chemistry to uncover other special features or gradation in chemical properties.

Potentiometric titration of adrenaline cation (2A; R = Me) affords two stoichiometric pK_a values, around 8.8 and 10.0, corresponding to two neutralisation points, but the assignment to particular sites of proton dissociation in the molecule is problematical. Making comparison with simpler molecules such as catechol (pK_a 9.4; Perrin, 1958) and phenylethanolamine (pK_a 8.9; Tuckerman et al., 1959), some authors attributed the lower pK_a to the $-NH_2{}^+R$ group (Leffler et al., 1951; Tuckerman et al., 1959) and the higher pK_a to the phenolic OH (Jameson and Neillie, 1965; Rajan et al., 1972), i.e. the implication being that the first dissociation occurred in the side-chain to give the uncharged molecule (2B), and subsequent dissociation occurred in the ring to afford the anion (2D), via the left-hand pathway shown in Scheme 1.6. However, using a UV method to determine the dissociation of the phenolic OH, such an assignment was shown to be in error and was reversed (Lewis, 1954; Kappe and Armstrong, 1965; Antikainen and Witikainen, 1973), i.e. the low pK_a was attributed to OH ionisation to afford the zwitterion (2C), via the right-hand pathway shown in Scheme 1.6. None of the above authors appeared to have considered that the measured pK_as are composite values. The acidities of the OH and $\overset{+}{N}H$ groups are very close, so that addition of one equivalent of alkali does not fully neutralise either site; both are partially neutralised. Thus it is not correct to assign pK_as to the specific

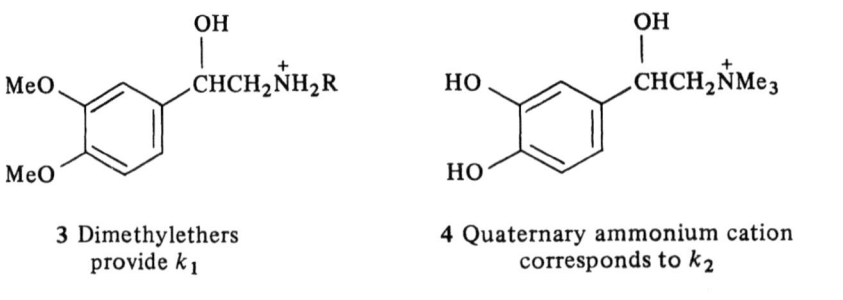

Scheme 1.6 Ionisation constants and species equilibria of catecholamines

sites of proton loss, unless they are resolved into the respective microscopic constants. To determine the microscopic constants (pk_1, pk_2, pk_3, pk_4) requires the use of special techniques, e.g. spectroscopic methods which permit the separate observation of each site, or the use of model compounds in which the problem is simplified by replacing the respective mobile protons with immobile groups, usually methyl. Such an analysis was published by Sinistri and Villa (1962a) but it seems to have escaped attention. Sinistri and Villa used appropriate methyl-substituted model analogues to analyse a series of catecholamines. The dimethyl ethers (3) provided the dissociation constant of the $-\overset{+}{N}HR$ group in the absence of phenolic dissociation, and this corresponds to the microscopic constant pk_1 in Scheme 1.6; in conjunction with the measured values for pK_{a_1}, pk_2 was calculated from Eq. (1.4). This reasoning involves the assumption that the methyl groups do not have a direct effect on pK_a; since the methyl groups are some distance from the respective ionisation sites, this seems likely to be a valid assumption, and it is supported by the excellent agreement obtained between the values of pk_2 and the value 8.90 determined by measurement from the quaternary ammonium model (4). The values of pk_3 and pk_4 follow from these results and the measured values of pK_{a_2} by use of Eq. (1.7). The difference between the values of pk_1 and pk_2 gives the equilibrium constant $\log K_t$ (from Eq. 1.5) which provides the ratio between the concentrations of the zwitterionic and uncharged forms. These two species are related tautomerically; they differ only in the siting of a proton and

Table 1.2 Dissociation constants at 25 °C for catecholamines in water, according to Sinistri and Villa (1962a)

$$HO-C_6H_3(OH)-CH(OH)CH_2\overset{+}{N}H_2R$$

	R	Macroscopic constants		Microscopic constants (defined in Scheme 1.6)			
		pK_{a_1}	pK_{a_2}	pk_1	pk_2	pk_3	pk_4
Noradrenaline	H	8.73	9.83	9.18	8.92	9.38	9.64
Adrenaline	Me	8.79	10.09	9.51	8.88	9.37	10.00
N-Ethylnoradrenaline	Et	8.86	10.19	9.61	8.94	9.44	10.11
Isoprenaline	^{i}Pr	8.83	10.19	9.58	8.91	9.44	10.11
N-tert-Butylnoradrenaline	^{t}Bu	8.82	10.37	9.73	8.88	9.46	10.31

pK_{a_1} and pK_{a_2} are the empirically determined macroscopic ionisation constants.
pk_1 is obtained by titration of the model compounds (3).
pk_2 is obtained from the equation: $K_{a_1} = k_1 + k_2$.
$pk_3 = pK_{a_1} + pK_{a_2} - pk_1$.
$pk_4 = pK_{a_1} + pK_{a_2} - pk_2$.

the consequent charge distribution. The respective constants determined by Sinistri and Villa are listed in Table 1.2, and it is apparent that the four microscopic ionisation constants are very close together. From these values we have calculated the relative populations of the various species at a given pH of the medium; results for the series of compounds at 25 °C and pH 7.4 are shown in Table 1.3. The cation is the main species in every case, to an extent greater than 95 per cent. There is a small proportion present as zwitterion and smaller amounts of the uncharged molecule and anion. At 37 °C the pK_a values would be lower (possibly by about 0.3 pK_a unit) and the proportion present as zwitterion would

Table 1.3 Species composition of catecholamines in water at pH 7.4 and 25°C, calculated from the data in Table 1.2

$$HO-C_6H_3(OH)-CH(OH)-CH_2\overset{+}{N}H_2R$$

	R	Cation	Zwitterion	Uncharged	Anion
Noradrenaline	H	95.1	2.9	1.6	0.4
Adrenaline	Me	95.9	3.2	0.7	0.2
N-Ethylnoradrenaline	Et	96.4	2.8	0.6	0.2
Isoprenaline	^{i}Pr	96.2	3.0	0.6	0.2
N-tert-Butylnoradrenaline	^{t}Bu	96.2	3.2	0.5	0.1

consequently be greater (about 5 - 6 per cent). At a higher pH of, say, 8.4 the amount of cation would fall to 50 - 60 per cent and the zwitterion rise to around 30 per cent. Changing the alkyl substituent R, on nitrogen, has almost no effect on pK_{a_1}, and a small effect on pK_{a_2} which increases slightly through the series from H, through Me, Et, ^{i}Pr, to ^{t}Bu. This has little effect on the populations of the two main species (cation and zwitterion), which appear to be almost constant over the series of compounds, but it does alter the populations of the minor forms. However, hidden in these values is a very interesting aspect which is revealed by examining K_t, which we obtain from the simple relationship K_t = antilog ($pk_1 - pk_2$), derived from Eq. (1.5). The values of K_t, the ratio of concentrations of zwitterion to uncharged form, given in Table 1.4 show a trend. For the monomethyl ether (Sinistri and Villa, 1962b), $K_t < 1$ and the uncharged form is favoured; the ratio reverses for noradrenaline and it increases going through the homologous series, up to the value 7 for the tert-butyl derivative.

Thus, if these data are correct, it appears that altering drug structure has altered the balance between the zwitterion and uncharged forms. It must be

Table 1.4 Relative concentrations (K_t) of zwitterionic to uncharged forms for catecholamines at 25 °C, calculated from the data in Table 1.2

$$K_t = \frac{\{\text{zwitterion: } O^-, O^-, H, \text{CHOH-CH}_2\text{-}\overset{+}{\text{NH}}_2R\}}{\text{HO-, HO-, CHOH-CH}_2\text{-NHR}}$$

	R	$K_t{}^a$
4-O-Methylnoradrenaline (5)[b]	H	0.7[c]
Noradrenaline	H	1.8
Adrenaline	Me	4.2
N-Ethylnoradrenaline	Et	4.7
Isoprenaline	^{i}Pr	4.7
tert-Butylnoradrenaline	^{t}Bu	7.1

^aK_t = antilog ($pk_1 - pk_2$).

[b] HO-, MeO-, CHOH-CH$_2\overset{+}{\text{NH}}_3$
540-Methylnoradrenaline

[c] Calculated from data published by Sinistri and Villa (1962b).

remembered that the pK_a values refer to an aqueous system; in reality, for compounds that act at receptors or on membranes, the medium may not be pure water but structured and partly lipoid; this would change the pK_as. Furthermore, we do not know exactly the pH that operates. Thus some of the differences seen with the compounds in water may become greatly magnified under non-aqueous conditions. However, taking these findings at face value, one may infer that *any mechanism of drug action involving proton transfer, during which time the zwitterion is transformed into the uncharged form, would be most favourable for noradrenaline and least favourable for the* tert-*butyl derivative*. This finding does not necessarily specify a molecular mechanism of drug action, but it is a possibility to be considered. An interesting question also arises as to the structure of the zwitterion, since there are two phenolic OH sites for proton dissociation. According to the results of Sinistri and Villa (1962b), there is little difference in the pK_a between respective O-monomethyl analogues, and this suggests that ionisation occurs about equally from the two sites. The structure of the anion and its relationship to internally H-bonded forms is still a matter for speculation.

Any suggestions for structure – activity implications based on the above observations are necessarily speculative, and it is also problematical to know what importance to attach to an analysis involving minor species. However, the point being made is that through examining the chemistry in detail of a series of drugs one may uncover quite marked structurally dependent effects that are not otherwise obvious. The gross changes in the macroscopic pK_as of these compounds are very small but, by assigning the sites of proton dissociation, we see that there are substantial changes in species ratio (i.e. their relative stabilities). Thus we have uncovered a structural effect that may have a mechanistic significance. Of course, it may be quite irrelevant but at least we can now look to see! A corollary to this is the further import for structure – activity considerations when one makes catecholamine analogues; if a powerful electron-withdrawing substituent were introduced into the catechol ring, it would have a substantial pK_a-lowering effect and would therefore considerably increase the zwitterion population; conversely, removal of one of the phenolic OH groups, through monomethylation, reduces the relative population of zwitterion.

Example 3: Species Equilibria for 3-Mercaptopicolinic Acid

3-Mercaptopicolinic acid (6) is of some interest as a hypoglycaemic agent; it has been described by Di Tullio *et al.* (1974) as an effective inhibitor of gluconeogenesis (glucose synthesis) capable of inducing hypoglycaemia in starved or alloxan-diabetic animals; derivatices and related analogues have been synthesised and tested and the results discussed by Blank *et al.* (1974). Considering the chemistry of 3-mercaptopicolinic acid in detail, it is apparent that it undergoes an extensive series of equilibria between different species (Scheme 1.7) involving three prototropic ionization sites, viz. on O, S and N. The situation is analogous to that obtaining with cysteine which has been analysed by Benesch and Benesch (1955), Grafius and Neilands (1955) and others (for further discussion see Rogers, 1969; Clement and Hartz, 1971; Walters and Leyden, 1974).

The pK_a values of the appropriate methyl-substituted model compounds required for estimating the microscopic ionisation constants of 3-mercaptopicolinic acid are not available, but consideration of the partial models in Table 1.5 suggests that the three stoichiometric pK_as are probably in the regions 1, 4 – 5 and 7, respectively. The main species at pH 7.4 would probably be the dianion (6C) and anionic zwitterion (6B). Although 3-mercaptopicolinic acid is written as (6A), less than one-millionth would be present in this form at pH 7.4. Structural analogues

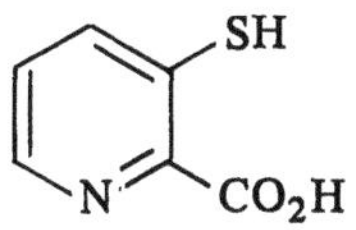

6A

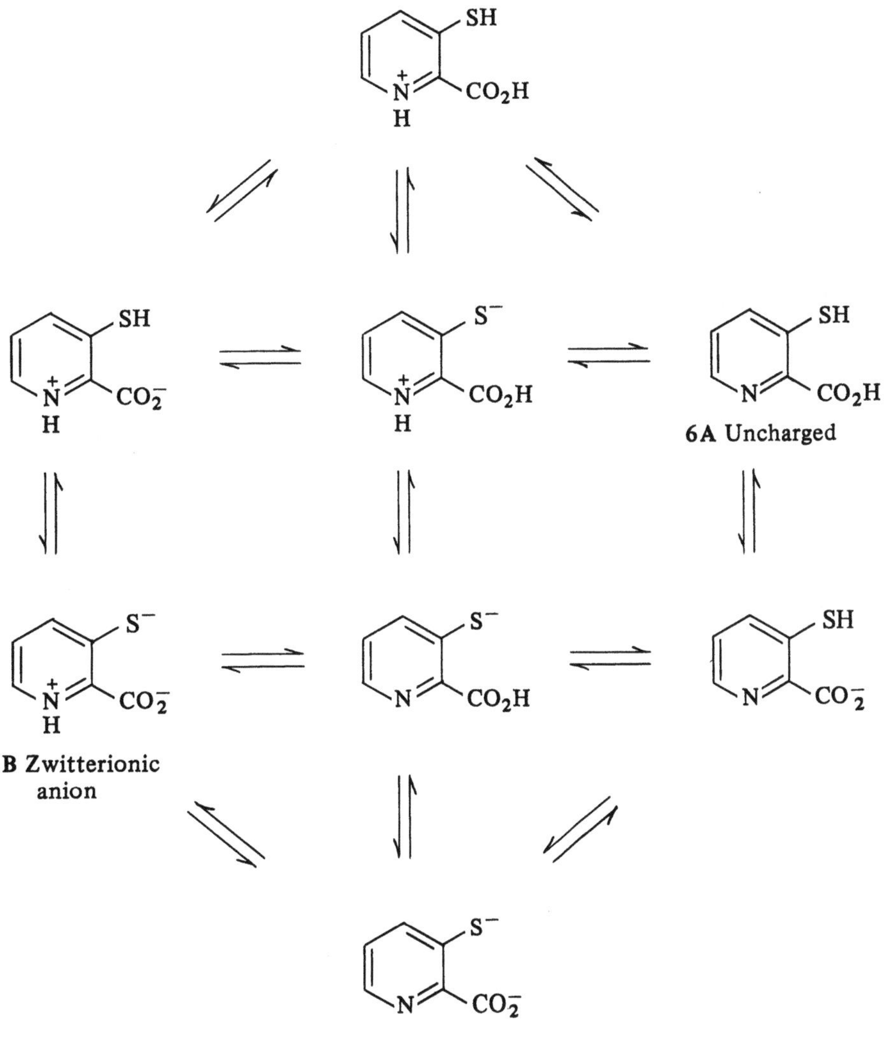

6C Dianion

Scheme 1.7 Species equilibria of 3-mercaptopicolinic acid

Table 1.5 pK_a values of partial-model compounds related to 3-mercaptopicolinic acid

Structure	pK_{a_1} (XH)[a]	pK_{a_2} ($\overset{+}{N}H$)	Reference
pyridinium (NH)	–	5.23	Albert and Barlin (1959)
pyridinium-2-CO$_2$H (NH)	1.01	5.32	Green and Tong (1956)
pyridinium-2-CO$_2$Me (NH)	–	2.21	Green and Tong (1956)
3-SH pyridinium (NH)	2.28	7.01	Albert and Barlin (1959)
3-SH pyridinium (N-Me)	2.27	–	Albert and Barlin (1959)
3-SMe pyridinium (NH)	–	4.45	Albert and Barlin (1959)

[a] X = O or S.

which altered ring basicity would have a considerable effect on the species populations; for example, incorporating an additional nitrogen atom in the ring to make a pyrimidine would suppress zwitterion formation. Such an effect could have considerable implications regarding mechanism of action if the zwitterion were the active form, not only does the zwitterion have a particular charge distribution, it also incorporates a special structural feature in the form of an NH group which could participate in H bonding. Clearly, when one considers structure-activity relationships, it would be necessary to take account of these effects.

Chemistry and Structure – Activity Analysis

Example 4: Functional Properties and Receptor Activity of Histamine

Histamine in aqueous solution is an equilibrium mixture of various ionic species, tautomers and conformers. Titration gives three stoichiometric pK_a values. Fully protonated histamine is a dication (7A; Scheme 1.8), and the first stoichiometric ionization constant (pK_{a_1} = 5.80 at 37 °C) corresponds to dissociation from the ring NH to give the monocation. The second ionisation constant (pK_{a_2} = 9.40 at 37 °C) corresponds to dissociation at the side-chain $-NH_3^+$ group to give the uncharged molecule. At high pH, the ring again ionises at NH (pK_{a_3} = 14) to give an anion (Paiva, Tominaga and Paiva, 1970). The relative populations of the species as a function of pH are shown graphically in Fig. 1.1. The curve for the monocation reaches a maximum in the pH range 7 - 8; since this is also the physiological range, it suggests (but does not prove) that the physiologically important species is the monocation. At pH 7.4, 96 per cent of histamine is present as the monocation; however, it must be remembered that the pH could be considerably lower in the vicinity of some membranes, and below pH 5.8 the dication predominates.

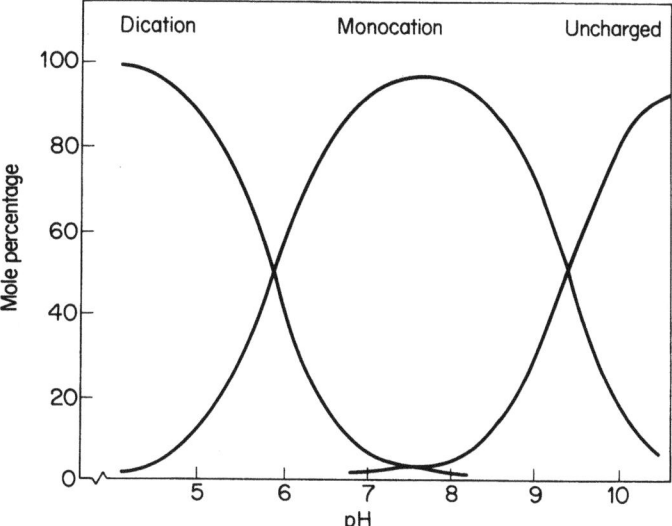

Figure 1.1 Species composition of histamine at 37°C in water as a function of pH, using the values pK_{a_1} = 5.80 and pK_{a_2} = 9.40

Although, for histamine, there is no difficulty in differentiating between proton ionisation from ring as opposed to side-chain, another problem arises because the imidazole ring possesses two nitrogen sites for proton dissociation, so that both monocation and uncharged forms are tautomeric mixtures; the full series of equilibria relating the various species is given in Scheme 1.8. To determine the relative populations of tautomers, one requires the microscopic dissociation constants, but these are not available from direct titration; they can be estimated by comparing the corresponding N-methyl or N-benzyl derivatives and this has

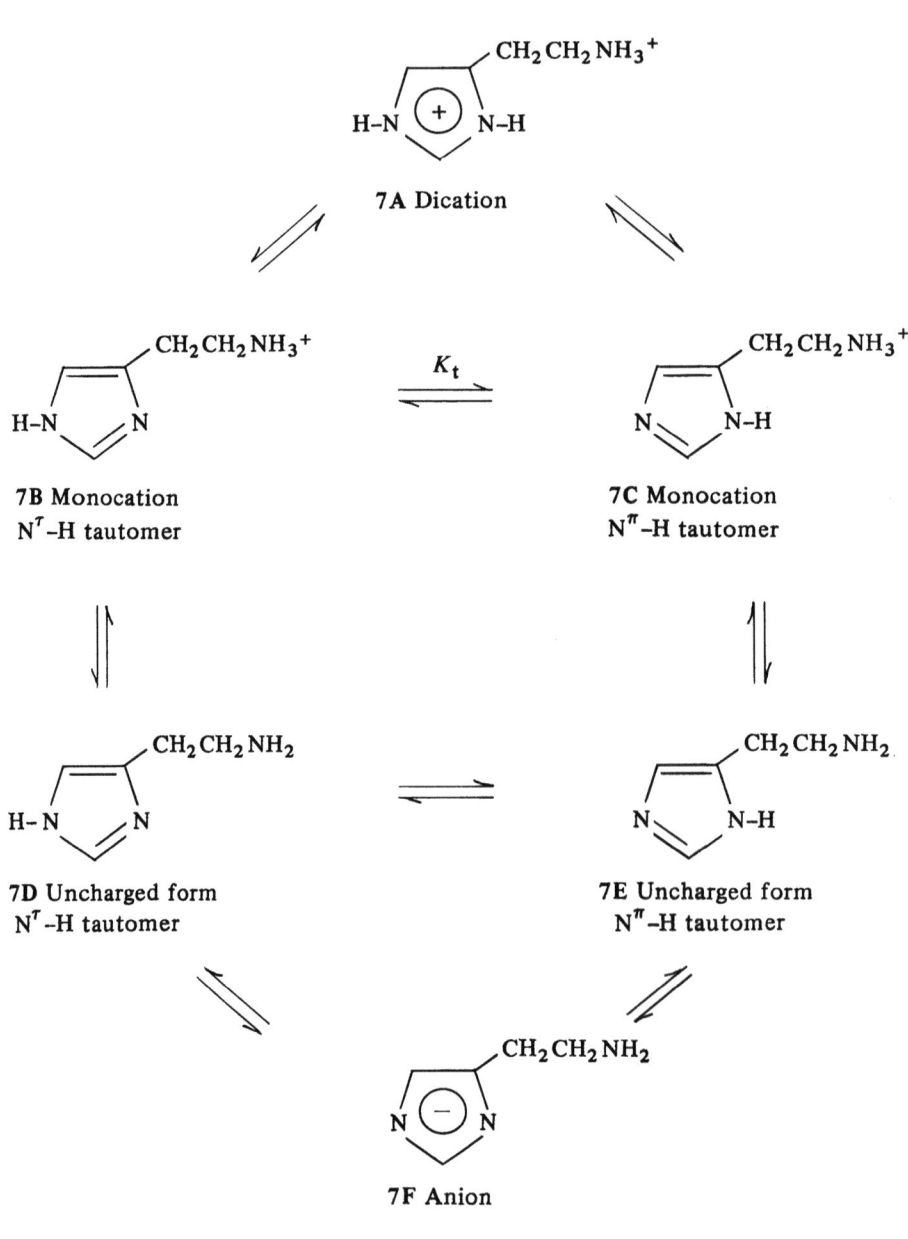

Scheme 1.8 Ionic and tautomeric equilibria between histamine species

$$\text{imidazole ring with substituent: } \overset{\beta}{CH_2}-\overset{a}{CH_2}-N^{\alpha}$$

positions labeled: 4, 2, N^{τ}, N^{π}

8. Histamine numbering according to Black and Ganellin (1974)

been done for the monocation (Ganellin, 1973a). The ratio of concentrations of the two monocation tautomers ([7B]/[7C]), given by the tautomeric equilibrium constant K_t, was found to be approximately 4.2. Thus, according to these measurements, about 80 per cent of histamine monocation in water is in the N^{τ} - H tautomeric form (for histamine numbering shown in formula 8, see Black and Ganellin 1974) and 20 per cent in the N^{π} - H form. The tautomeric equilibrium constant for the uncharged molecule is unknown; an attempt has been made to calculate the relative tautomer stabilities by molecular orbital procedures but substantiation of the result by physical measurement is still required (Kang and Chou, 1975). The conformational equilibria for the various ionic species have been widely studied using nuclear magnetic resonance spectroscopy and molecular orbital calculations (Kier, 1968; Margolis, Kang and Green, 1971; Ganellin et al., 1973a; Ham, Casy and Ison, 1973; see Pullman and Port, 1974, for further references).

Having characterised the species equilibria of histamine, one may try to identify which aspects are involved in the biological activity of histamine. Pharmacologically, the actions of histamine are considered to be mediated by at least two distinct classes of receptor. One receptor type, designated H_1 by Ash and Schild (1966), mediates histamine-induced contraction of smooth muscle of the small intestine and bronchi. A second receptor type, designated H_2 and characterised by Black et al. (1972), mediates the action of histamine in vivo in stimulating gastric acid secretion, and in vitro in increasing the rate of beating of the guinea-pig atrium. Many other actions of histamine have also been shown to involve H_1 or H_2 receptors but they need not concern us here (for a recent review see Chand and Eyre, 1975). The receptors are defined pharmacologically from the antagonists which selectively block the responses of the tissues to histamine stimulation. The differentiation is also reflected in the relative agonist activities of certain histamine analogues, and this raises the interesting question of whether the chemical mechanism of histamine interaction differs at the two types of receptor. Thus it is necessary to identify which chemical properties of histamine differentiate its action at H_1 and H_2 receptors.

As an approach to identifying the properties of histamine critical for activity, a number of closely related structural analogues of histamine have been investigated; the approach requires one to define the chemical consequences of modifying drug structure and subsequently to establish which changes in chemical properties may have affected biological activity. A series of methyl-substituted histamines were studied with respect to their conformational properties and receptor selectivities

Table 1.6 Histamine receptor activities, ring pK_a values and mole percentages of dicationic species at pH 7.4 and 5.4 of some histamine analogues

Structure	Ring pK_a	Mole percentage of dication at pH		Receptor activity	
		7.4	5.4	$H_1{}^a$	$H_2{}^b$
histamine (imidazole-$CH_2CH_2NH_3{}^+$)	5.80	2.5	71	100%	100%
1,2,4-triazolylethylamine	1.4^c	10^{-4}	0.01	12.7^c	13.7^c
2-thiazolylethylamine	$<2^d$	$<4 \times 10^{-4}$	<0.04	26^c	0.3^c
4-chlorohistamine	3.1^e	0.005	0.5	1.7^c	12^c

[a] Agonist activity as an H_1-receptor stimulant determined[c] *in vitro*, on guinea-pig ileum, in the presence of atropine.
[b] Agonist activity as an H_2-receptor stimulant determined[c] *in vivo* for stimulation of gastric acid secretion in the anaesthetised rat.
[c] Durant, Ganellin and Parsons (1975a).
[d] Holmes and Jones (1960) report pK_a 1.68 for the isomeric compound 4-thiazolylethylamine.
[e] Ganellin (1974).

(Ganellin, Port and Richards, 1973b), and it was suggested that the dramatic receptor selectivity of 4-methyl histamine (which has 40 per cent of the potency of histamine as an H_2-receptor stimulant but only 0.2 per cent at H_1 receptors) could be accounted for in the difference between its conformational properties and those of histamine (Ganellin, 1973b); this permitted the definition of an 'H_1-essential' conformation, i.e. a conformation essential to drug activity which has to be adopted by histamine at some stage during interaction at the H_1-receptor site. In another approach, heterocyclic analogues and substituted histamines of low ring pK_a were studied; in these compounds (Table 1.6) dication formation is very low at pH values above 5, and since the compounds have at least 10 per cent of the potency of histamine at either H_1 or H_2 receptors, it seems most unlikely for the dication to be the biologically active species. From this and other arguments it was inferred that the monocation is the active form of histamine (Durant et al., 1975a) at both H_1 and H_2 receptors.

Although histamine is tautomeric, it is probable that imidazole tautomerism is not functionally involved in H_1-receptor stimulation. This follows from the finding that 2-pyridylethylamine (9) (Walter, Hunt and Fosbinder, 1941; Hunt and Fosbinder, 1942) and 2-thiazolylethylamine (10) (Lee and Jones, 1949), which cannot tautomerise, have histamine-like activity in stimulating contractions of the guinea-pig ileum (an H_1-receptor system). The activity of these compounds, taken together with the inactivity of their isomers (3-pyridylethylamine and 5-thiazolylethylamine), also suggests that the N^τ-H tautomer of histamine monocation is the active form at H_1 receptors (Durant et al., 1975a).

9. 2-Pyridylethylamine cation

10. 2-Thiazolylethylamine cation

These non-tautomeric heterocyclic ethylamines are only weakly active at H_2 receptors, however, and it appears that effective H_2-receptor agonists are compounds which can undergo a 1,3-prototropic tautomerism (Durant et al., 1975a). Further indications of the importance of tautomerism for H_2-receptor agonist activity comes from a comparison of the activities of 4-substituted histamine derivatives (Table 1.7). 4-Methylhistamine (11) is about half as active as histamine; r plsacement of methyl by electron-withdrawing substituents reduces activity. Thus 4-chloro- and 4-bromohistamine (12 and 13) have about one-tenth and 4-nitrohistamine (14) has less than one-hundredth of the activity of histamine. Electron-withdrawing substituents in the 4 position of the imidazole ring change the relative tautomer concentrations since they alter the electron densities at the nitrogen atoms and affect proton acidities; the effect is more pronounced at the nearer nitrogen atom, so that the relative stabilities of the tautomers change in comparison with histamine and can be estimated by application of the Hammett equation (Charton, 1965a; Ganellin, 1974). The population of the N^τ-H tautomer of 4-methylhistamine is similar to that of histamine but is reduced by one order of

Table 1.7 Tautomer concentration ratios, K_t, percentage mole fractions of N^τ-H tautomer, and H_2-receptor agonist activities (relative to histamine = 100) of 4-substituted histamine monocations

$$K_t = \frac{\text{[R-imidazole with H-N, N; }CH_2CH_2NH_3^+\text{ at 4-position]}}{\text{[R-imidazole with N, N-H; }CH_2CH_2NH_3^+\text{ at 4-position]}}$$

Compound number	R	$K_t{}^a$	Percentage mole fraction[b] N^τ-H	H_2-receptor agonist activity (%)[c]
Histamine	H	2.4	71	100
11	CH_3	4.1	80	43[d]
12	Cl	0.13	12	11
13	Br	0.11	10	9[e]
14	NO_2	0.009	0.9	0.6

[a] $K_{t,R}$ = antilog [3.4 $(\sigma_{m,CH_2CH_2NH_3^+} - \sigma_{m,R})$]
$\sigma_{m,CH_2CH_2NH_3^+}$ taken as + 0.11 (Ganellin, 1974).
[b] Mole fraction of monocation – not the mole fraction of total species which would be pH-dependent.
[c] Activities determined *in vitro* on guinea-pig right atrium, in the presence of propranolol, expressed relative to histamine = 100 (R. C. Blakemore in Ganellin, 1974).
[d] 95 per cent fiducial limits 40–46.
[e] 95 per cent fiducial limits 7.4–10.1.

magnitude for 4-chlorohistamine and by two orders of magnitude for 4-nitrohistamine (Table 1.7). These reductions in populations of the N^τ-H tautomer approximately parallel the changes in H_2-receptor agonist activities. Of course the tautomeric effect may not be the only factor affecting receptor activity; the substituent will exert other effects, e.g. steric, polarity and lipid-water distribution. However, the results are suggestive and one is led to the speculative deduction either that the N^τ-H tautomer is the biologically active form of histamine at the H_2 receptor or that the free-energy difference between the two tautomers must be small for effective biological activity. This latter observation suggests that tautomerism (or proton transfer) might be involved in the H_2-receptor action of histamine (Ganellin, 1974).

(1) H₁ receptors

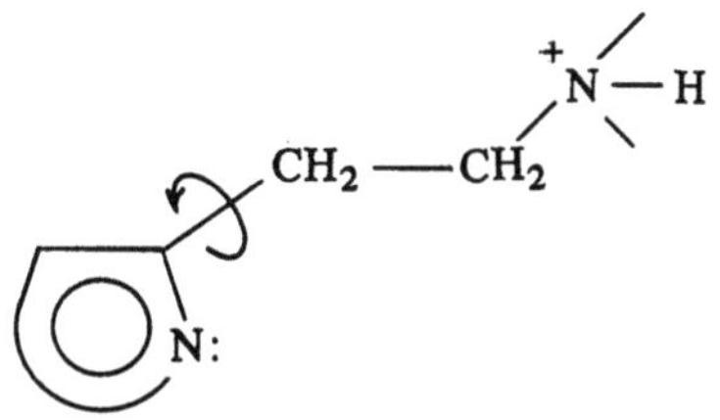

indicating (i) side-chain cation and $\overset{+}{N}$-H
(ii) heterocyclic ring with basic N:
(with lone pair of electrons) in *ortho* position
(iii) ring rotation or possible 'essential' conformation

(2) H₂ receptors

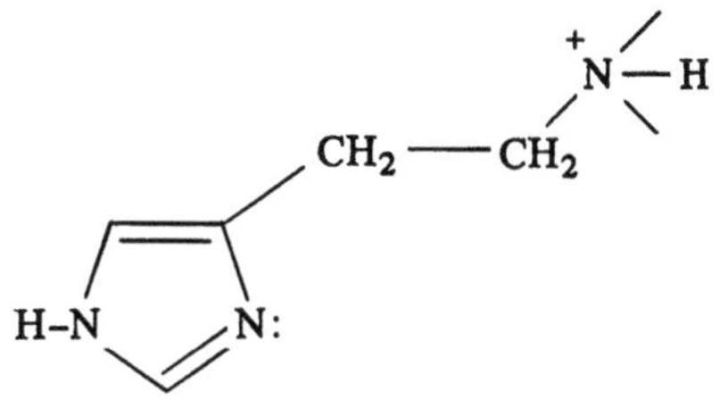

indicating (i) side-chain cation and $\overset{+}{N}$-H
(ii) N^τ-H tautomer and amidine system
(iii) possible function as a proton transfer agent;

thus:

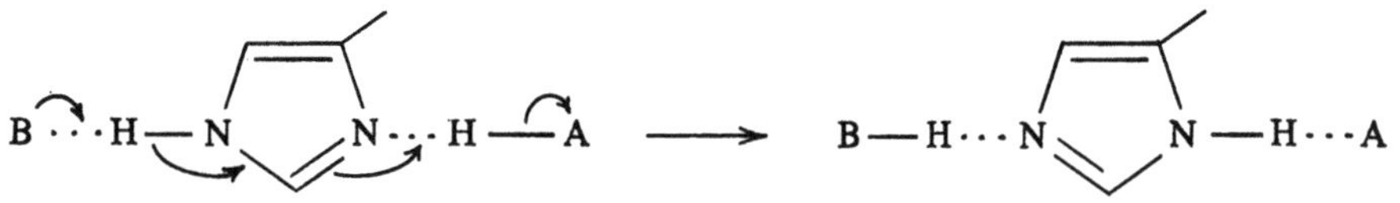

B···H—N⟨⟩N···H—A → B—H···N⟨⟩N—H···A

Scheme 1.9 Functional requirements of agonists at histamine receptors

Thus the active form of histamine for both receptors is likely to be the N^τ-H tautomer of the monocation (7B), which is also the most prevalent species in water at around neutrality. However, different chemical properties of histamine may be associated with interactions at the two receptor types (Scheme 1.9). At the H₁ receptor, imidazole tautomerism is not a functional requirement, but the ammonium-ethyl group should be *ortho* to a heterocyclic nitrogen atom. The ring may also need to be able to freely rotate or at least to achieve coplanarity with the side-chain (Ganellin, 1973b). At the H_2 receptor, the tautomeric property of the imidazole ring of histamine appears to be of importance and histamine might be involved as a proton-transfer agent. Pictorially, one can envisage the imidazole ring catalysing the transfer of a proton from site A to site B, and perhaps a catalytic mechanism of some kind may be involved in the events leading to an effective H_2-receptor response (Durant *et al.*, 1975a).

Example 5: Considerations of Prototropic Equilibria in the Development of Histamine H_2-receptor Antagonists

Development of metiamide

We defined burimamide (15; Table 1.8) as a histamine H_2-receptor antagonist (Black *et al.*, 1972) and, although we investigated its properties in man, it seemed desirable to have a more active compound in order to explore the therapeutic potential of this new type of drug action. In aqueous solution burimamide is a

Table 1.8 Structures of histamine H_2-receptor antagonists

15	Burimamide	imidazole–$CH_2CH_2CH_2CH_2NH$–$C(=S)$–$NHCH_3$
16	Metiamide	4-methylimidazole–$CH_2SCH_2CH_2NH$–$C(=S)$–$NHCH_3$
17		4-methylimidazole–$CH_2SCH_2CH_2NH$–$C(=\overset{+}{N}H_2)$–$NHCH_3$
18	Cimetidine	4-methylimidazole–$CH_2SCH_2CH_2NH$–$C(=N-CN)$–$NHCH_3$

mixture of many chemical species in equilibrium. There are four possible configurational isomers of the thioureido group, various *trans* and *gauche* rotamer combinations of the side-chain CH_2 — CH_2 bonds, and the prototropic equilibria of the imidazole ring. One of the chemical aspects which we examined in detail was concerned with the imidazole ring species.

In aqueous solution at physiological pH (7.4) burimamide exists as an equilibrium mixture of mainly three different imidazole species: the two uncharged tautomers B and C, and the cation A (Scheme 1.10; R = —$(CH_2)_4 NHCSNHCH_3$).

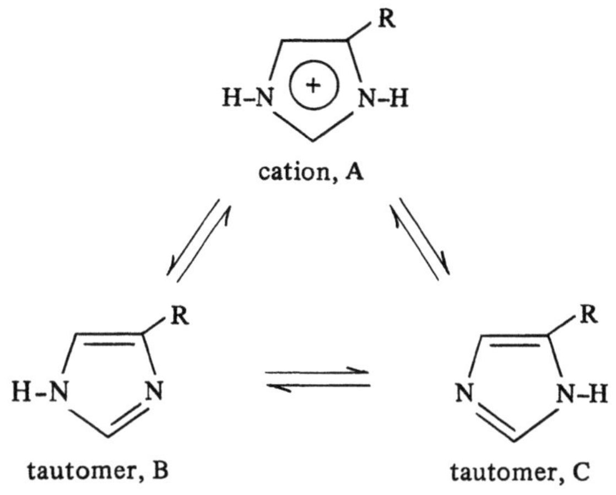

Scheme 1.10 Three species of imidazole with a side-chain R at position 4 (5)

If only one of these forms were active, its relative population could determine the amount of drug required for a given effect. The populations of these species were estimated from the electronic influence of the side chain. The substituent R alters the electron densities at the ring nitrogen atoms and affects proton acidity (Katritzky and Lagowski, 1963b). Its effect is more marked at the nearer nitrogen atom, so that if R is an electron-releasing group, tautomer C should predominate; if it is an electron-withdrawing group, B should predominate. The fraction present as cation A is determined by the ring pK_a of the solution. The electronic influence of the side-chain was assessed from the measured ring pK_a using the Hammett equation: $pK_{aR} = pK_{aH} + \rho\sigma_m$ (Charton, 1965a). The pK_a values of relevant compounds are given in Table 1.9.

For histamine the ammonium-ethyl side-chain (R = —$CH_2 CH_2 NH_3^+$) lowers the pK_a of the imidazole ring; it withdraws electrons and favours tautomer B to the extent that approximately 80 per cent of histamine molecules are in this form (see above). For burimamide the ring pK_a is greater than for imidazole; therefore

Table 1.9 Apparent pK_a values of substituted imidazole cations at 37°C and their mole percentages at pH 7.4

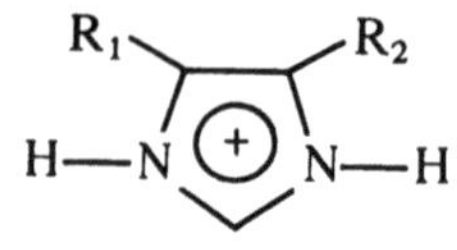

$$\text{H—N}\overset{R_1 \quad R_2}{\underset{\oplus}{\diagdown\diagup}}\text{N—H}$$

Compound	R_1	R_2	pK_a	Preferred tautomer[a]	Mole % of cation A at pH 7.4
Methylburimamide	CH_3	—$(CH_2)_4$NHCSNHCH$_3$	7.80		72
4(5)-Methylimidazole	H	—CH_3	7.40	C	50
Burimamide	H	—$(CH_2)_4$NHCSNHCH$_3$	7.25	C	40
Imidazole	H	—H	6.80		20
Metiamide	CH_3	—$CH_2SCH_2CH_2$NHCSNHCH$_3$	6.80	B	20
Thiaburimamide	H	—$CH_2SCH_2CH_2$NHCSNHCH$_3$	6.25	B	7
Histamine	H	—$CH_2CH_2NH_3^+$	5.90	B	3

[a]Structures in Scheme 10; R_2 = R.
pK_a determined potentiometrically at 25°C on 0.005 M solutions in 0.1 M KCl by titration against HCl, corrected to 37°C by subtracting 0.0225 units per degree for values in the range 7.5–7.0 (Datta and Grzybowski, 1966), and 0.02 for the range 6.5–6.0 (Paiva et al., 1970) and rounded off to the nearest 0.05 unit (Black et al., 1974).

the side-chain (R = —$(CH_2)_4$NHCSNHCH$_3$) is electron-releasing and tautomer C should be favoured. Electronically the side-chain must resemble a methyl group since the pK_a is close to that of 4(5)-methylimidazole. At pH 7.4 the cation is one of the main species (about 40 per cent) and tautomer B should be the least favoured.

Thus, although both histamine and burimamide are mono-substituted imidazoles, the structural similarity is misleading in that the predominant species of the respective imidazole rings are chemically different. If the active form of the antagonist were species B, the form most preferred for histamine, then activity might be enhanced by increasing its relative population. This could be done by converting the antagonist side-chain into an electron-withdrawing group, for example, by incorporating an additional electronegative atom in the side-chain, preferably near to the ring. The disturbance to other molecular properties, such as stereochemistry and lipid-water partition, should, however, be kept minimal. This was achieved by isosteric replacement of a methylene group (—CH_2—) by a thioether linkage (—S—) in burimamide at the carbon atom next but one to the ring to give the compound 'thiaburimamide' (R = —$CH_2SCH_2CH_2$NHCSNHCH$_3$) (Black et al., 1974). The electronic influence of the modified side-chain, shown by the ring pK_a, is similar in magnitude but in the opposite direction to that of a methyl group. The main species should be tautomer B, although its population may not be as large as it is in histamine because the electronic effect of the side-chain is not as marked.

Table 1.10 H_2-receptor antagonist activities determined *in vitro* on guinea-pig atrium and rat uterus. The dissociation constant (K_B) was calculated from the equation $K_B = B/(x - 1)$, where x is the respective ratio of concentrations of histamine needed to produce half-maximal responses in the presence and absence of different concentrations (B) of antagonist, and $-\log K_B = pA_2$ (Black *et al.* 1974)

	Atrium K_B (95% limits) $\times 10^{-6}$ M	Uterus K_B (95% limits) $\times 10^{-6}$ M
Metiamide	0.92 (0.74 – 1.15)	0.75 (0.40 – 1.36)
Thiaburimamide	3.2 (2.5 – 4.5)	3.2 (2.5 – 4.5)
Burimamide	7.8 (6.4 – 9.6)	6.6 (4.9 – 8.3)
Methylburimamide	8.9 (5.6 – 15)	10.7 (4.5 – 31)

To further increase the population of tautomer B, methyl as an electron-releasing substituent was introduced into the vacant 4(5)-position of the ring (since electron-releasing groups favour the form with the hydrogen atom on the adjacent nitrogen) to give the compound metiamide (16) (Black *et al.*, 1974). The two ring substituents in metiamide are seen to have electronic effects of equal magnitude but of opposite direction. They should combine to favour tautomer B but oppose in their effect on ring pK_a; indeed, they must exactly cancel since the pK_as of metiamide and imidazole are identical. This means that at pH 7.4 the main species should be tautomer B, as for histamine, although there would still be a substantial proportion of cation present (about 20 per cent). In comparison with burimamide, the ratio of tautomers is reversed for metiamide and the proportion of cation is decreased.

The pharmacological consequences of these manipulations are shown in Table 1.10. The effectiveness of each compound as an H_2-receptor histamine antagonist was compared by estimating the dissociation constant, K_B, (with 95 per cent confidence limits) for the drug-receptor complex on two systems *in vitro*, viz. guinea-pig atrium and the rat uterus. The results obtained on the two tissues are in good agreement and, taken together, show that the metiamide *in vitro* is three to four times more active than thiaburimamide and eight to nine times more active than burimamide.

Thus it can be seen that modifying the side-chain in burimamide by isosteric replacement of —CH_2— by —S— favours tautomer B, reduces the ring pK_a and gives a more active compound (thiaburimamide). Introducing a 4(5)-methyl group to give metiamide increases further the preference for tautomer B but decreases the combined populations of the uncharged tautomers (B and C) through raising the ring pK_a. But although these are opposing effects, the net result is that metiamide is more active still. By contrast, the analogous structural modification of burimamide, viz. incorporation of a ring 4(5)-methyl group to give 'methylburimamide', does not increase activity. In this case the two ring substituents have nearly equal electronic effects in the same direction; the methyl group counterbalances the electronic influence of the side-chain on tautomerism, so that the two tautomers become equally populated, but it raises the ring pK_a to 7.80, so that at pH 7.4 the predominant species is the cation A (about 72 per cent). This illustrates one of the problems of attempting to manipulate the biological properties of drug molecules through altering their chemical structures. Although the methyl group was introduced to increase the tautomer ratio, it also increases the amount of cation; this may be disadvantageous, and one has to discover the optimum balance of opposing influences. One does not know what the optimum will be until one tests it out experimentally.

Development of cimetidine

Metiamide (above) was first described by Black et al. (1973) and shown to be highly effective clinically in reducing hypersecretion of gastric acid (Wyllie and Hesselbo, 1973; Milton-Thompson et al., 1974). In chronic toxicity tests, using daily doses of metiamide at least twenty times the orally effective dose in the dog,

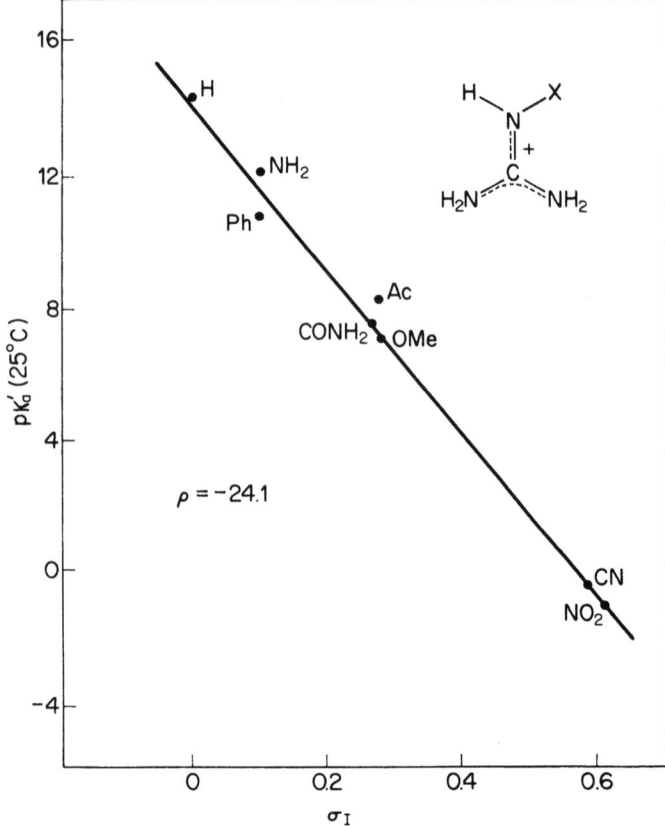

Figure 1.2 Apparent pK_a values at 25°C of N-substituted guanidinium cations plotted against σ_I substituent constants. Data mainly from Charton (1965b). The line corresponds to the equation $pK_a' = 14.20 - 24.1\, \sigma_I$

some animals developed kidney damage and agranulocytosis (Black et al., 1973; Brimblecombe, Duncan and Walker, 1973). The possibility existed that the toxic effects were related to the presence of a thioureido group in metiamide and it appeared to be worthwhile, therefore, to investigate a non-thiourea antagonist.

When we thought about alternatives to a thiourea, we considered replacing S by NH to give a guanidine (e.g. 17; Table 8) because H_2-antagonist activity had previously be demonstrated with guanidines (Durant, Parsons and Black, 1975b; Parsons et al., 1975). However, guanidines were not sufficiently active. It occurred to us that one problem may be the basicity of the guanidino group. Guanidine is an extremely strong base ($pK_a > 13$), i.e. it is much more basic than most amines, and in aqueous solution at physiological pH it is almost exclusively present as the cation; however, the pK_a is very susceptible to substituent effects. The basicity of guanidines can be markedly reduced by substituting electron-withdrawing groups at the N atoms. Charton (1965b) investigated the relationships between substituent effect and guanidine pK_a using the Hammett equation and obtained a good correlation

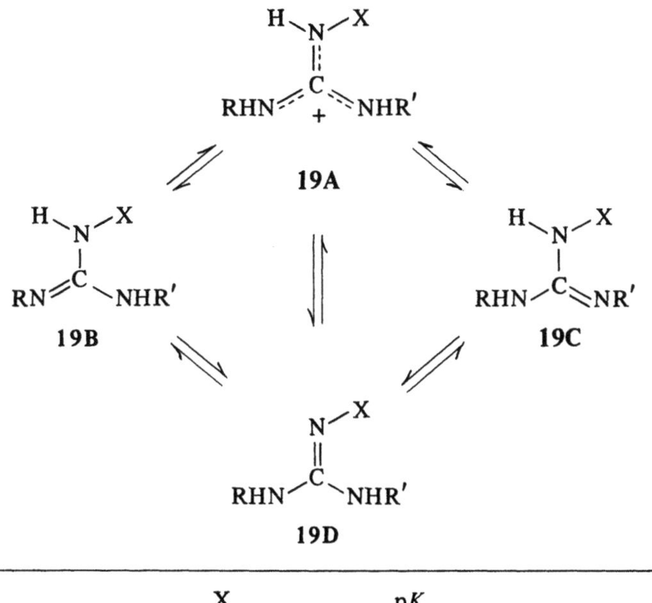

X	pK_a
H or CH_3	> 13
$-COCH_3$	~ 7.5
$-CN$	< 0

Scheme 1.11 Equilibria between substituted guanidine species (cation and three conjugate bases)

with the inductive substituent constant σ_I. The plot of pK_a against σ_I for a series of monosubstituted guanidines is shown in Fig. 1.2; the ρ value of -24 indicates the extreme sensitivity of pK_a to substituent effects in guanidines. The cyano and nitro groups reduce pK_a by over 14 units, to values < 0.

The substituted guanidinium cation (19A) is in equilibrium with three conjugate bases (19B, C, D in Scheme 1.11), since proton dissociation may occur from each of the three nitrogen atoms. When X = H or Me, the $pK_a > 13$ and the cation is overwhelmingly favoured at pH 7; an electron-withdrawing group such as X = COCH$_3$ lowers the pK_a to about 7.5 (when R = R' = CH$_3$; Matsumoto and Rapoport, 1968), giving a more equal mixture of species. With a very powerful electron-withdrawing group, such as X = CN, $pK_a < 0$ and the most intense effect is exerted on the N atom carrying the group X; proton dissociation gives rise almost exclusively to the imino form of the conjugate base (19D).

Incorporating the cyanoguanidino group into the antagonist structure (i.e. replacing thione C=S by cyanoimino C=N—C≡N) afforded the drug cimetidine (18; Table 1.8) (Tagamet®) (Brimblecombe et al., 1975). As an H$_2$-receptor antagonist, cimetidine is very similar to metiamide and has a slightly enhanced potency *in vivo*. This biological similarity is reflected in the chemical similarities between thiourea and cyanoguanidine shown in Table 1.11. Cyanoguanidine and

Table 1.11 Some physicochemical properties of cyanoguanidines and thioureas

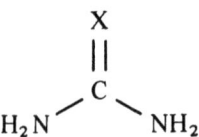

		X = NCN cyanoguanidine	X = S thiourea
Geometry	: C—N bond length (Å)	1.33[a]	1.34[b]
Basicity	: pK_a (proton gained)	-0.4[c]	-1.2[d]
Acidity	: pK_a (proton lost)	14[e]	15[f]
Polarity	: Dipole moment in dioxane, μ(D)	8.16[g]	4.89[h]
Hydrophilicity	: partition (37°C), $P = \dfrac{C_{octanol}}{C_{water}}$	0.07[i]	0.09[i]

[a]Hughes (1940).
[b]Truter (1967).
[c]Hirt et al. (1961).
[d]Janssen (1962).
[e]Kameyama (1921).
[f]Herlem (1965).
[g]Schneider (1950).
[h]Kumler and Fohlen (1942).
[i]Determined by Dr R. C. Mitchell and reported in Brimblecombe et al. (1975).

thiourea have many chemical properties in common. They have similar geometries, they are planar structures and are weakly amphoteric (very weakly basic and acidic), so that in the pH range 2 - 12 they are un-ionised; both are very polar and hydrophilic: thus they have high dipole moments (μ), low octanol - water partition coefficients (P), and are reasonably soluble in water. The physicochemical properties of cimetidine and metiamide reflect these characteristics of cyanoguanidine and thiourea (Brimblecombe *et al.*, 1975).

SUMMARY

Drug molecules must exert their effects through interactions at the molecular level. *Molecular interactions* involve the *size* and *shape* of molecules and the *electron distribution* and *polarisabilities* within molecules. In *structure - activity analysis* we modify chemical features by *changing drug structure*, and we have to consider the effects on chemical properties that are sensitive to structure, i.e. *constitutive properties*.

However, drug molecules often consist of different *species in equilibrium*, and in such cases we should employ an approach of *dynamic structure - activity analysis* (DSAA). We need to characterise the drug, chemically, in terms of its *conformational equilibria* and *prototropic equilibria*. We may then consider the effect of structural modification on the species equilibria and try to relate this to effects on biological activity. It may be possible to then infer something about the chemical mechanism of drug action and the analysis may provide a method for drug design.

The basis of prototropic equilibria is proton acidity, i.e. pK_a. It is not enough, however, to simply measure empirical pK_as — one must *identify the sites of ionisation* and consider the implications. In this way one may uncover fundamental chemical changes that were otherwise not at all obvious. It is necessary to identify the relative species *populations*, and the *properties* of these species. Some examples of DSAA have been given which hint at the usefulness, or potential use, of such an approach, viz. the site of protonation in thiamine, the relationship between zwitterionic and uncharged forms of catecholamines, species equilibria for 3-mercaptopicolinic acid, functional properties and receptor activity of histamine, and considerations of prototropic equilibria in the development of the histamine H_2-receptor antagonists, metiamide and cimetidine. Many other examples could have been considered; for instance, studies of prototropic equilibria have been published dealing with morphine (Schill and Gustavi, 1964), tyrosine (Martin *et al.*, 1958), DOPA and tyramine (Martin, 1971), tetracycline (Rigler *et al.*, 1965) and pyridoxal (Metzler and Snell, 1955; Williams and Neilands, 1954). Zwitterions occur ubiquitously in nature as amino acids, and tautomerism is a feature of the nucleotide bases. Clearly, prototropic equilibria have a fundamental importance in biology.

ACKNOWLEDGEMENTS

The author gratefully acknowledges his debt to his colleagues, Drs J. C. Emmett and R. C. Young, for many helpful and enlightening discussions of problems concerning structure-activity analysis.

REFERENCES

Ahlquist, R. P. (1948). *Am. J. Physiol.*, **153**, 586
Albert, A. (1952). *Pharmacol. Rev.*, **4**, 136
Albert, A. (1966). *The Acridines*, 2nd edn, London, Arnold, Ch. 20
Albert, A. (1968). *Selective Toxicity*, 4th edn, London, Methuen
Albert, A. and Barlin, G. B. (1959). *J. Chem. Soc.*, 2384
Albert, A., Goldacre, R. and Phillips, J. (1948). *J. Chem. Soc.*, 2240
Albert, A. and Serjeant, E. P. (1971). *The Determination of Ionization Constants*, 2nd edn, London, Chapman and Hall
Antikainen, P. J. and Witikainen, U. (1973). *Acta Chem. Scand.*, **27**, 2075
Ash, A. S. F. and Schild, H. O. (1966). *Br. J. Pharmacol. Chemother.*, **27**, 427
Barlow, R. B. (1964). *Introduction to Chemical Pharmacology*, 2nd edn, London, Methuen
Bell, P. H. and Roblin, R. O. (1942). *J. Am. Chem. Soc.*, **64**, 2905
Benesch, R. E. and Benesch, R. (1955). *J. Am. Chem. Soc.*, **77**, 5877
Black, J. W., Duncan, W. A. M., Durant, G. J., Ganellin, C. R. and Parsons, M. E. (1972). *Nature (London)*, **236**, 385
Black, J. W., Duncan, W. A. M., Emmett, J. C., Ganellin, C. R., Hesselbo, T., Parsons, M. E. and Wyllie, J. H., (1973). *Agents and Actions*, **3**, 133
Black, J. W., Durant, G. J., Emmett, J. C. and Ganellin, C. R. (1974). *Nature (London)*, **248**, 65
Black, J. W. and Ganellin, C. R. (1974). *Experientia*, **30**, 111
Blank, B., Di Tullio, N. W., Miao, C. K., Owings, F. F., Gleason, J. G., Ross, S. T., Berkoff, C. E., Saunders, H. L., Delarge, J. and Lapiere, C. L. (1974). *J. Med. Chem.*, **17**, 1065
Breslow, R. (1958). *J. Am. Chem. Soc.*, **80**, 3719
Brimblecombe, R. W., Duncan, W. A. M., Durant, G. J., Emmett, J. C., Ganellin, C. R. and Parsons, M. E. (1975). *J. Int. Med. Res.*, **3**, 86
Brimblecombe, R. W., Duncan, W. A. M. and Walker, T. F. (1973). *International Symposium on Histamine H_2-Receptor Antagonists* (ed. C. J. Wood and M. A. Simkins), London, Smith Kline and French, p. 53
Brittain, R. T., Jack, D. and Ritchie, A. C. (1970). *Adv. Drug Res.*, **5**, 197
Brown, D. J., Hoerger, E. and Mason, S. F. (1955). *J. Chem. Soc.*, 4035
Bruice, T. C. and Benkovic, S. (1966). *Bio-organic Mechanisms*, Vol. 2, New York, Benjamin, Ch. 8
Buckingham, A. D. (1975). *Phil. Trans. R. Soc. London. B*, **272**, 5
Burger, A. (1970). *Medicinal Chemistry*, 3rd edn, New York, Wiley-Interscience
Cammarata, A. and Allen, R. C. (1967). *J. Pharm. Sci.*, **56**, 640
Chand, N. and Eyre, P. (1975). *Agents and Actions*, **5**, 277
Charton, M. (1965a). *J. Org. Chem.*, **30**, 3346
Charton, M. (1965b). *J. Org. Chem.*, **30**, 969
Clement, G. E. and Hartz, T. P. (1971). *J. Chem. Ed.*, **48**, 395
Craig, P. N. (1971). *J. Med. Chem.*, **14**, 680
Datta, S. P. and Grzybowski, A. K. (1966). *J. Chem. Soc. B*, 136

Di Tullio, N. W., Berkoff, C. E., Blank, B., Kostos, V., Stack, E. J. and Saunders, H. L. (1974). *Biochem. J.*, 138, 387
Durant, G. J., Ganellin, C. R. and Parsons, M. E. (1975a). *J. Med. Chem.*, 18, 905
Durant, G. J., Parsons, M. E. and Black, J. W. (1975b). *J. Med. Chem.*, 18, 830
Frieden, E. (1975). *J. Chem. Ed.*, 52, 754
Ganellin, C. R. (1973a). *J. Pharm. Pharmacol.*, 25, 787
Ganellin, C. R. (1973b). *J. Med. Chem.*, 16, 620
Ganellin, C. R. (1974). In *Molecular and Quantum Pharmacology; Proceedings of the 7th Jerusalem Symposium On Quantum Chemistry and Biochemistry* (ed. E. D. Bergman and B. Pullman), Dordrecht, Reidel, p. 43
Ganellin, C. R., Pepper, E. S., Port, G. N. J. and Richards, W. G. (1973a). *J. Med. Chem.*, 16, 610
Ganellin, C. R., Port, G. N. J. and Richards, W. G. (1973b). *J. Med. Chem.*, 16, 616
Gill, E. W. (1965). Drug receptor interactions. In *Progress in Medicinal Chemistry* (ed. G. P. Ellis and G. B. West), Vol. 4, London, Butterworths, p. 39
Goodford, P. J. (1973). *Adv. Pharmacol. Chemother.*, 11, 51
Grafius, M. A. and Neilands, J. B. (1955). *J. Am. Chem. Soc.*, 77, 3389
Green, J. P., Johnson, C. L. and Kang, S. (1974). *Ann. Rev. Pharmacol.*, 14, 319
Green, R. W. and Tong, H. K. (1956). *J. Am. Chem. Soc.*, 78, 4896
Ham, N. S., Casy, A. F. and Ison, R. R. (1973). *J. Med. Chem.*, 16, 470
Hansch, C. (1969). *Acc. Chem. Res.*, 2, 232
Hansch, C. (1976). *J. Med. Chem.*, 19, 1
Hansch, C., Deutsch, E. W. and Smith, R. N. (1965). *J. Am. Chem. Soc.*, 87, 2738
Hansch, C., Leo, A. and Nikaitani, D. (1972). *J. Org. Chem.*, 37, 3090
Hansch, C., Leo, A., Unger, S. H., Kim, K. H., Nikaitani, D. and Lien, E. J. (1973a). *J. Med. Chem.*, 16, 1207
Hansch, C., Unger, S. H. and Forsythe, A. B. (1973b). *J. Med. Chem.*, 16, 1217
Herlem, M. (1965). *Bull. Soc. Chim. France*, 3329
Higuchi, T. and Davis, S. S. (1970). *J. Pharm. Sci.*, 59, 1376
Hine, J. and Mookerjee, P. K. (1975). *J. Org. Chem.*, 40, 292
Hirt, R. C., Schmitt, R. G., Strauss, H. L. and Koren, J. G. (1961). *J. Chem. Eng. Data*, 6, 610
Holmes, F. and Jones, F. (1960). *J. Chem. Soc.*, 2398
Hopmann, R. F. W. and Brugnoni, G. P. (1973). *Nature New Biology*, 246, 157
Hughes, E. W. (1940). *J. Am. Chem. Soc.*, 62, 1258
Hunt, W. H. and Fosbinder, R. J. (1942). *J. Pharmacol. Exp. Ther.*, 75, 299
Ing, H. R. (1964). In the Foreword to Barlow (1964)
Jaffe, H. H. and Jones, H. L. (1964). *Adv. Heterocyclic Chem.*, 3, 256
Jameson, R. F. and Neillie, W. F. S. (1965). *J. Chem. Soc.*, 2391
Janssen, M. J. (1962). *Rec. Trav. Chim. Pays-Bas Belg.*, 81, 650
Kameyama, N. (1921). *J. Chem. Ind. (Japan)*, 24, 1263; *Chem. Abstr.*, 16, 2247 (1922)
Kang, S. and Chou, D. (1975). *Chem. Phys. Lett.*, 34, 537
Kappe, T. and Armstrong, M. D. (1965). *J. Med. Chem.*, 8, 368
Katritzky, A. R. and Lagowski, J. M. (1963a). *Adv. Heterocyclic Chem.*, 1, 312
Katritzky, A. R. and Lagowski, J. M. (1963b). *Adv. Heterocyclic Chem.*, 2, 32
Kellie, G. M. and Riddell, F. G. (1975). *J. Chem. Soc. Perkin*, 11, 740
Kier, L. B. (1968). *J. Med. Chem.*, 11, 441
Korolkovas, A. (1970). *Essentials of Molecular Pharmacology*, New York, Wiley-Interscience
Korte, F. and Weitkamp, H. (1959). *Annalen*, 622, 121
Krampitz, L. O. (1969). *Ann. Rev. Biochem.*, 38, 213
Kraut, J. and Reed, H. J. (1962). *Acta Cryst.*, 15, 747
Kumler, W. D. and Fohlen, G. M. (1942). *J. Am. Chem. Soc.*, 64, 1944

Lee, H. M. and Jones, R. G. (1949). *J. Pharmacol. Exp. Ther.*, **95**, 71
Leffler, E. B., Spencer, H. M. and Burger, A. (1951). *J. Am. Chem. Soc.*, **73**, 2611
Leo, A., Hansch, C. and Church, C. (1969). *J. Med. Chem.*, **12**, 766
Lewis, G. P. (1954). *Br. J. Pharmacol. Chemother.*, **9**, 488
Lien, E. J. (1969). *Am. J. Pharm. Ed.*, **33**, 368
Liler, M. (1975). *Adv. Phys. Org. Chem.*, **11**, 267
Margolis, S., Kang, S. and Green, J. P. (1971). *Int. J. Clin. Pharmacol. Ther. Toxicol.*, **5**, 279
Martin, R. B. (1971). *J. Phys. Chem.*, **75**, 2657
Martin, R. B., Edsall, J. T., Wetlaufer, D. B. and Hollingworth, B. R. (1958). *J. Biol. Chem.*, **233**, 1429
Matsumoto, K. and Rapoport, H. (1968). *J. Org. Chem.*, **33**, 552
Metzler, D. E. and Snell, E. E. (1955). *J. Am. Chem. Soc.*, **77**, 2431
Milton-Thompson, G. J., Williams, J. G., Jenkins, D. J. A. and Misiewicz, J. J. (1974). *Lancet*, **I**, 693
Nemethy, G. (1969). *Ann. N. Y. Acad. Sci.*, **155**, Art.2, 492
Nys, G. G. and Rekker, R. F. (1973). *Chim. Therap.*, 521
Osborn, A. R., Schofield, K. and Short, L. N. (1956). *J. Chem. Soc.*, 4191
Paiva, T. B., Tominaga, M. and Paiva, A. C. M. (1970). *J. Med. Chem.*, **13**, 689
Parsons, M. E., Blakemore, R. C., Durant, G. J., Ganellin, C. R. and Rasmussen, A. C. (1975). *Agents and Actions*, **5**, 464
Perrin, D. D. (1958). *Nature (London)*, **182**, 741
Pletcher, J. and Sax, M. (1972). *J. Am. Chem. Soc.*, **94**, 3998
Pullman, B. and Port, J. (1974). *Mol. Pharmacol.*, **10**, 360
Purcell, W. P., Bass, G. E. and Clayton, J. M. (1973). *Strategy of Drug Design*, New York, Wiley
Rajan, K. S., Davis, J. M., Colburn, R. W. and Jarke, F. H. (1972). *J. Neurochem.*, **19**, 1099
Richardson, M. F., Franklin, K. and Thompson, D. M. (1975). *J. Am. Chem. Soc.*, **97**, 3204. I thank Professor Richardson for personal communication of her unpublished results on the structure of thiamine iodide hydroiodide and thiamine bromide hydrobromide
Rigler, N. E., Bag, S. P., Leyden, D. E., Sudmeier, J. L. and Reilley, C. N. (1965). *Anal. Chem.*, **37**, 872
Risinger, G. E., Gore, W. E. and Pulver, K. (1974). *Synthesis*, 659
Roberts, G. C. K. (1974). In *Molecular and Quantum Pharmacology, Proceedings of the 7th Jerusalem Symposium On Quantum Chemistry and Biochemistry* (ed. E. D. Bergman and B. Pullman), Dordrecht, Reidel, p. 77
Rogers, S. J. (1969). *J. Chem. Ed.*, **46**, 239
Rouvray, D. H. (1975). *J. Chem. Ed.*, **52**, 768
Schill, G. and Gustavi, K. (1964). *Acta Pharm. Suec.*, **1**, 24
Schneider, W. C. (1950). *J. Am. Chem. Soc.*, **72**, 761
Sexton, W. A. (1963). *Chemical Constitution and Biological Activity*, 3rd edn, London, Spon
Seydel, J. K. (1968). *J. Pharm. Sci.*, **57**, 1455
Silipo, C. and Hansch, C. (1975). *J. Am. Chem. Soc.*, **97**, 6849
Sinistri, C. and Villa, L. (1962a). *Farmaco, Ed. Sci.*, **17**, 949
Sinistri, C. and Villa, L. (1962b). *Farmaco, Ed. Sci.*, **17**, 967
Tolstoouhov, A. V. (1955). *Ionic Interpretation of Drug Action in Chemotherapeutic Research*, New York, Chemical Publishing Co.
Topliss, J. G. and Costello, R. J. (1972), *J. Med. Chem.*, **15**, 1066
Truter, M. (1967). *Acta. Cryst.*, **22**, 556
Tuckerman, M. M., Mayer, J. R. and Nachod, F. C. (1959). *J. Am. Chem. Soc.*, **81**, 92
Tute, M. S. (1970). *J. Med. Chem.*, **13**, 48
Viscontini, M., Bonetti, G., Ebnother, C. and Karrer, P. (1951). *Helv. Chim. Acta*, **34**, 1388
Walter, L. A., Hunt, W. H. and Fosbinder, R. J. (1941). *J. Am. Chem. Soc.*, **63**, 2771
Walters, D. B. and Leyden, D. E. (1974). *Anal. Chim. Acta*, **72**, 275

Watanabe, A. and Asahi, Y. (1955). *Yakugaku Zasshi*, 75, 1046
Williams, R. R. and Ruehle, A. E. (1935). *J. Am. Chem. Soc.*, 57, 1856
Williams, V. R. and Neilands, J. B. (1954). *Arch. Biochem. Biophys.*, 53, 56
Wootton, R., Cranfield, R., Sheppey, G. C. and Goodford, P. J. (1975). *J. Med. Chem.*, 18, 607
Wyllie, J. H. and Hesselbo, T. (1973). *International Symposium on Histamine H_2-Receptor Antagonists* (ed. C. J. Wood and M. A. Simkins), London, Smith Kline and French, p. 371

2
Calculation of essential drug conformations and electron distributions

W. G. Richards (Stanford Magnetic Resonance Laboratory, Stanford University, California, USA)†

INTRODUCTION

What would the molecular pharmacologist really like to know? It may seem arrogant for a theoretician to pose and attempt to answer this question, but it is necessary if the full value of theoretical calculations is to be appreciated.

The conventional wisdom is that drug action at a molecular level involves the interaction of the drug, a small molecule, with a macromolecular receptor. Ideally what is sought is the topography of nuclei and electrons in both binding partners in the active environment. This being too Utopian, the crystal structure of the receptor molecule — and, in particular, its binding site — seems to be the next most fundamental type of information. Some progress has been made in this direction, but detailed information about receptors remains elusive.

In consequence, most molecular information comes from studying the small molecule partner: the neurotransmitters, hormones and drugs. Experimental structural studies have been made on these species in the crystalline state and in solution, but the results of such experiments are not necessarily relevant to the essential interaction with the receptor. The outworn analogy of drug and receptor resembling a key fitting a lock is too facile. Although it is possible to build up a picture of a lock by studying keys which fit and keys which do not, the same cannot be done by studying a range of agonists and antagonists binding to the same receptor. The small molecules, unlike keys, are generally flexible. The idea of induced changes in conformation or electron distribution on binding is widespread in molecular biology and it seems eminently possible that drug molecules use their flexibility when binding. This could be the mechanism whereby individual neurotransmitters bind to distinctly different receptors.

Because of this possibility of shape alteration, theoretical calculations are of value in supporting and extending experimental structural studies such as X-ray crystallography and nuclear magnetic resonance spectroscopy. Calculations can indicate which conformations are likely in addition to those found in equilibrium measurements. If done with care and acknowledging all the problems involved, calculations can, in addition to extending experimental studies, add a detailed description of the electron distribution in the small molecule while the nuclei

†Permanent address: Physical Chemistry Laboratory, South Parks Road, Oxford, UK.

are in the conformation essential for binding to the receptor. Most molecular pharmacology has concentrated on molecular shape in terms of nuclear conformation. However, in any interaction or recognition process it is the electrons on the binding partners which provide the forces. A drug receptor will experience the effects of the electron clouds of the approaching small molecule.

Theoretical calculations should be capable of providing two types of information to supplement experimental studies: the range of possible non-equilibrium conformations which must include the unique conformation essential for binding and the electron distribution in that configuration.

THEORETICAL CALCULATIONS

It is well known that the exact solution of the Schrödinger equation,

$$H\psi = E\psi$$

is only possible for some idealised model systems and hydrogen-like atoms. The development of powerful modern computers, however, has permitted the use of brute force iterative methods which can provide solutions of an approximate form of the equation to an arbitrary level of accuracy.

For any molecule with up to about twenty atoms it is possible to solve the equation for a given conformation of the atomic nuclei providing as input only the atomic numbers of the various nuclei and their Cartesian coordinates in some reference system of axes. The solution will yield the energy of the system of nuclei and electrons, E, and more importantly the molecular wave function, ψ. From the wave function the mean value of any physical observable can be computed, including the electron distribution.

Calculations of this type are called *ab initio* calculations. Although they suffer from some well-known defects (Richards and Horsley, 1970), these may be eliminated if sufficient trouble is taken, so that very accurate wave functions are available for small isolated molecules. The isolated molecule is a reasonable approximation to the situation pertaining in interstellar space and in many gas-phase molecular physics experiments. Although it may be more expensive to do the calculations than to perform the experiments, the problems of gas-phase molecular physics are essentially solved.

Molecules of similar size in biology present many problems which are not solved, but the isolated molecule is not a suitable model. The effects of solvent water molecules and ions may be incorporated in an approximate manner either by including a first hydration shell as part of the isolated molecule (Pullman and Pullman, 1975) or by treating the solvent as a dielectric continuum (Beveridge, Kelly and Radna, 1974). Neither approach is totally satisfactory and may not be directly relevant if we are interested in the small molecule in its receptor-binding environment rather than in pure water. This environment is largely unknown and may contain counter-ions, lipid molecules and a membrane surface as well as receptor and water.

For any study, theoretical or experimental, the only way to proceed to an understanding of the essentials for productive binding is to study a series of physically and chemically similar molecules with a variety of biological potencies and to concentrate on differences between members of the series, assuming that the receptor environment produces a constant effect.

The use of a series of molecules, together with the fact that each member must be studied in a variety of ionic, tautomeric and conformational forms, multiplies the number of individual theoretical calculations. For this reason it may not be possible to use the more accurate *ab initio* Hartree-Fock methods. There are a variety of approximations to the pure methods which incorporate some empirical data and neglect some of the integrals implied by the rigorous approach. These methods are listed in Figure 2.1 with quality, as regards isolated molecule calculations, increasing as the figure is read from bottom to top and from left to right.

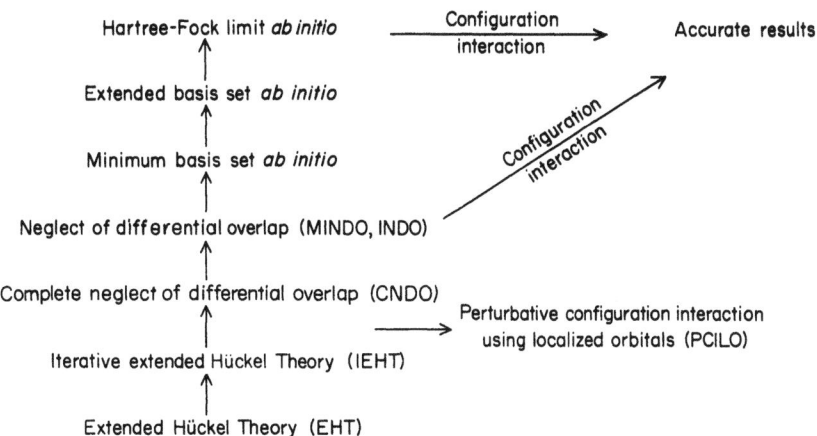

Figure 2.1 The approximate molecular orbital methods in ascending order of reliability for isolated molecule calculations. Accuracy increases going from bottom to top of the figure and left to right

When these approximate theoretical methods are applied to a biological problem, it is imperative that they be checked against some experimental observations. The results should be in harmony with crystallographic structures and solution conformer populations produced by NMR spectroscopy.

CONFORMATIONAL STUDIES

The first stage in studying the conformational properties of any molecule is to build a molecular model, preferably one of the space-filling type. In such models where the atoms are represented by hard spheres the conformational forms which are highly energetic and improbable may be ruled out.

A slightly more realistic picture may be given by theoretical calculations which do not rely upon quantum mechanics but rather on empirical atom–atom potentials. Although there is no sound theoretical basis for doing so, it is possible to represent the internal energy of a molecule as a sum of atom–atom potentials of the form

$$U = Ae^{-Br} + Cr^{-6}$$

Since forces are not pairwise additive and dispersion forces only have an inverse sixth power dependence between charge distributions which are spherically symmetric, the values of the disposable constants A, B and C have no physical significance. Rather this approach should be considered as a method of introducing soft edges to the atoms in a model. These calculations can be performed rapidly and inexpensively and are very useful in conformational problems, provided they are not treated as genuine physically based studies.

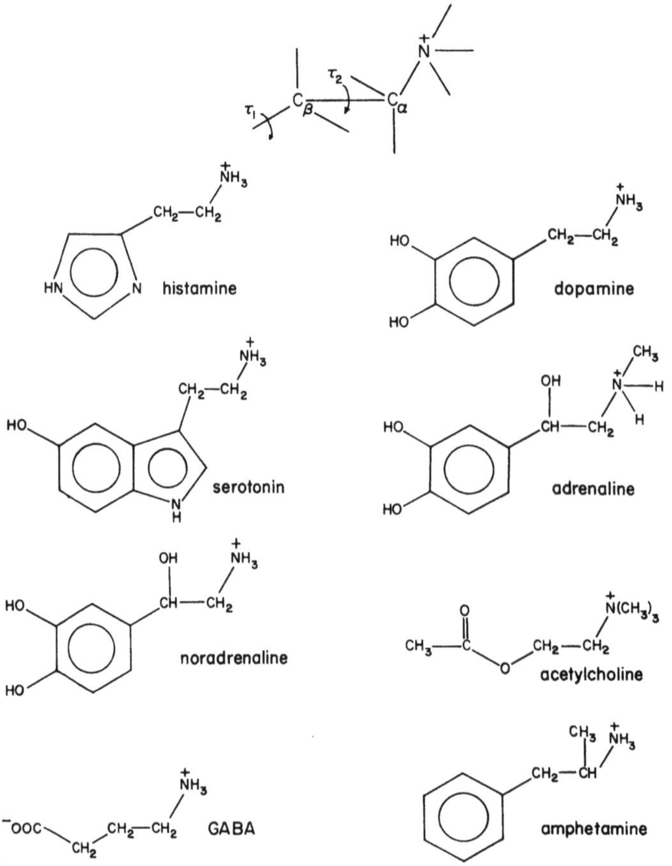

Figure 2.2 Twist angles defining conformation of molecules with two variable angles and some examples of species which are in this category

Alternatively, conformational studies can be performed with quantum mechanical methods. These are based on physics and can cope with purely quantum mechanical phenomena such as delocalisation. Possibly the most effective course is to use first the empirical methods followed by molecular orbital calculations, particularly as the latter will provide not only conformational energies, but also the wave function.

It is an interesting fact that most of the putative neurotransmitters and many drugs can have their conformations defined by two twist angles, τ_1 and τ_2. This is illustrated in Fig. 2.2.

The species illustrated in this figure are in the monocationic form, which is the most prevalent at physiological pH and which is generally believed to be the form involved in the binding to the receptor.

In order to compute the conformational potential energy for any conformer defined by a fixed τ_1 and τ_2, all the other bond length and bond angle data must be supplied. Preferably these should come from X-ray crystallographic sources; otherwise standard values have to be employed (Sutton, 1958, 1965). As a first approximation all bond lengths and angles may be held constant while τ_1 and τ_2 are varied systematically in steps of perhaps $5°$.

For the wide range of compounds which have two variable angles the resulting energies may be presented as maps with contours joining equal energies. The

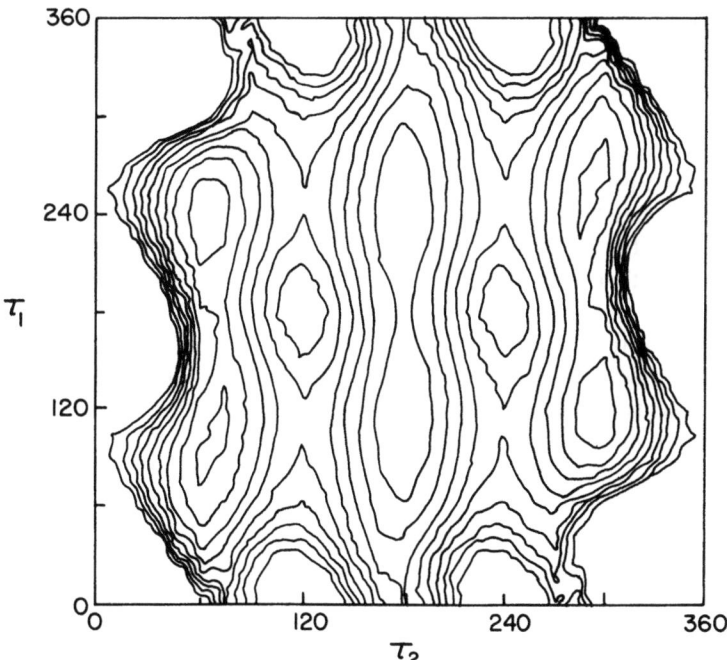

Figure 2.3 Conformational potential energy map for the histamine monocation. The global minimum is at the position $\tau_1 = 120°$ and $\tau_2 = 180°$. The contours are separated by 0.05 eV

case of the histamine monocation is shown in Fig. 2.3. This ion will be used as an illustration throughout this article. It has been the subject of a series of papers (Ganellin, 1973; Ganellin et al., 1973 a; Ganellin, Port and Richards, 1973b; Farnell, Richards and Ganellin, 1975).

On potential energy maps such as this, valleys represent stable forms. The validity can be checked by noting that crystallographic studies give a single point on such a diagram. The point should be at or near a minimum. Solution conformation studies by NMR coupling constant measurements yield populations of stable conformers and, hence, free energy differences between these forms. The diagrams also give free energy differences, provided entropy effects are also included (Farnell, Richards and Ganellin, 1974). This may be done by first computing a Boltzmann factor exp $[E(\tau_1, \tau_2)/kT]$ for each point (τ_1, τ_2) and the appropriate temperature (37°C). The surface illustrated shows three areas of low energy corresponding to two *gauche* (syn-clinal) and one *trans* (antiperiplanar) form of the side-chain.

The definition of a particular region as *trans* or *gauche* is arbitrary, but if a boundary in terms of internal energy is chosen, then conformational partition functions, Z, may be found for each form by summing the Boltzmann factors within the regions. Then

$$\Delta G^\circ = -kT \ln (Z_{trans}/Z_{gauche})$$

assuming no volume change on altering conformation.

In the case under discussion the conformational preferences of a series of methyl-substituted histamine molecules were studied, and free energy differences computed in this way were in accord with NMR solution measurements to approximately 5 per cent in *trans*: *gauche* population ratios, despite the fact that the original potential surfaces were based on simple extended Hückel calculations (Richards et al., 1975).

The set of methyl-substituted histamines have a range of biological activities which could vary owing to differences in conformational freedom, especially since by all indications their electronic properties are not very different (Ganellin, 1974).

Drawing distinctions between conformational potential maps for a series of a dozen members is complicated by the fact that the energy surfaces contain so much information. A clearer picture may be gained from probability maps where a single contour delineates that region of space which contains a prescribed percentage of molecules. Figure 2.4 is an example where the shaded region is the conformational space incorporating 99 per cent of the molecules at 37°C.

These population maps are computed from the Boltzmann factors (Farnell et al., 1975) and show at a glance just how flexible a given molecule is and over precisely what regions of conformation this flexibility is exercised. The whole procedure from the provision of crystallographic data from which atomic coordinates are derived to variations of twist angles and plotting of potential energy and probability maps is completely programmed and takes a few minutes per molecule.

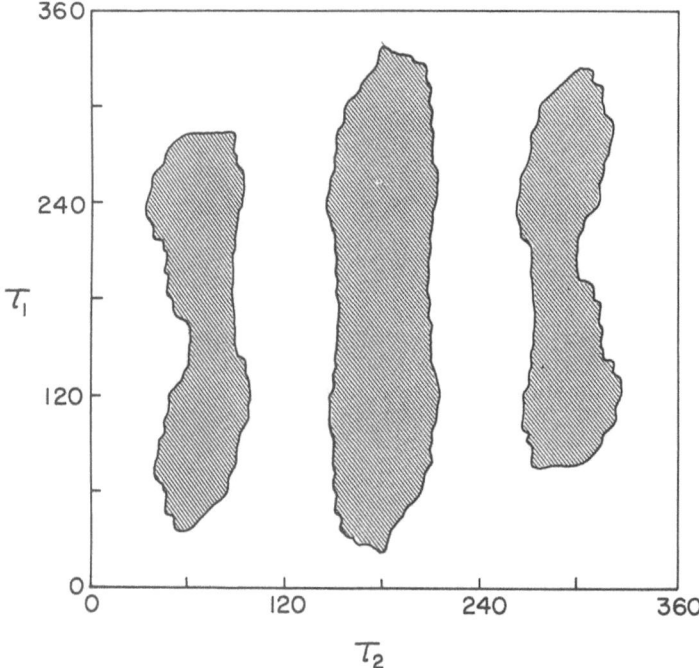

Figure 2.4 Conformational percentage map for the histamine monocation. The shaded area indicates the conformational space incorporating 99 per cent of the molecules at 37°C

ESSENTIAL CONFORMATIONS FOR ACTIVITY

As an illustration of the variation of conformational preference exhibited by three of the members of the series of methyl-substituted histamines, Fig. 2.5 shows maps for N,N-dimethyl histamine, 4-methyl histamine and α-methyl histamine, which may be compared with the unsubstituted ion shown in Fig. 2.4.

Most striking is the difference between the diagrams for histamine and the 4-methyl compound which is substituted in the imidazole ring at the position adjacent to the side-chain. The 4-methyl histamine exhibits about half the activity of histamine at H_2 receptors but only 1/500th of the activity at H_1 receptors. This led to the suggestion (Ganellin, 1973) that possibly the methyl group, in reducing conformational flexibility, precludes the ion from adopting a conformation which is essential for H_1 activity.

Ab initio calculations (Richards *et al.*, 1975) show that there is a very high barrier to internal rotation about the ring-carbon β bond (τ_1) in the substituted molecule, while superposition of the percentage maps for the two species reveals regions of space available to the active compound but denied to the less active agonist. This superposition is illustrated in Fig. 2.6.

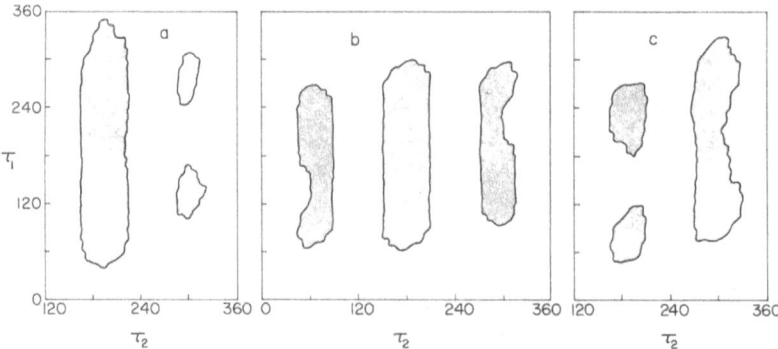

Figure 2.5 Conformational percentage maps indicating 99 per cent probability conformations at 37° for: (a) N,N-dimethyl histamine (H_1 activity 44 relative to histamine 100); (b) 4-methyl histamine (H_1 activity $\sim$ 0); (c) α-methyl histamine (H_1 activity $\sim$ 0)

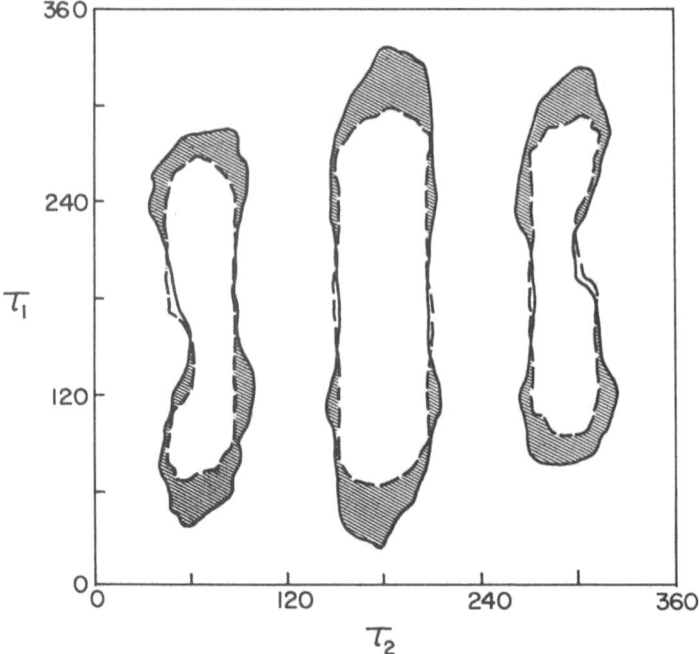

Figure 2.6 Superposition of 99 per cent probability contours of histamine (unbroken line) and 4-methyl histamine (dotted line) to reveal as shaded areas possible H_1 essential conformations

The shaded areas indicate possible conformations which may be essential for activity. This essential conformation can be further specified by incorporating data from other members of the series such as those referred to in Fig. 2.5. In this way one is led to the definition of the activity-essential conformation as a *trans* form which is not a stable form found in either the solid state or in solution. It has $\tau_1 = 300°$ and $\tau_2 = 180°$.

The defined essential conformation may be 'essential' for one of two reasons: it could merely represent an unstable conformation through which the active molecule must pass in order to gain access to the receptor; equally it might represent the precise conformation required to bind to the receptor site in the active environment.

If the second possibility is correct, then we are close to learning about the nature of the receptor site by studying its partner, but if the flexibility is needed to gain access, then the situation is more complex and the receptor site remains elusive. In either case by defining the essential conformation of nuclei we are only part way towards providing the ideal information for the molecular pharmacologist: we may know about the nuclei, but what about the electrons?

ELECTRON DISTRIBUTIONS

Among the experimental techniques which yield information on electron distributions are dipole moments, ^{13}C NMR shifts, X-ray photoelectron shifts and X-ray diffraction. None of these gives a simple indication of the electron density at a defined point in space, and they give no information at all for a conformation which is not an equilibrium form.

The electronic wave function is in principle capable of providing just this information, since the value of ψ^2 (or $\psi^*\psi$ if ψ is complex) at any point is a probability or charge density. The value of $\int \psi^2 \, dv$ integrated over a volume v should give the number of electrons within that volume.

This direct approach to the use of wave functions to provide charge densities has not been employed until recently for molecules as complex as those of interest to the medicinal chemist. Instead a crude but easily programmed population analysis is generally produced (Mulliken, 1955). Population analyses have well-known defects: all the charge in a molecule is assigned to the various nuclei; charge in a bond is divided evenly between the bound nuclei; and, above all, the results are not invariant to changes of basis set within one of the molecular orbital techniques. For these reasons the results have not been considered worthy of detailed study, although they are useful in a comparative fashion.

The recent advance (Dean and Richards, 1975) is based upon the fact that molecular orbital wave functions can now be computed very rapidly. The difficulty in integrating ψ^2 is only severe when the volume element is not simply related to the Cartesian axes defining the molecular geometry. For spheres centred at the origin of the axes, integration is relatively easy. Thus, in order to compute the charge within a sphere centred at a particular nucleus, one only has to choose that atom as the co-ordinate origin. Each successive nucleus may be treated in this way in turn and the wave function computed very rapidly, since the result is known after the first computation. The choice of what radius of sphere to take remains arbitrary, but whatever value is chosen, the charge within that sphere may be calculated very accurately with wave functions of small basis set *ab initio* quality. In trial calculations physical plausibility was demonstrated by a linear relationship between the computed charges and X-ray photoelectron shifts.

Being able to define precisely where one is considering the charge highlights the looseness of phrases such as 'the charge on an atom' when it is the 'charge near to an atom' which is implied. As a relevant test case the charges within a sphere of covalent radius of the nitrogen atom in substituted ammonium ions was taken. The results are given in Table 2.1

Table 2.1 Number of electrons within a sphere of covalent radius centred on the nitrogen atom of substituted ammonium ions

Molecule	Charge within sphere
NH_4^+	5.189
$CH_3 \cdot NH_3^+$	4.919
$C_2H_5 \cdot NH_3^+$	4.932
$(CH_3)_2 \cdot NH_2^+$	4.646
$CH_3 \cdot NH_2^+ \cdot C_2H_5$	4.656
$CH_3 \cdot NH_2^+ \cdot i\text{-}C_3H_7$	4.664
$CH_3 \cdot NH_2^+ \cdot n\text{-}C_3H_7$	4.654

The most obviously striking aspect of these figures is that they vary in a sense quite contrary to naïve notions of the inductive effect. Replacing a proton in NH_4^+ by an alkyl group actually decreases the charge around the nitrogen atom. These conclusions, which are supported by gas-phase studies of basicities (Brauman and Blair, 1969; Brauman, Riveros and Blair, 1971), underline the fact that many previously held ideas of electronic distribution may be erroneous.

With this soundly based method we are now in a position to investigate the charge distribution of the histamine cation in the conformation which has been defined as essential for H_1 activity.

ESSENTIAL ELECTRON DISTRIBUTION

The actual molecular geometry and conformation of the histamine cation in its 'essential' conformation is shown in Fig. 2.7. With the nuclei held in this conformation, *ab initio* molecular wave functions were computed using the Gaussian '70 program (Hehre, Stewart and Pople, 1969) and a basis set of STO3G quality. Since charge densities depend on the square of a wave function at a point, with no consequent problems due to cancelling of positive and negative regions of the function, this should be satisfactory to give a good indication of electron distribution.

Drug Conformations and Electron Interactions

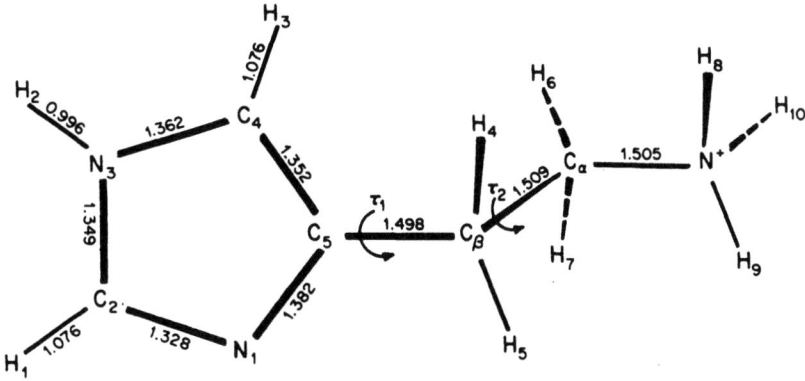

Figure 2.7 Molecular geometry of histamine monocation used in calculations of the essential electron distribution. Angles refer to $C_4 - C_5 - C_\beta$ as $0°$; unless stated C–H distance is 1.073 Å, N–H distance is 1.032 Å; $\tau_1 = 300°$ and $\tau_2 = 180°$

Table 2.2 Total charge density within spheres of radius r centred on atoms of histamine monocation in its 'essential' conformation

r(Å)	0.77	0.70	0.68	0.65	0.63	0.33	0.30
Atom							
N_1		4.631		4.318	4.190		
C_2	3.824	3.478	3.384				
N_3		4.638		4.312	4.180		
C_4	3.843	3.508	3.416				
C_5	3.507	3.256	3.184				
C_β	3.918						
C_α	3.902						
N^+		4.947					
H_1						0.089	0.073
H_2						0.067	0.054
H_3						0.090	0.074
H_4						0.088	0.073
H_5						0.083	0.069
H_6						0.081	0.067
H_7						0.079	0.065
H_8						0.054	0.044
H_9						0.054	0.044
H_{10}						0.054	0.044

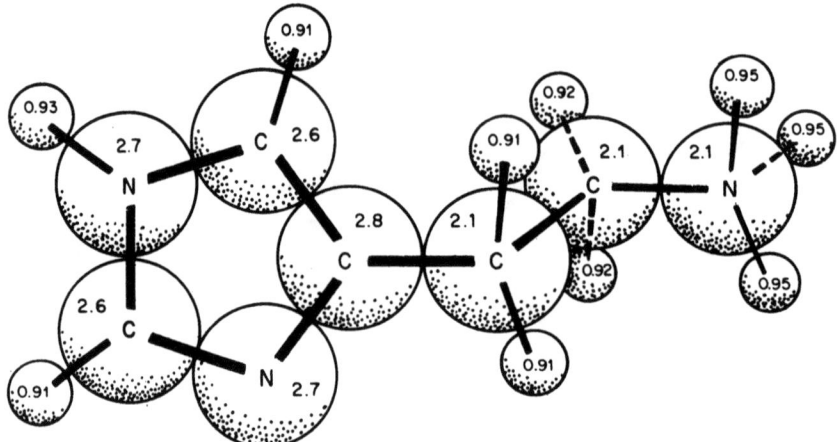

Figure 2.8 Net positive charges within spheres centred on atoms of the histamine monocation. The conformation and geometry is as indicated in Figure 2.7. Radii of spheres correspond to the underlined values in Table 2.2

Table 2.2 summarises some of the resulting data. In this table the charges within spheres of a variety of radii are given for some of the nuclei where it is not immediately obvious what is the most appropriate covalent radii to choose. The values underlined are those which allow adjacent spheres to touch but not to overlap and take cognisance of the differences in bonding of atoms in the imidazole ring and in the side-chain.

Figure 2.8 illustrates this charge distribution with the net positive charges being given for each sphere (that is, the nuclear charge with the number of electrons in the sphere subtracted).

Although these calculations do not include any solvent or counter-ion, the very uniform distribution of the positive charge makes it unlikely that the surrounding medium would produce dramatic changes.

The very important result is the uniform distribution of positive charge over the molecular skeleton. The nitrogen atom conventionally written with a positive sign alongside it is no more positive than other nuclei, and even the protons attached to it are scarcely more positive than others in the molecule.

This charge picture emphasises the futility of drawings so commonly produced of schematic receptor sites in which there are highly localised centres of negative charge which are supposed to bind equally localised positive centres. In reality it seems that the overall positive ion is attracted to a negative site but that details of short-range binding depend on dispersion forces.

DISCUSSION

There are two aspects to the use of quantum mechanical calculations in investigating the binding of drugs to receptors. The first is conformational and the second is the provision of submolecular electron distributions.

The role of theoretical calculations in conformational studies is clearest in the extension of experimental data to cover conformations which are not equilibrium forms but attainable without the provision of significant amounts of energy. Many studies, both experimental and, particularly, theoretical, concentrate on the stable conformers which can exist in free space or in solution. The justification for this is sometimes referred to as the 'weak binding approximation' (Kier and Truitt, 1970). In essence this idea rejects the analogy of drug plus receptor being likened to substrate plus enzyme, since the binding to drug receptors is not normally covalent and wash-out reversal is easy. Although it may be true that a drug can be capable of producing a perturbation in the receptor before being tightly bound, it is hard to understand the degree of structural specificity demanded by receptors if intimate binding is not an essential prerequisite of efficacy.

Theoretical computations cannot stand on their own, but if supported by crystallographic and spectroscopic studies, they may be capable of indicating the range of possible conformations of active molecules that are plausible for binding. A comparative study of a well-chosen series of compounds with variable activity may then reveal an increasingly well-defined essential conformation for potency.

Given the defined essential conformation, the wave function appropriate for that disposition of nuclei can be used to compute accurate values of the charge distribution. In the case studied here, the histamine monocation is revealed as having no localised positive centre. This probably rules out simplified pictures of the receptor with localised anionic sites.

The nature of the charge distribution is also suggestive as to the nature of the essential conformation. If the cationic head had a localised positive charge, it would seem probable that the binding process would consist of long-range coulombic attraction of the positive nitrogen, which would be bound first, followed by a step-wise attachment of the rest of the molecule. The essential conformation would then more likely refer to one through which the molecule had to pass to achieve effective binding involving several parts of the molecule.

Since the charge is not localised, it seems more likely that the initial recognition process would involve coulombic attraction in a quite unspecific manner. At short range the steeper dispersion forces would provide binding and, above all, discrimination between molecules. The initial attraction not involving any isolated local attachment makes it more likely that the hypothesis that the essential conformation is the one needed to bind is the correct alternative.

It is difficult to prove this contention, but if it is true, then the calculations are indeed providing a part of the answer to the molecular pharmacologist's question. They are revealing not only where nuclei must be situated in order to produce an effective interaction, but also, more importantly, what the electron distribution must be.

ACKNOWLEDGEMENTS

The author would like to thank the Science Research Council for a grant of computing time and generous support from the Lord Dowding Fund for Humane Research.

REFERENCES

Beveridge, D. L., Kelly, M. M. and Radna, R. J. (1974). *J. Am. Chem. Soc.*, **96**, 3769
Brauman, J. I. and Blair, L. K. (1969). *J. Am. Chem. Soc.*, **91**, 2126
Brauman, J. I., Riveros, J. M. and Blair, L. K. (1971). *J. Am. Chem. Soc.*, **93**, 3914
Dean, S. M. and Richards, W. G. (1975). *Nature (London)*, **256**, 473
Farnell, L., Richards, W. G. and Ganellin, C. R. (1974). *J. Theoret. Biol.*, **43**, 389
Farnell, L., Richards, W. G. and Ganellin, C. R. (1975). *J. Med. Chem.*, **18**, 662
Ganellin, C. R. (1973). *J. Med. Chem.*, **16**, 620
Ganellin, C. R. (1974). In *Molecular and Quantum Pharmacology* (ed. E. Bergmann and B. Pullman), Dordrecht, Reidel, p. 43
Ganellin, C. R., Pepper, E. S., Port, G. N. J. and Richards, W. G. (1973a). *J. Med. Chem.*, **16**, 610
Ganellin, C. R., Port, G. N. J. and Richards, W. G. (1973b). *J. Med. Chem.*, **16**, 616
Hehre, W. J., Stewart, R. F. and Pople, J. A. (1969). *J. Chem. Phys.*, **51**, 2657
Kier, L. B. and Truitt, E. B. (1970). *J. Pharm. Exp. Ther.*, **174**, 94
Mulliken, R. S. (1955). *J. Chem. Phys.*, **23**, 1833
Pullman, A. and Pullman, B. (1975). *Quart. Rev. Biophys.*, **7**, 505
Richards, W. G., Hammond, J. and Aschman, D. G. (1975). *J. Theoret. Biol.*, **51**, 237
Richards, W. G. and Horsley, J. (1970). *Ab Initio Molecular Orbital Calculations for Chemists*, Oxford, Clarendon Press
Sutton, L. E. (1958, 1965). *Tables of Interatomic Distances and Configurations in Molecules and Ions*, London, Chem. Soc. Special Publ. No. 11; Supplement No. 18

3
The conformation of hormonal peptides in solution

J. Feeney (Division of Molecular Pharmacology, National Institute for Medical Research, Mill Hill, London, UK)

INTRODUCTION

For large hormonal peptides such as insulin it seems reasonable to assume that the molecules will have a fairly well-defined three-dimensional structure in solution where the groups are organised, to a large extent, into a conformation suitable for a favourable interaction with its receptor. When one considers much smaller hormonal peptides such as the linear peptides thyrotropin releasing factor (TRF), gastrin tetrapeptide and luteinising hormone releasing hormone (LH - RH) and the cyclic neurohypophysial hormones, oxytocin and lysine vasopressin, it is of interest to ask if these molecules also exist in some strongly preferred conformation in solution. Some workers have argued that the most populated conformation of the hormone will bind with the highest affinity to the receptor, although there is no *a priori* reason for believing this to be the case. At the present time there are no available data on hormone conformations in hormone - receptor complexes on which to examine these claims. However, the X-ray structures of several enzyme - coenzyme and enzyme - inhibitor complexes indicate that conformational changes often occur on complex formation. If there is a conformational change when the hormonal peptides bind to their receptors, then it will be necessary to define the conformational state for both the free and bound peptides if we are to fully understand the energetics of the hormone - receptor interaction.

Theoretical potential energy calculations for several hormonal peptides have been made and these provide us with information about the fractional populations of the different conformations. On the experimental side, nuclear magnetic resonance (NMR) spectroscopy can be used (sometimes in conjunction with the potential energy calculations) to estimate the fractional populations of the conformers. When the lifetimes (τ) of the conformers are short on the NMR time scale ($\tau \ll 1/2\, \pi v$, where v is the shift difference between the same nucleus in different conformers), the observed NMR spectrum is an averaged spectrum. The coupling constants and chemical shifts in such a spectrum are the averaged values of the parameters in the contributing conformers weighted according to their fractional populations. If we can measure the values of the coupling constants and chemical shifts in the component conformers, then it is often possible to calculate the fractional populations of the conformers from the observed averaged coupling constants and chemical shifts.

It is also of interest to study how the conformations of hormonal peptides are influenced by different solvents. This not only gives us some insight into the range of accessible conformational states, but can also uncover interactions which become favoured in hydrophobic environments (of possible relevance to the hormone in its hormone - receptor complex). For example, the NMR method can sometimes identify specific NH protons which are involved in intramolecular hydrogen bonding in some solvents (DMSO) but not in others (H_2O).

The purpose of this present paper is to indicate the different kinds of conformational information obtainable from NMR measurements on hormonal peptides, to summarise the experimental findings for some small linear and cyclic hormones and, finally, to consider whether or not this information helps us to understand how the hormones bind to their receptors.

CONFORMATIONAL INFORMATION FROM NMR MEASUREMENTS

The conformations of the neurohypophysial hormones oxytocin (1) and lysine vasopressin (2) have been extensively studied in several laboratories (Johnson, Schwartz and Walter, 1969; Urry, Ohnishi and Walter, 1970; Feeney *et al.*, 1971; Urry and Walter, 1971; Walter, 1971; Kotelchuck, Scheraga and Walter, 1972; Von Dreele *et al.*, 1972; Brewster and Hruby, 1973; Brewster *et al.*, 1973; Smith *et al.*, 1973; Walter and Glickson, 1973; Walter *et al.*, 1973; Bradbury *et al.*, 1974; Deslauriers and co-workers, 1974 b) and it is convenient to use the NMR results for these molecules to illustrate the kinds of conformational information which are available.

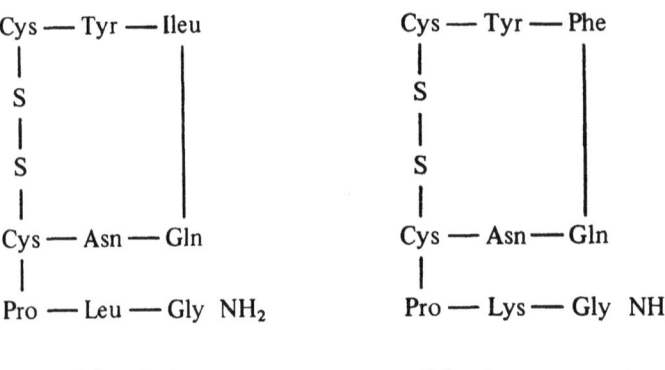

1 Oxytocin　　　　　　　　2 Lysine vasopressin

The Conformation of Hormonal Peptides in Solution

Spectral Assignments

The first stage is to record and assign the high-resolution NMR ^{1}H spectra of the molecules. Most assignments have been made by using data from model peptides and by applying spin decoupling techniques to connect the more securely assigned βCH_2 protons with their αCH and NH protons (Brewster and Hruby, 1973). Unequivocal assignments can best be made by examining isotopically labelled analogues (Brewster and Hruby, 1973; Bradbury et al., 1974). For example, if the nitrogen in the peptide bond is replaced by ^{15}N (spin number $I = \frac{1}{2}$), then the coupling between the ^{15}N nucleus and the NH proton gives rise to a large doublet splitting ($^1J_{^{15}N-^1H} \approx 93$ Hz) on the NH proton absorption which leads to an unambiguous assignment of the labelled NH resonance: thus a study of 2-[^{15}N Tyr]-oxytocin and 3-[^{15}N-Ileu] oxytocin gave unequivocal assignments for the Tyr and Ileu NH absorptions, respectively (Bradbury et al., 1974). Deuterium-substituted compounds can also be used to assist in making assignments: for example, replacement of an αCH proton by deuterium results in the loss of an αCH resonance in the spectrum, converts the doublet NH absorption into a broad singlet and simplifies the βCH_2 multiplets, thus leading to unequivocal assignments for all these protons (Brewster and Hruby, 1973; Bradbury et al., 1974)

Intramolecular Hydrogen Bonding Involving NH Protons

In H_2O solutions it is possible to observe ^{1}H signals for all the NH protons in a molecule such as oxytocin (see Fig. 3.1). A study of the temperature dependence of the NH chemical shifts can provide information about the presence of intramolecular hydrogen bonding involving the NH protons (Urry et al., 1970). Normally the NH protons are hydrogen bonded to the solvent molecules; when the temperature is raised, the number of hydrogen-bonded species in the equilibrium is decreased, and the NH signal moves towards the high-field chemical shift position expected for non-hydrogen-bonded NH protons. For aqueous

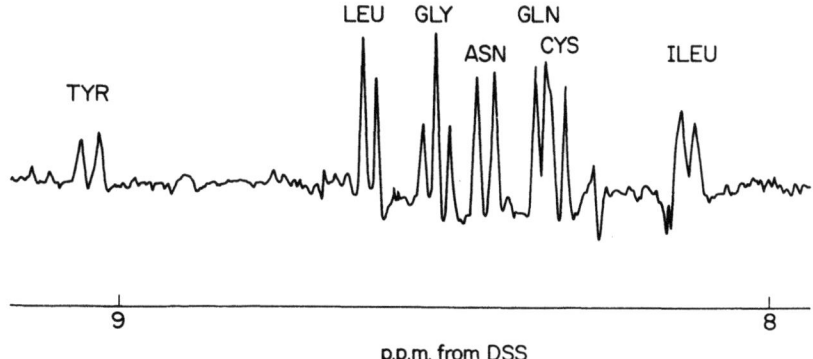

Figure 3.1 The peptide NH region of the 270 MHz proton NMR spectrum of oxytocin hydrochloride in aqueous (H_2O) solution

Table 3.1 The $^3J_{\alpha CHNH}$ coupling constants (Hz) and temperature/chemical shift coefficients for oxytocin and lysine vasopressin (H$_2$O solutions at pH 3.7)

Residue	J_{NC} (Hz)		NH temp. coeff. (p.p.m. x 10^3 deg^{-1})	
	Oxytocin	Vasopressin	Oxytocin	Vasopressin
Tyr	7.6	7.1	6.5	6.5
Ileu (Phe)	7.0	6.5	7.0	6.3
Gln	4.9	5.2	5.5	4.3
Asn	8.2	8.7	5.0	6.0
Cys (6)	7.0	6.2	5.5	7.0
Leu (Lys)	6.5	7.0	9.5	9.0
Gly	5.5	5.5	7.0	7.5

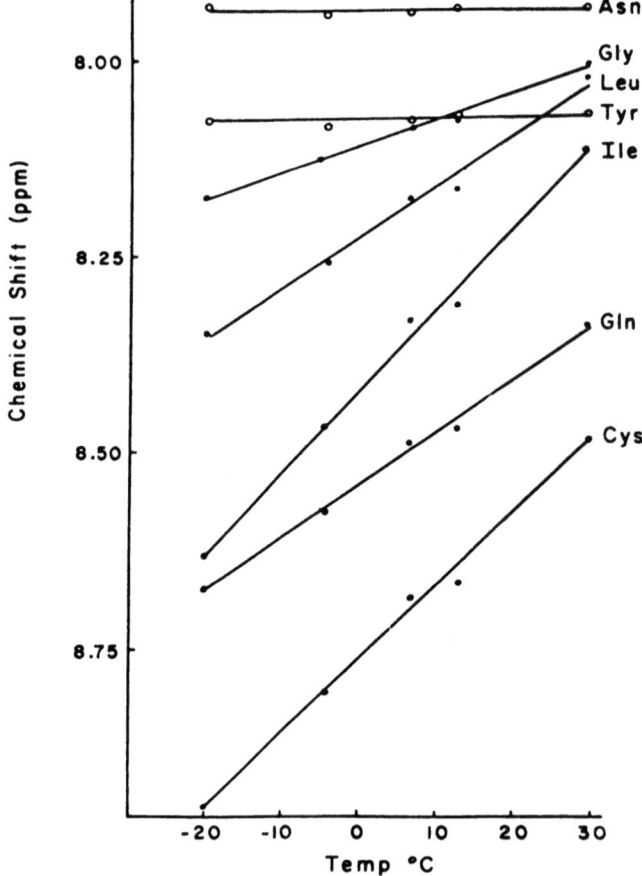

Figure 3.2 The temperature dependence of the peptide NH proton chemical shifts for deamino oxytocin in dimethylsulphoxide/methanol solution. Reproduced with permission from Urry et al. (1970)

solutions of oxytocin and lysine vasopressin all the NH signals have appreciable temperature/chemical shift coefficients (see Table 3.1), indicating that they are all hydrogen bonded to solvent water molecules. Urry and co-workers had previously carried out similar measurements in dimethylsulphoxide/methanol solution, where they found that the Asn NH had a zero temperature/chemical shift coefficient for both oxytocin and lysine vasopressin. They interpret this finding as a strong evidence for an intramolecular hydrogen bond involving the Asn NH proton. We will see later that there is good evidence to indicate that the ring structure has a different conformation from that in water. For deamino oxytocin the same workers used this method to demonstrate the presence of two intramolecular hydrogen bonds (Fig. 3.2) involving the Asn NH and the Tyr NH. From consideration of other data ($J_{\alpha CHNH}$ spin coupling constants) they were able to deduce that the Asn NH proton was intramolecularly hydrogen bonded to the Tyr peptide CO oxygen and the Tyr NH proton hydrogen bonded to the Asn peptide CO oxygen (see Fig. 3.3).

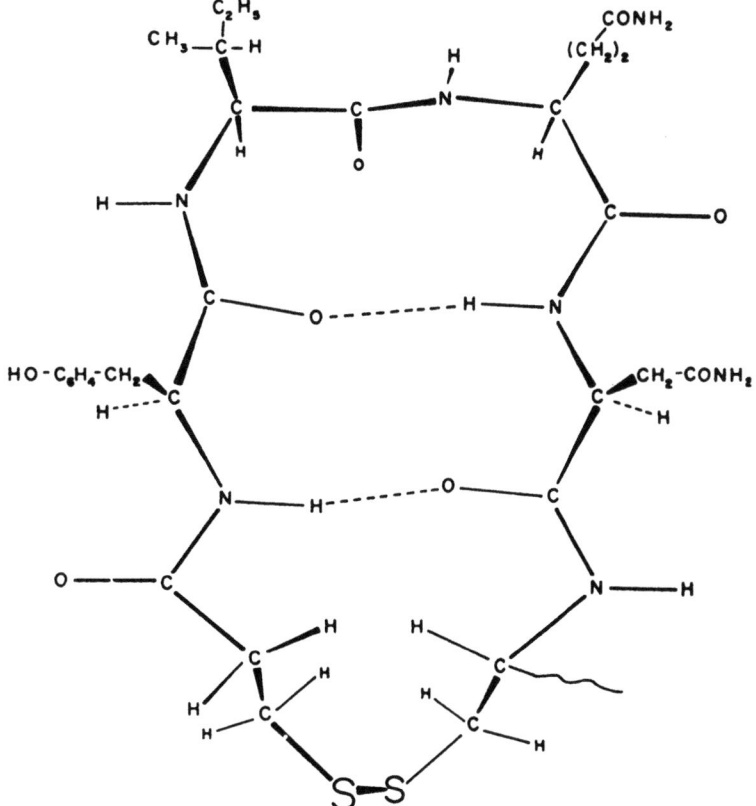

Figure 3.3 Proposed structure of deamino oxytocin in dimethylsulphoxide solution. Reproduced with permission from Urry et al. (1970)

If an intramolecular hydrogen bond is suspected on the basis of temperature/chemical shift measurements, then experiments at different peptide concentrations need to be undertaken to eliminate the possibility of contributions from intermolecular hydrogen bonds in self-associated complexes (Higashijima, Tasumi and Miyazawa, 1975). There is also the possibility that a low temperature/shift coefficient can be associated with a solvent-inaccessible NH proton which is not necessarily involved in an intramolecular hydrogen bond. However, the finding of large temperature/chemical shift coefficients (as for oxytocin and lysine vasopressin in water) can be confidently interpreted as indicating the absence of intramolecular hydrogen bonds involving the NH protons.

Conformational Information from Three-bond Spin–Spin Coupling Constants

The backbone and side-chain conformations in a peptide can be defined in terms of the torsional angles ϕ, ψ and ω (backbone) and χ_1, χ_2 (side-chain) as illustrated in Fig. 3.4.

NMR conformational studies of peptides mainly depend on using established relationships between the observed three-bond coupling constants in fragments $^1H-X-Y-{}^1H$ or $^1H-X-Y-{}^{13}C$ and the dihedral angle for rotation about the various X–Y bonds in peptides (Bystrov, 1976; Feeney, 1975).

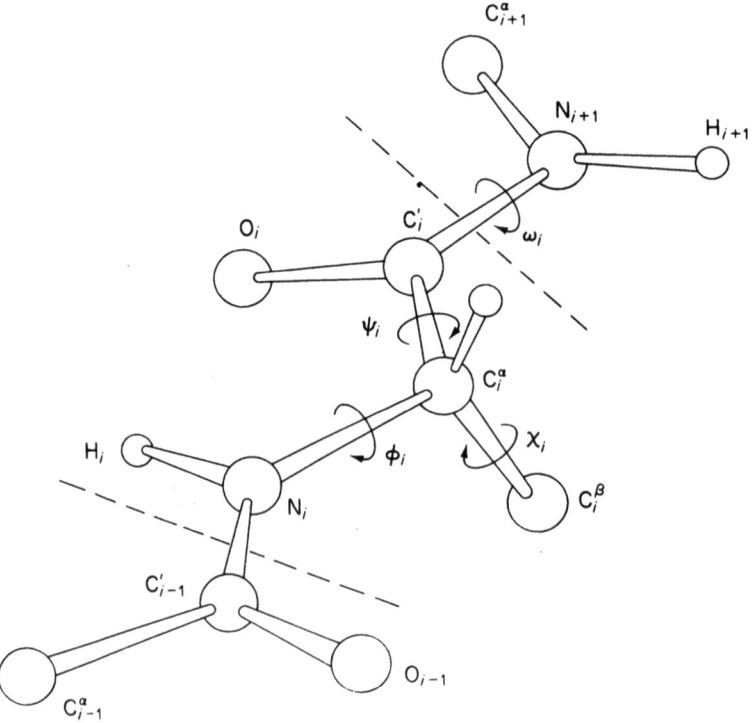

Figure 3.4 The torsional angles ϕ, ψ, ω and χ_1 used to define the conformation of a residue within a peptide

Backbone conformations

The φ torsion angle

Bystrov *et al.* (1973) have set up a Karplus-type curve (Fig. 3.5) relating the three-bond coupling constant between the α-CH proton and the NH proton with the dihedral angle ϕ. The curve has two maxima and one can see immediately that there is a problem in relating a measured coupling constant to a particular dihedral angle. For example, a $^3J_{\alpha CHNH}$ coupling constant of 7 Hz could arise from any one of four possible dihedral angles or be an averaged value from different conformations in rapid exchange with each other. Some of these ambiguities can be resolved either (1) by considering the results of potential energy calculations (Gibbons *et al.*, 1970) or (2) by studying $^{13}C-^1H$ three-bond coupling constants (Bystrov, 1976; Hansen, Feeney and Roberts, 1975) such as $^3J_{NHCO}$, where the relevant Karplus curve is out of phase with that shown in Fig. 3.5. However, it is always a difficult problem trying to decide whether one is dealing with a single conformation or a rapidly interconverting mixture of conformers.

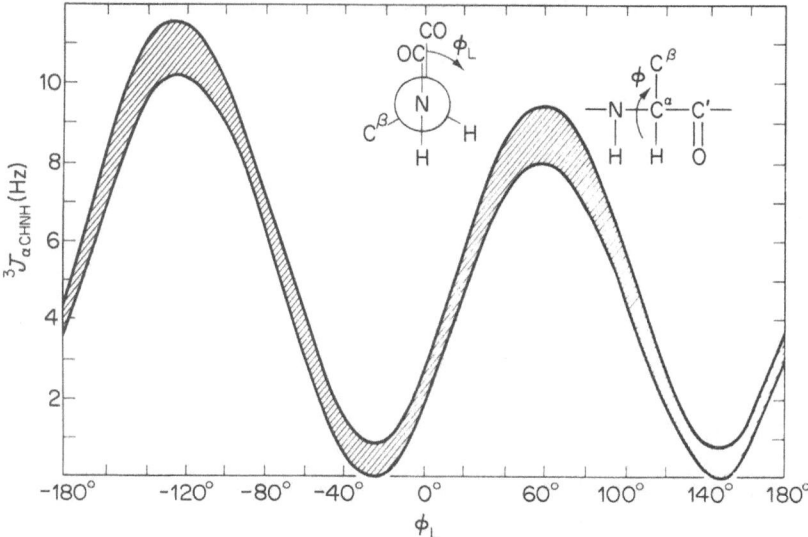

Figure 3.5 The dependence of the $^3J_{\alpha CHNH}$ coupling constant on the ϕ dihedral angle. Reproduced with permission from Bystrov (1976)

Even without a detailed interpretation of the coupling constants, it is often possible to use these conformationally sensitive parameters to compare conformations in related compounds such as oxytocin and lysine vasopressin. Figure 3.6 shows the NH absorption bands for these cyclic peptides and also for their reduced open-chain forms: clearly there are dramatic spectral differences between the oxidised and reduced forms (Feeney *et al.*, 1971). The $^3J_{\alpha CHNH}$ coupling constants can be measured directly from the multiplet splittings on the NH bands,

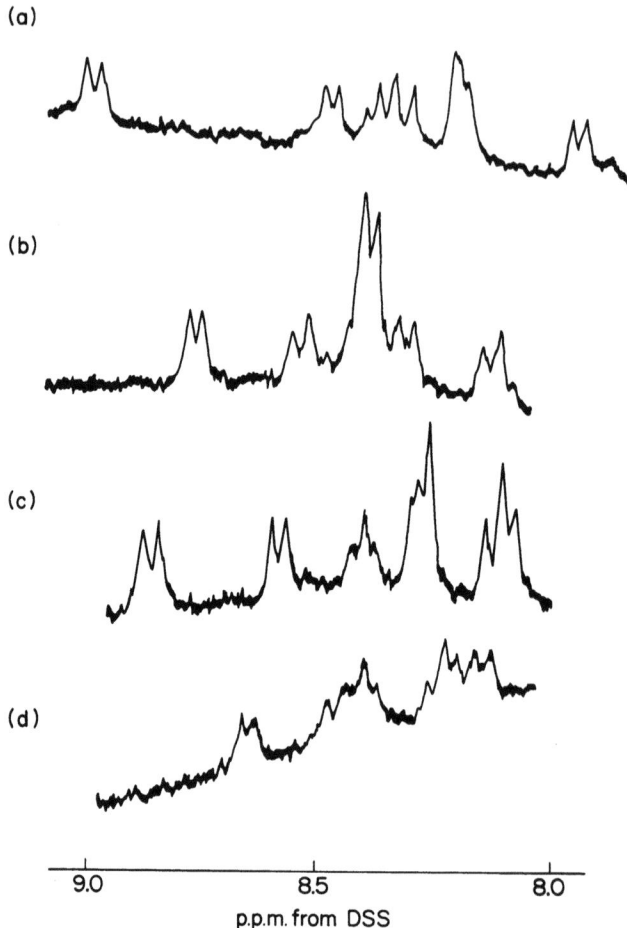

Figure 3.6 The peptide NH proton signals at 220 MHz in aqueous (H$_2$O) solution at 22°C for (a) oxytocin, (b) reduced oxytocin, (c) lysine vasopressin, (d) reduced lysine vasopressin. Reproduced with permission from Feeney et al. (1971)

and these are given in Table 3.1. When we compare the coupling constants in oxytocin with those in lysine vasopressin, we see a close 1:1 correspondence for the values at the corresponding residues in the two molecules. We have taken this as good evidence that the ring structures of oxytocin and lysine vasopressin are similar in aqueous solution. There is also a degree of correspondence for the NH temperature/chemical shift coefficients at the same residue positions in the two molecules. The $^3J_{\alpha CHNH}$ coupling constants for the reduced forms of the peptides are appreciably larger than in the parent hormone and are the values expected for random coil peptides (6 - 8 Hz). Several workers (Tonelli and Bovey, 1970; Scott and Scheraga, 1966; Nemethy, 1975) have calculated the ψ/ϕ two-dimensional potential energy maps for various dipeptides, and one can use these to calculate the distribution of molecules over the different conformational states. The fractional population for each value of ϕ_i and ψ_j is given by

$$P_{ij} = \frac{\exp[-(E_{ij}-E_0)/RT]}{\sum_{ij}\exp[-(E_{ij}-E_0)/RT]}$$

where E_{ij} is the energy of the molecule in this particular conformation and E_0 is the minimum potential energy value. With this information it is possible to compute the expected coupling constant from a curve as shown in Fig. 3.5, since

$$J = \sum_i P_{\phi_i} J_{\phi_i}$$

where $P_{\phi_i} = \sum_j P_{ij}$.

We have also used coupling constant data to compare the conformation of oxytocin with that of oxytocinoic acid (3) to see whether the absence of the Gly amide group or the presence of a charged carboxylate group perturbs the conformation (Boicelli, Bradbury and Feeney, 1976). Again there is very good agreement between the coupling constants at corresponding residues in the two compounds, indicating that the molecules have similar conformations.

Potential-energy calculations for oxytocin and related analogues in aqueous solution (Kotelchuck et al., 1972) indicate that the molecules probably exist as a mixture of several interconverting conformers and thus it is not possible to relate the observed $J_{\alpha\, CHNH}$ values to particular ϕ angle values. For oxytocin in dimethylsulphoxide solution (where a hydrogen bond has been found between the Asn NH hydrogen and the Tyr peptide CO oxygen) the molecule will probably have less ring flexibility, and Urry and co-workers (1970) have used the observed $J_{\alpha CHNH}$ values and the intramolecular hydrogen-bonding information to postulate a β-turn involving the Tyr – Gln – Asn fragment. This is not maintained in aqueous solutions, since the $J_{\alpha CHNH}$ coupling constants change and the intramolecular Asn NH hydrogen bond no longer exists (Feeney et al., 1971).

The ψ torsion angle
It is very difficult to obtain conformational information about the ψ dihedral angle because it is not readily characterised by three-bond coupling constants. Some studies have been reported using $J_{15\, NH\alpha CH}$ in isotopically labelled compounds (Bystrov, 1976; Gibbons et al., 1970; Sogn, Gibbons and Randall, 1973). However, the range of observed values is small and the requirement for isotopically labelled compounds considerably limits the general applicability of this approach.

The ω torsion angle
The ω dihedral angle can be characterised by observing the three-bond coupling constant $^3J_{13\, CO-NH}$: for the usual *trans* CONH conformation the coupling constant is 7.1 Hz, while for the *cis* CONH conformation the value is 0 Hz

(Dorman and Bovey, 1973). However, *cis* peptide bonds occur most frequently in X - Pro- and N - Me-substituted peptides where there is no NH proton to participate in coupling. Fortunately, the ^{13}C chemical shifts of the Pro ring carbons in X - Pro peptides have different values in the *cis* and *trans* conformations (Thomas and Williams, 1972; Deslauriers, Walter and Smith, 1972; Smith *et al.*, 1973; Wüthrich, Tun-kyi and Schwyzer, 1972; Dorman and Bovey, 1973), and such measurements have been used to show that in oxytocin the Pro is in the *trans* CONH form. For smaller peptides where the Pro is nearer to the N terminus there is often a *cis - trans* mixture: thus for benzoyloxycarbonyl-Pro - Leu - Gly NH$_2$ in dimethylsulphoxide solution there are almost equal amounts of the *cis* and *trans* forms, giving rise to two distinct ^{13}C NMR spectra for the Pro ring carbons in each form (Deslauriers *et al.*, 1972).

Side-chain conformations
Side-chain conformational information is obtained by relating the observed $J_{\alpha CH \beta CH}$ coupling constants with the χ_1 dihedral angles (Kopple *et al.*, 1972; Deslauriers *et al.*, 1974 a; Pachler, 1964; Feeney, 1976). Model compound studies (Feeney, 1976) show that the relationships can be expressed as

$$^3J_{\alpha CH \beta CH} = 9.9 \cos^2 \chi_1 + 1.6 \, (0 < \chi_1 < 180°) \tag{3.1}$$

$$^3J_{\alpha CH \beta CH} = 12.3 \cos^2 \chi_1 - 0.8 \, (180 < \chi_1 < 360°) \tag{3.2}$$

where χ_1 is the dihedral angle between the planes $H - C^\alpha - C^\beta$ and $C^\alpha - C^\beta - H$. The three-bond coupling constants can be calculated readily from the βCH_2 multiplets in the peptide ^1H spectrum.

We have measured the $J_{\alpha CH \beta CH}$ coupling constants for oxytocin, oxytocinoic acid (3) and tocinoic acid (4) and used these values to compare their side-chain conformations (Boicelli *et al.*, 1976).

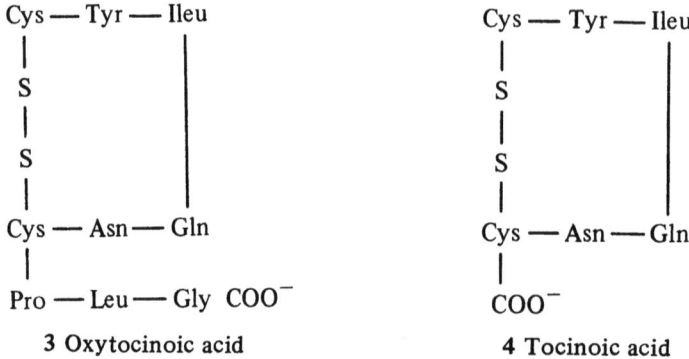

3 Oxytocinoic acid   4 Tocinoic acid

Examination of the data given in Table 3.2 reveals the excellent correspondence between the coupling constants measured at the same residue position in the different compounds, indicating that the side-chain conformations are similar in all

Table 3.2 The $^3J_{\alpha CH \beta CH}$ coupling constants (Hz) for oxytocin, tocinoic acid and oxytocinoic acid in D_2O solution

Residue	$J_{\alpha\beta}$ (Hz)	Oxytocinoc	Oxytocic acid	Tocinoic acid
Cys (1)	$\alpha\beta_1$	5.5	5.4	5.4
	$\alpha\beta_2$	6.5	6.5	5.4
Tyr	$\alpha\beta_1$	7.1	6.5	7.3
	$\alpha\beta_2$	9.5	9.5	8.2
Ileu	$\alpha\beta$	6.0	6.3	6.6
Gln	$\alpha\beta_1$	6.8	7.0	6.9
	$\alpha\beta_2$	8.2	8.6	7.4
Asn	$\alpha\beta_1$	6.6	(7.7)	5.7
	$\alpha\beta_2$	9.9	(7.7)	8.3
Cys (6)	$\alpha\beta_1$	3.8	3.8	3.9
	$\alpha\beta_2$	9.5	9.5	8.5
Leu	$\alpha\beta_1$	5.2	4.5	–
	$\alpha\beta_2$	8.7	8.9	–

the compounds. Clearly neither the presence of charged carboxylate groups nor the absence of the Pro - Leu - Gly NH_2 tail is perturbing the side-chain conformations. To get a more detailed conformational picture we need to know whether or not we are dealing with unique conformations or with a rapidly interconverting mixture of conformers. Deslauriers and co-workers (1974a) have made detailed ^{13}C relaxation time studies of oxytocin and related molecules, and their findings indicate that there is a high degree of flexibility in the side-chains of all the residues except the Cys (1) - Cys (6) fragment which forms part of the oxytocin ring. If we attempt to use the observed $J_{\alpha CH \beta CH}$ coupling constant for the Cys (1) - Cys (6) fragment to predict χ_1 angles using Eqs. (3.1) and (3.2), it is not possible to find a single conformation which fits all the data, suggesting that some conformational averaging is taking place. The coupling constants are consistent with averaging of rotamers with χ_1 angles within $\pm 10°$ of any of the following values:

χ_1 (Cys 1) 53°, 122°, 227°, 313°

χ_1 (Cys 6) 65°, 115°, 236°, 304°

Of course one cannot exclude the possibility that more extreme conformations are contributing to the observed coupling constants.

For the flexible side-chains such as Tyr, Ileu, Gln and Asn, it is usual to consider that there is a mixture of the three minimum energy rotameric forms (I), (II) and (III).

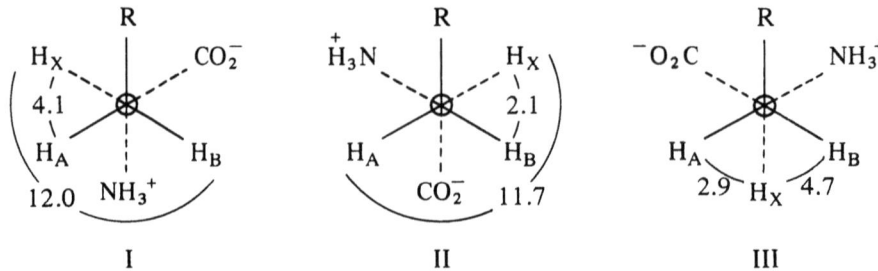

The component coupling constants indicated on these rotamers have been estimated from model compounds (Feeney, 1976). If the fractional populations are p_I, p_{II} and p_{III}, then the averaged $J_{\alpha CH \beta CH}$ coupling constants are

$$J_{AX} = 4.1 \, p_I + 11.7 \, p_{II} + 2.9 \, p_{III} \tag{3.3}$$

$$J_{BX} = 12.0 \, p_I + 2.1 \, p_{II} + 4.7 \, p_{III} \tag{3.4}$$

where

$$p_I + p_{II} + p_{III} = 1 \tag{3.5}$$

From the measured values of J_{AX} and J_{BX} the fractional populations of the rotamers can be calculated using Eqs. (3.3)-(3.5). Thus for Tyr the values indicate that only two of the rotameric states are populated ($p_I = 0.70$, $p_{II} = 0.30$, $p_{III} = 0.0$). It is more difficult to get detailed information when only one $J_{\alpha CH \beta CH}$ coupling constant can be meausred (Ileu) or when only the sum of the two three-bond coupling constants is available (Gln); it has been shown that all three rotamer populations are obtainable for such systems if the three-bond $J_{13_{CO-\beta CH}}$ are also measured, since these are similarly related to the χ_1 dihedral angle (Hansen et al., 1975).

Use of Paramagnetic Probes

If it is possible to bind a paramagnetic lanthanide ion to a well-defined binding site in a molecule, then one can study the molecular conformation by analysing the observed induced shift and relaxation effects at the different magnetic nuclei in the molecule. Williams and co-workers (Barry et al., 1971; Levine and Williams, 1975) have shown how this method can be used for conformational analysis of various molecules including nucleotides and peptides. For peptides such as tocinoic and oxytocinoic acid, lanthanide ions will bind selectively to the free carboxylate groups and thus provide a possible method of extracting further conformational information.

Levine and Williams (1975) have shown that when a lanthanide ion binds to a peptide carboxylate group, the induced chemical shifts are pseudocontact in origin for all protons except the αCH protons. In cases where there is effective axial symmetry the pseudocontact shift contribution is given by

$$\frac{\Delta v}{\Delta v_0} = D \frac{(3\cos^2 \theta_i - 1)}{r_i^3}$$

where D is a constant, r_i is the distance between the metal ion and a specific nucleus and θ_i is the angle between the principal symmetry axis of the complexed ion and the distance vector r_i.

The dipolar relaxation contributions from the paramagnetic ion are proportional to r_i^{-6}.

It is usual to express the induced chemical shift and relaxation effects as ratios referenced to the nucleus giving the largest effect. Computer programs have been written (BURLESK) which search for unique conformations that give theoretical shift and relaxation ratios in agreement (within a preset tolerance) to the measured values (Barry et al., 1971). For molecules which exist as rapidly interconverting mixtures of conformers, the lanthanide-induced shifts and relaxation data can sometimes be used to estimate the populations of the low-energy conformers contributing to the equilibrium (Birdsall et al., 1975; Birdsall, Feeney and Guiliani, 1976). The lanthanide-induced shift and relaxation parameters are first calculated for each of the expected low-energy conformations and then one finds the mixtures of conformations which give good fits for the averaged experimental values.

When Eu^{3+} ions bind to oxytocinoic acid, the main pseudocontact shifts are observed for the Pro αCH, with smaller shifts for the Cys (1) - Cys (6) protons. Clearly the tail of the molecule spends some time over this part of the ring in oxytocinoic acid (Boicelli et al., 1976).

For tocinoic acid the Eu^{3+} ion paramagnetic probes mainly affect the αCHβCH$_2$ protons of the Cys (1) - S - S - Cys (6) fragment, and when the data are analysed in conjunction with the $J_{\alpha CH\beta CH}$ values, it can be shown that the molecules are averaging over a range of conformations centred on the conformation in which the Cys (6) has the carboxylate group *gauche* to both βCH$_2$ protons and the Cys (1) has the C^α - N bond almost eclipsed with the C^β - S bond. Because oxytocin and oxytocinoic acid have similar conformations to that of tocinoic acid, these results will also be valid for the former molecules.

Use of ^{13}C Relaxation Times to Monitor Conformational Flexibility

^{13}C spin lattice relaxation times, T_1, can provide a useful indication of the molecular motion in the various fragments of the molecule. For proton-bearing carbons in systems with rapid isotropic motion the product NT_1, where N is the number of protons directly bonded to the carbon, is proportional to the rotational diffusion rate of the ^{13}C atom; thus for small molecules such as oxytocin, large values of NT_1 correspond to rapid molecular motion. Deslauriers and co-workers (1974a) have reported the NT_1 values for oxytocin and their interesting results

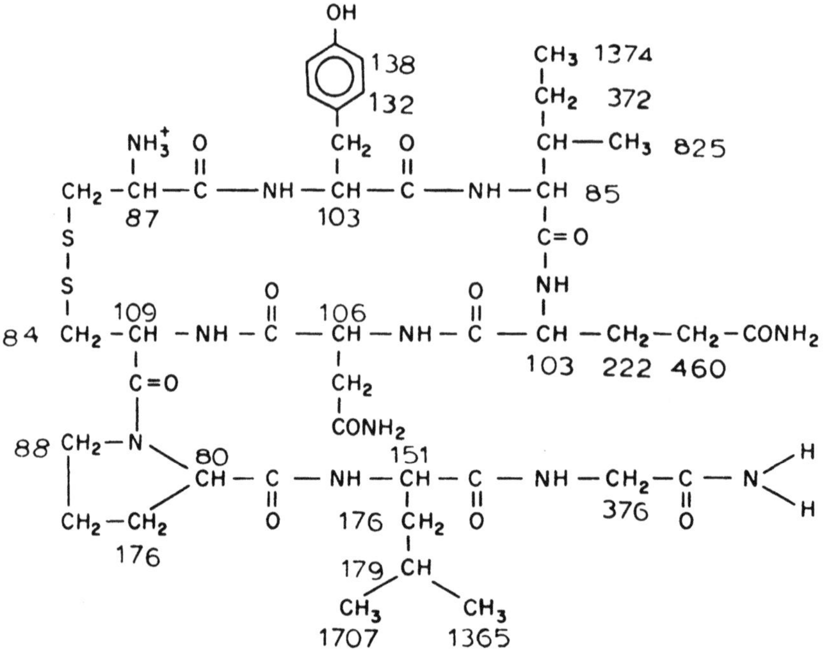

68   J. Feeney

```
                    OH
                    |
                    ⌬ 138
                    | 132              CH₃  1374
                    |                  |
       NH₃⁺  O      CH₂  O             CH₂   372
        |    ||     |    ||            |
      CH₂—CH—C —NH—CH—C —NH—CH—CH₃  825
        |   87         103        |
        S                         CH  85
        |                         |
        S         O         O     C=O
        | 109     ||  106   ||    |
    84 CH₂—CH—NH—C —CH—NH—C —CH—CH₂—CH₂—CONH₂
              |         |         NH
              C=O       CH₂       103  222  460
              |         |
   88 CH₂—N   CONH₂
       |    \  80   151                           H
       |     CH—C—NH—CH—C —NH—CH₂—C —N
      CH₂—CH₂  ||       |    ||       376 ||    \
        176    O    176 CH₂  O                    H
                        |
                    179 CH
                       /  \
                     CH₃   CH₃
                    1707  1365
```

Figure 3.7 The NT_1 values for the ^{13}C nuclei in oxytocin in aqueous solution. T_1 is the measured spin–lattice relaxation time and N the number of protons directly bonded to the carbon under investigation. Reproduced with permission from Deslauriers *et al.* (1974b)

are presented in Fig. 3.7. The smallest values are found for the α carbons within the oxytocin ring and correspond to an overall rotational correlation time of 5×10^{-10} s. In the side-chains the NT_1 values become progressively larger for carbons further removed from the oxytocin ring, indicating the rapid segmental motion in side-chains of the various residues. Similar results are obtained for carbon atoms in the tail of oxytocin, which eliminates the possibility that the tail exists predominantly in a single conformation with a strong interaction between the tail and the ring in aqueous solution. However, the relaxation time of the Gly αC in lysine vasopressin is longer than that in oxytocin, which indicates that the oxytocin tail has restricted motion in some of its conformational states. The relaxation time data also can be used to show the presence of a rapid intracyclic motion within the Pro ring (Deslauriers *et al.*, 1974a).

Glasel and co-workers (1973) have made deuterium (^{2}H) relaxation measurements on selectively deuterated oxytocin analogues with similar findings to those of Deslauriers and co-workers (1974a).

In summary, it can be concluded that even in these cyclic peptides there is a high degree of flexibility and the molecules clearly exist as a mixture of rapidly interconverting conformers rather than as a unique conformation.

CONFORMATIONS OF LINEAR HORMONAL PEPTIDES

Linear hormonal peptides such as gastrin tetrapeptide (Trp - Met - Asp - PheNH$_2$) (Feeney et al., 1972), thyrotropin releasing factor (TRF; [Glu - His - ProNH$_2$) (Burgess, Momany and Scheraga, 1973; Feeney, Roberts and Burgen, 1974a; Feeney, Bedford and Wessels, 1974b) and luteinising hormone releasing hormone ([Glu - His - Trp - Ser - Tyr - Gly - Leu - Arg - Pro - Gly NH$_2$; LH-RH) (Wessels et al., 1973; Deslauriers et al., 1975) have been studied by NMR methods, and in every case the molecules can be shown to exist as mixtures of rapidly interconverting conformers. Relaxation time measurements on LH-RH (Deslauriers et al., 1975, 1976) indicate a high degree of flexibility in the molecule. From studies of the $\alpha CH \beta CH$ coupling constants the side-chain rotamer populations have been estimated for many of the side-chains : the fractional populations are similar to those normally observed in small peptides containing the same residues. Some backbone conformation can be obtained from studying the $NH - \alpha CH$ coupling constants. The observed values are all within the range 7 ± 1 Hz, which are the values expected for a random-coil distribution of conformers as predicted for simple dipeptides. Furthermore, the temperature dependence of the NH chemical shifts, in every case, is typical of NH protons hydrogen bonding to the solvent molecules with no intramolecular hydrogen bonds. Thus, in general, it appears that small linear hormonal peptides exist as mixtures of random-coil conformations in solution with no structure-forming intramolecular hydrogen bonding* (Feeney et al., 1972, 1974 a, b; Wessels et al., 1973).

HOW DOES THE HORMONE PEPTIDE BIND TO ITS RECEPTOR?

We must now ask whether or not this conformational information tells us anything about how a small flexible hormone might bind to its receptor. At the present time the answer to this question is that it tells us very little. Clearly we cannot deduce any of the conformational features of the binding site from the conformation of the free hormone, since the bound conformation could be quite different from the most populated conformation in solution.

Given that we have a mixture of hormone conformations in solution and that the hormone has a unique conformation when bound to its receptor, we might speculate on how this conformational selection process takes place. In the so-called 'lock and key' model, it is considered that the only molecules which bind to the receptor are those which have the correct conformation to fit the binding site (see Fig. 3.8A). This model predicts that the association rate constant would be much less than the diffusion-controlled value because of the precise orientational and conformational requirements. An alternative model (Feeney et al., 1974a; Burgen, Feeney and Roberts, 1975), illustrated in Fig. 3.8B proposes that the

---

*Angiotensin II amide could be an exception to this in that there appears to be some hydrogen bonding in concentrated solutions at pH 4.0 (Bleich et al., 1973); the possibility of intermolecular hydrogen bonds has not been excluded at the present time.

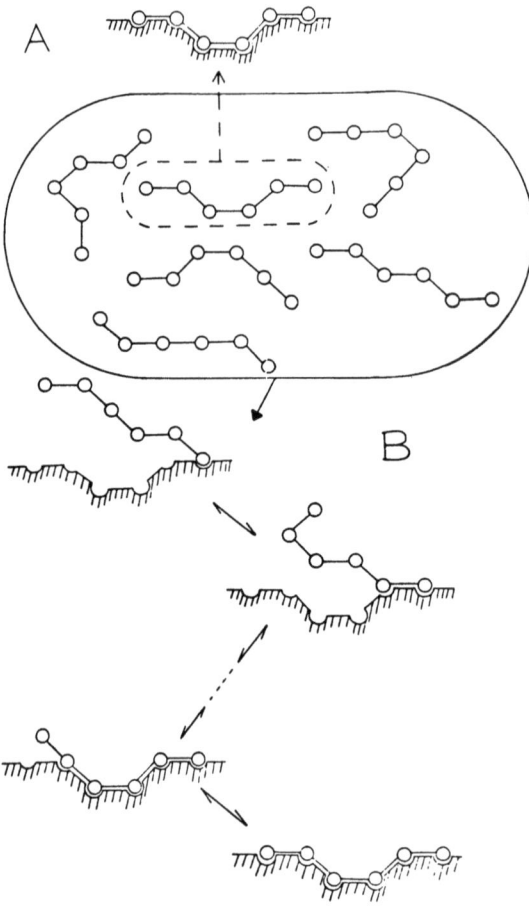

Figure 3.8 Schematic representation of (A) the 'Lock and key' and (B) the 'zipper' models discussed in the text. Reproduced with permission from Burgen et al. (1975)

flexible hormone binds to form a nucleation complex by interaction of a single segment of the ligand with a subsite on the receptor and that the hormone then reorganises its conformation so that the other segments bind to their subsites on the receptor. Thus the hormone would bind itself in a step-wise or 'zipper' process in which it would also be much easier for the receptor protein to modify its conformation to its optimum arrangement during the binding process. This 'zipper' mechanism would lead to faster association and dissociation rate constants. Direct evidence for such a binding process will only come from kinetic measurements of the complex formation, which are not yet available. However, such a mechanism is perfectly feasible, because even with a modest binding energy of 1 kcal/mol for the initial nucleation complex a life-time of 10^{-7} s is expected and during this time many bond rotations at rates of $10^{10} - 10^{12} s^{-1}$ are possible. This 'zipper mechanism' provides an attractive method by which flexible molecules with several recognition sites (needed for high specificity) can interact with their receptors with the required rapid association and dissociation rate constants (Feeney et al., 1974; Burgen et al., 1975).

REFERENCES

Barry, C. D., North, A. C. T., Glasel, J. A., Williams, R. J. P. and Xavier, A. V. (1971). *Nature (London)*, 232, 236
Birdsall, B., Birdsall, N. J. M., Feeney, J. and Thornton, J. (1975). *J. Am. Chem. Soc.*, 97, 2845
Birdsall, B., Feeney, J. and Guiliani, A. M. (1977). In *Metal-Ligand Interactions in Organic and Biochemistry* (ed. B. Pullman)
Bleich, H. E., Galardy, R. E. and Printz, M. P. (1973). *J. Am. Chem. Soc.*, 95, 2041
Boicelli, C. A., Bradbury, A. F. and Feeney, J. (1977). *J. Chem. Soc.*, 477.
Bradbury, A. F., Burgen, A. S. V., Feeney, J., Roberts, G. C. K. and Smyth, D. G. (1974). *FEBS Lett.*, 42, 179
Brewster, A. I. and Hruby, V. J. (1973). *Proc. Nat. Acad. Sci. U.S.A.*, 70, 3806
Brewster, A. I., Hruby, V. J., Glasel, J. A. and Tonelli, A. E. (1973). *Biochemistry*, 12, 5294
Burgen, A. S. V., Feeney, J. and Roberts, G. C. K. (1975). *Nature (London)*, 253, 753
Burgess, R. W., Momany, F. A. and Scheraga, H. A. (1973). *Proc. Nat. Acad. Sci. U.S.A.*, 70, 1456
Bystrov, V. F. (1976). In *Progress in Nuclear Magnetic Resonance Spectroscopy*, Vol. 10 (ed. J. W. Emsley, J. Feeney and L. H. Sutcliffe), Oxford, Pergamon Press.
Deslauriers, R., Levy, G. C., McGregor, W. H., Sarantakis, K. and Smith, I. C. P. (1975). *Biochemistry*, 14, 4335
Deslauriers, R. and Somorjai, R. L. (1976). *J. Am. Chem. Soc.*, 98, 1931
Deslauriers, R., Smith, I. C. P. and Walter, R. (1974a). *J. Am. Chem. Soc.*, 96, 2289
Deslauriers, R., Walter, R. and Smith, I. C. P. (1972). *Biochem. Biophys. Res. Comm.*, 48, 854
Deslauriers, R., Walter, R. and Smith, I. C. P. (1974b). *Proc. Nat. Acad. Sci. U.S.A.*, 71, 265
Dorman, D. E. and Bovey, F. A. (1973) *J. Org. Chem.*, 38, 1719
Feeney, J. (1975). *Proc. R. Soc. London A*, 345, 61
Feeney, J. (1976). *J. Mag. Res.*, 21, 473
Feeney, J., Bedford, G. R. and Wessels, P. L. (1974b). *FEBS Lett.*, 42, 347
Feeney, J., Roberts, G. C. K., Brown, J. P., Burgen, A. S. V. and Gregory, H. (1972). *J. Chem. Soc. II*, 601
Feeney, J., Roberts, G. C. K. and Burgen, A. S. V. (1974a). In *Molecular and Quantum Pharmacology* (ed. E. Bergmann and B. Pullman), Dordrecht, Reidel, pp. 301-312
Feeney, J., Roberts, G. C. K., Rockey, J. H. and Burgen, A. S. V. (1971). *Nature (London)*, 232, 108
Gibbons, W. A., Nemethy, G., Stern, A. and Craig, L. C. (1970). *Proc. Nat. Acad. Sci. U.S.A.*, 67, 239
Glasel, J. A., Hruby, V. J., McKelvy, J. F. and Spatola, A. F. (1973). *J. Mol. Biol.*, 79, 555
Hansen, P. E., Feeney, J. and Roberts, G. C. K. (1975). *J. Mag. Res.*, 17, 249
Higashijima, T., Tasumi, M. and Miyazawa, T. (1975). *FEBS Lett.*, 57, 175
Johnson, L. F., Schwartz, I. L. and Walter, R. (1969). *Proc. Nat. Acad. Sci. U.S.A.*, 64, 1269
Kopple, K. D., Go, A., Logan, R. H. and Savoda, J. (1972). *J. Am. Chem. Soc.*, 94, 973
Kotelchuck, D., Scheraga, H. A. and Walter, R. (1972). *Proc. Nat. Acad. Sci. U.S.A.*, 69, 3629

Levine, B. A. and Williams, R. J. P. (1975). *Proc. R. Soc. London A*, **345**, 5
Nemethy, G. (1975). *Biochimie*, **57**, 471
Pachler, K. G. R. (1964). *Spectrochim. Acta*, **20**, 581
Scott, R. A. and Scheraga, H. A. (1966). *J. Chem. Phys.*, **45**, 2091
Smith, I. C. P. (1975). Varian Application Note, NMR 75-2
Smith, I. C. P., Deslauriers, R., Saito, H. and Walter, R. (1973). *Ann. N. Y. Acad. Sci.*, **222**, 597
Smith, I. C. P., Deslauriers, R. and Walter, R. (1972). In *Chemistry and Biology of Peptides* (ed. J. Meienhofer), Ann Arbor Sci. Publ. Inc., p. 29
Sogn, J. A., Gibbons, W. A. and Randall, E. W. (1973). *Biochemistry*, **12**, 2100
Thomas, W. A. and Williams, M. K. (1972). *Chem. Commun.*, 994
Tonelli, A. E. and Bovey, F. A. (1970). *Macromolecules*, **3**, 410
Urry, D. W., Ohnishi, M. and Walter, R. (1970). *Proc. Nat. Acad. Sci. U.S.A.*, **66**, 111
Urry, D. W. and Walter, R. (1971). *Proc. Nat. Acad. Sci. U.S.A.*, **68**, 956
Von Dreele, P. H., Scheraga, H. A., Dyckes, D. F., Ferger, M. F. and du Vigneaud, V. (1972). *Proc. Nat. Acad. Sci. U.S.A.*, **69**, 3322
Walter, R. (1971). In *Structure Activity Relationships of Protein and Polypeptide Hormones* (ed. M. Margoulies and F. C. Greenwood), Amsterdam, Excepta Medica, pp. 181-193
Walter, R. and Glickson, J. D. (1973). *Proc. Nat. Acad. Sci. U.S.A.*, **70**, 1199
Walter, R., Prasad, K. U., Deslauriers, R. and Smith, I. C. P. (1973). *Proc. Nat. Acad. Sci. U.S.A.*, **70**, 2086
Wessels, P. L., Feeney, J., Gregory, H. and Gormley, J. J. (1973). *J. Chem. Soc. II*, 1671
Wüthrich, K., Tun-kyi, A. and Schwyzer, R. (1972). *FEBS Lett.*, **25**, 104

4
Structure and function of carbonic anhydrase: comparative studies of sulphonamide binding to human erythrocyte carbonic anhydrases B and C

K. K. Kannan, I. Vaara, B. Notstrand, S. Lövgren, A. Borell, K. Fridborg and M. Petef (Department of Molecular Biology, Wallenberg Laboratory, Uppsala University, Uppsala, Sweden)

INTRODUCTION

Soon after the discovery of carbonic anhydrase from bovine erythrocytes (E.C.4.2.1.1), which catalyses the reaction

$$CO_2 + H_2O \rightleftharpoons HCO_3^- + H^+$$

by Meldrum and Roughton (1932) it was shown by Mann and Keilin (1940) that certain sulphonamides were specific and potent inhibitors of this enzyme. It has been well documented (see Maren, 1967, for an extensive review on inhibition and physiology, and Lindskog et al., 1971, and Coleman, 1971, for general reviews on carbonic anhydrases) that aromatic and heterocyclic sulphonamides with unsubstituted $R-SO_2NH_2$ groups constitute a class of powerful inhibitors, while aliphatic sulphonamides are poor inhibitors of the carbonic anhydrases.

Nyman (1961) succeeded in isolating two distinct forms of carbonic anhydrases from human erythrocytes with differing chemical composition and catalytic activity towards substrates and inhibitors. The low-activity enzyme was denoted as the B form (HCAB) and that with high activity the C form (HCAC).

The crystallisation of the isoenzymes HCAB and HCAC has been reported by Kannan et al. (1972) and Strandberg et al. (1962), respectively. The three-dimensional structures (Kannan et al., 1971; Liljas et al., 1972; Kannan et al., 1975; Notstrand, Vaara and Kannan, 1975) and complete amino acid sequences (Andersson et al., 1972; Kuang-Tzu and Deutsch, 1973; Marriq et al., 1973; Henderson et al., 1973; Henrikson, 1975) have been established. In an effort to understand the inhibition of carbonic anhydrases by sulphonamides we have determined the crystal structures of the enzyme – sulphonamide complexes for the human isoenzymes HCAB and HCAC, respectively. A knowledge of the three-dimensional structures and complete amino acid sequence of HCAB and HCAC has been very valuable in establishing the interaction of the inhibitors with the isoenzymes. Here we report a comparative study of the sulphonamide binding to these isozymes at the molecular level.

MATERIAL AND METHODS

Human erythrocyte carbonic anhydrase forms B and C were prepared by a mild purification method according to Armstrong *et al.* (1966). Crystals of HCAB were prepared by the seeding technique described by Kannan *et al.* (1972). The crystals of the C enzyme were prepared by the method of Strandberg *et al.* (1962). Acetazolamide, purchased from American Cyanamid Company, New York, was used without further purification. The aromatic sulphonamide, believed to be 3-acetoxymercury-4-aminobenzene sulphonamide, was prepared by the late B. Tilander and was used without further purification. The isoenzyme – sulphonamide inhibitor complexes were prepared by soaking or dialysing the HCAB or HCAC native enzyme crystals in 2.3 M ammonium sulphate, 0.05 M tris-HCl and 10^{-3} M of the inhibitor at pH 8.7 or 8.5, respectively.

Photographic diffraction data were collected on a Buerger – Supper precession camera using Ni-filtered CuK_α radiation. The diffraction intensities were measured on an automatic microdensitometer constructed by Mr V. Klimecki in collaboration with our group and the data were processed on an IBM 370/155 computer with the programs described by Järup *et al.* (1970) after suitable modifications. The electron density maps were calculated with a program kindly provided by Dr G. N. Reeke Jr, Rockefeller University, New York, and plotted on a Benzon microfilm plotter using a contouring program written by Dr R. Hoge, University of British Columbia, and kindly provided by Dr C. E. Nordman, University of Michigan, Ann Arbor, Michigan.

Two types of electron density maps were calculated:

$$\rho_1(x,y,z) = \frac{1}{V} \sum_{h} \sum_{k} \sum_{l} m \times (|F_D| - |F_P|) \exp[-i\{2\pi(hx+ky+lz)-\alpha_p\}] \quad (4.2)$$

$$\rho_2(x,y,z) = \frac{1}{V} \sum_{h} \sum_{k} \sum_{l} m \times (2|F_D| - |F_P|) \exp[-i\{2\pi(hx-ky-lz)-\alpha_p\}] \quad (4.3)$$

where F_P and F_D are the observed amplitudes of the reflexion $(h\ k\ l)$ for the protein and the sulphonamide-protein complex, respectively, m is the figure of merit and α_p the centroid phase angles for the protein, calculated on the basis of the multiple isomorphous replacement method (Blow and Crick, 1959; Dickerson,

Kendrew and Strandberg, 1961). The electron density maps were superimposed on the native enzyme maps and interpreted by fitting Kendrew – Watson skeletal model parts to the electron density in an optical comparator (Richards, 1968). The atomic co-ordinates were measured from the model and plotted using the ORTEP program (Johnson, 1965).

THE STRUCTURE OF CARBONIC ANHYDRASE

Notstrand *et al.* (1975) have discussed the gross structural similarities of human erythrocyte carbonic anhydrase isozymes B and C on the basis of their three-dimensional structures and postulated that the structures of carbonic anhydrases from other species would be very similar to the human enzymes. A detailed description of the similarities and differences between the two isozyme structures

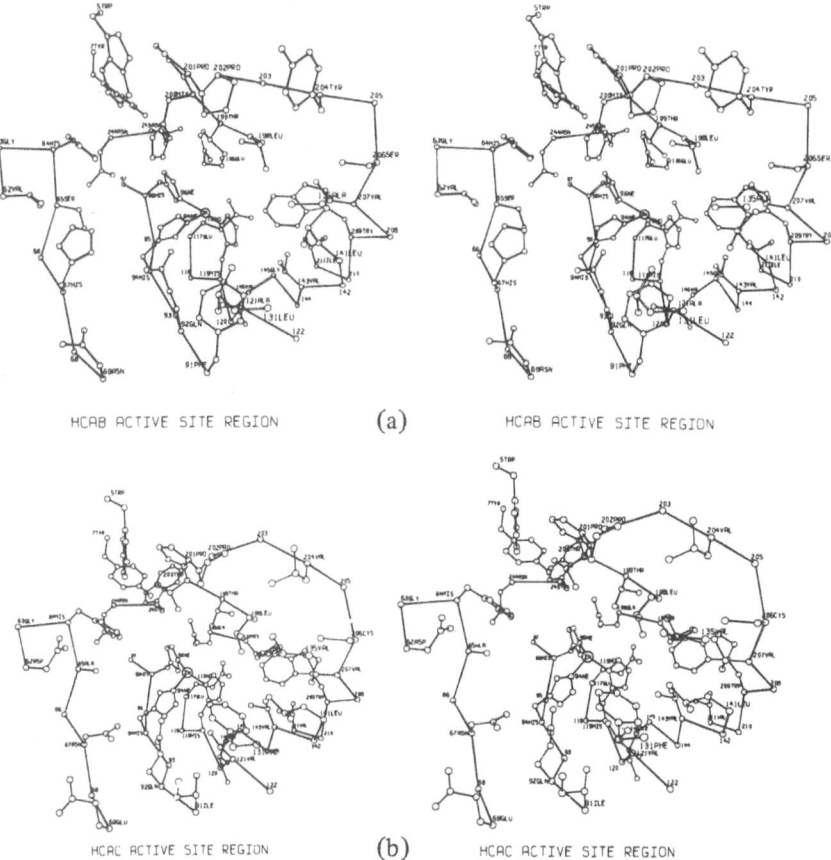

Figure 4.1 ORTEP drawing of the residues in the active site region of (a) HCAB and (b) HCAC

has been given by them and only a short account of the essential features of the two isoenzymes will be given here.

The carbonic anhydrase molecule is a compact ellipsoid of dimensions about 41 × 42 × 55 Å. A large twisted β structure consisting of 10 chain segments forms the central feature of the molecular folding. There are both parallel and antiparallel chain segments in the pleated sheet structure. About 35 per cent of the residues are in β pleated sheet conformation and about 20 per cent in helical conformation. There are also ten bends occurring at the same points in the three-dimensional structures of HCAB and HCAC. The three-dimensional structures are stabilised by these secondary structures and also by the aromatic clusters and hydrophobic interactions in the interior of the molecule.

The active sites of HCAB and HCAC (Figs. 4.1a and 4.1b) are conical cavities about 12 Å deep formed mainly by chain segments 3–6 of the central pleated sheet and two extra loops consisting of residues 128–135 and 196–202. The essential zinc ion is located at the bottom of this cavity. His 94, 96 and 119 and a solvent molecule give the zinc ion a distorted tetrahedral co-ordination. The solvent molecule is hydrogen-bonded to the O^γ atom of Thr 199, which is in turn hydrogen-bonded to the carboxyl group of Glu 106. All these residues are invariant in all carbonic anhydrases for which sequence information is available (Tashian, 1975).

The active site cavity is further characterised by its divisibility into a hydrophobic half-cone and a hydrophilic half. The amino acid residues located in the active sites of HCAB and HCAC are listed in Table 4.1. There are a number of differences in the active site residues in the two isoenzymes, especially in the hydrophobic half. The presence of His 67 and His 200 in HCAB instead of Asn 67 and Thr 200 in HCAC in the hydrophilic half of the active site also tends to reduce the available volume of the active site cavity in the immediate vicinity of the zinc

Table 4.1 Amino acids located in the active site of HCAB and HCAC

HCAB	HCAC if different	HCAB	HCAC if different
Polar residues		Non-polar residues	
Tyr 7		Ser 65	Ala
Asn 61		Phe 91	Ile
His 64		Ala 121	Val
His 67	Asn	Leu 131	Phe
Asn 69	Glu	Leu 141	
Gln 92		Val 143	
His 94		Gly 145	
His 96		Pro 201	
Glu 106		(cis)Pro 202	
His 119		Val 207	
Thr 199		Trp 209	
His 200	Thr	Ile 211	Val

ion in HCAB compared with HCAC. The only common free histidyl residue (His 64) in the active site of the carbonic anhydrase isozymes is very accessible in the case of HCAC, while it is partially shielded by His 67 and His 200 in HCAB.

SULPHONAMIDE INTERACTION WITH CARBONIC ANHYDRASE

Acetazolamide

Acetazolamide (Fig. 4.2), a heterocyclic sulphonamide, is a powerful inhibitor of the carbonic anhydrases and has been extensively used as a drug in the treatment of glaucoma.

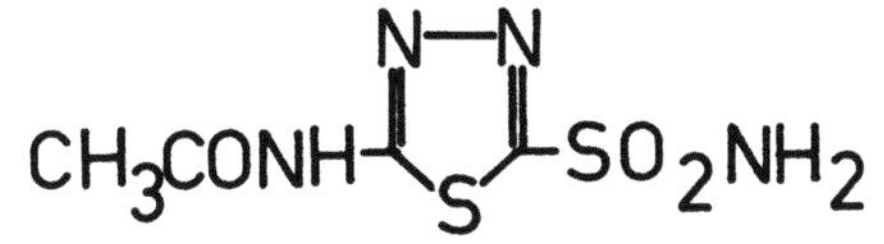

$$CH_3CONH-\underset{S}{\overset{N-N}{\diagdown\diagup}}-SO_2NH_2$$

Figure 4.2 The chemical formula of acetazolamide

In the crystallographic investigations the two sulphur atoms could easily be located in the difference Fourier maps and the co-ordinates improved by least squares refinement in conjunction with the isomorphous replacement method (Bergstén *et al.*, 1972, and Kannan *et al.*, 1975). The two sulphur atoms in the

Table 4.2 Atomic co-ordinates of the acetazolamide inhibitor in the HCAB – acetazolamide complex (Å)

	x	y	z
S_1	38.1	41.5	−39.3
O_1	38.0	40.3	−38.2
O_2	37.6	42.8	−38.6
N_1	39.6	41.5	−39.3
C_1	37.5	41.7	−40.3
N_2	37.1	41.8	−42.4
N_3	37.5	42.4	−41.6
C_2	36.2	40.6	−42.3
S_2	36.2	40.4	−40.7
N_4	35.9	40.1	−43.5
C_3	36.5	39.2	−44.2
O_3	37.8	39.1	−43.9
C_4	35.8	38.2	−45.0
Zn ion	40.1	40.8	−36.6

Matrix and translation parameters to convert HCAB co-ordinates into HCAC orientation:

M = 0.024 81   −0.861 29   0.507 50
      0.674 65   0.389 05   0.627 29
     −0.737 72   0.326 82   0.590 72

T = (43.37   13.26   55.80)

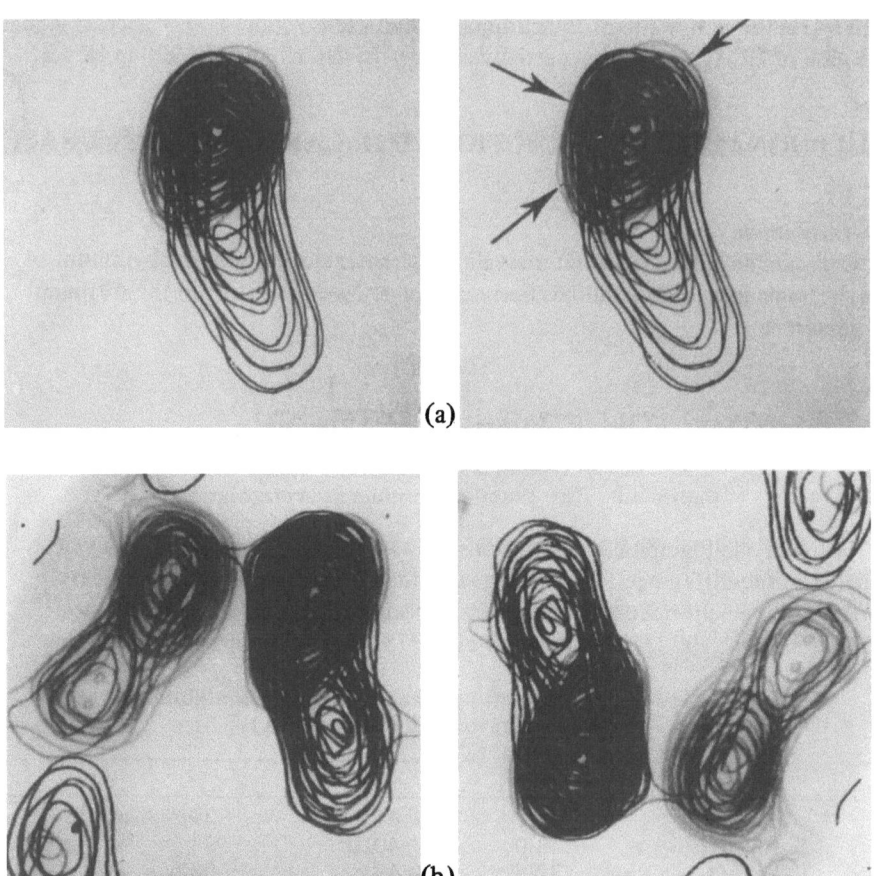

Figure 4.3 Electron density maps, in stereo, of the HCAB – acetazolamide complex (a) according to Eq. (4.2) and (b) according to Eq. (4.3). The arrow markings indicate the oxygen and nitrogen atoms of the sulphonamide group. Only the relevant part of the active site region is presented here

difference electron density maps guide the orientation of the heterocyclic ring (Figs. 4.3a, b, 4.4a, b). In the electron density maps the whole acetazolamide molecule is also well defined. The atoms in the $SO_2 NH_2$ group are also identifiable by projections of density, indicated by arrow markings from the sulphur atom (Figs. 4.3a, 4.4a). The difference electron density maps for the HCAB – acetazolamide complex and the HCAC – acetazolamide complex are given in Figs. 4.3a, b and 4.4a, b, and their interpretation in Figs. 4.3c and 4.4c, respectively. Preliminary crystallographic co-ordinates of the non-hydrogen atoms of the inhibitor are given in Tables 4.2 and 4.3 together with the co-ordinates of the

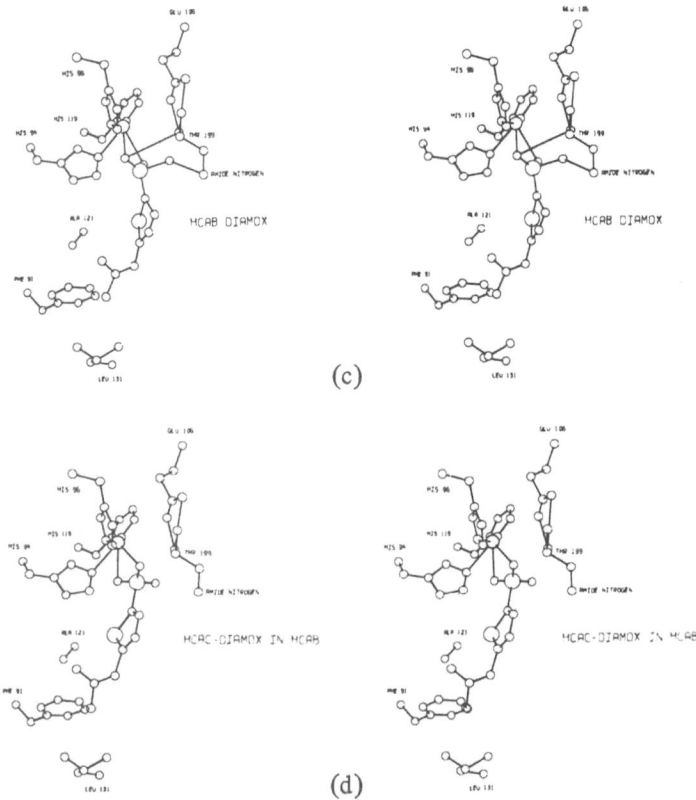

Figure 4.3(c) ORTEP drawing of acetazolamide binding to HCAB as interpreted from the electron density maps, but not in the same orientation as the maps

Figure 4.3(d) ORTEP drawing of the acetazolamide molecule bound to HCAC drawn in the active site of HCAB. The co-ordinates of the inhibitor molecule interpreted from HCAC electron density maps were rotated and translated to the orientation of the HCAB molecule and drawn in the active site of HCAB. The difference in the orientation of the sulphonamide group is evident. The heterocyclic ring has a similar orientation

zinc ion. The amino acids in the immediate neighbourhood of the inhibitor are listed in Table 4.4.

Even though the individual atoms of the SO_2NH_2 group can be located in the electron density maps, one cannot distinguish between the nitrogen and the oxygen atoms. A reasonable interpretation would, however, be that the nitrogen atom binds to the zinc ion replacing the solvent molecule co-ordinated to the metal in the native enzyme. The O^γ atom of Thr 199 is hydrogen-bonded to this nitrogen. The O^γ atom of Thr 199 is also hydrogen-bonded to Glu 106 as in the

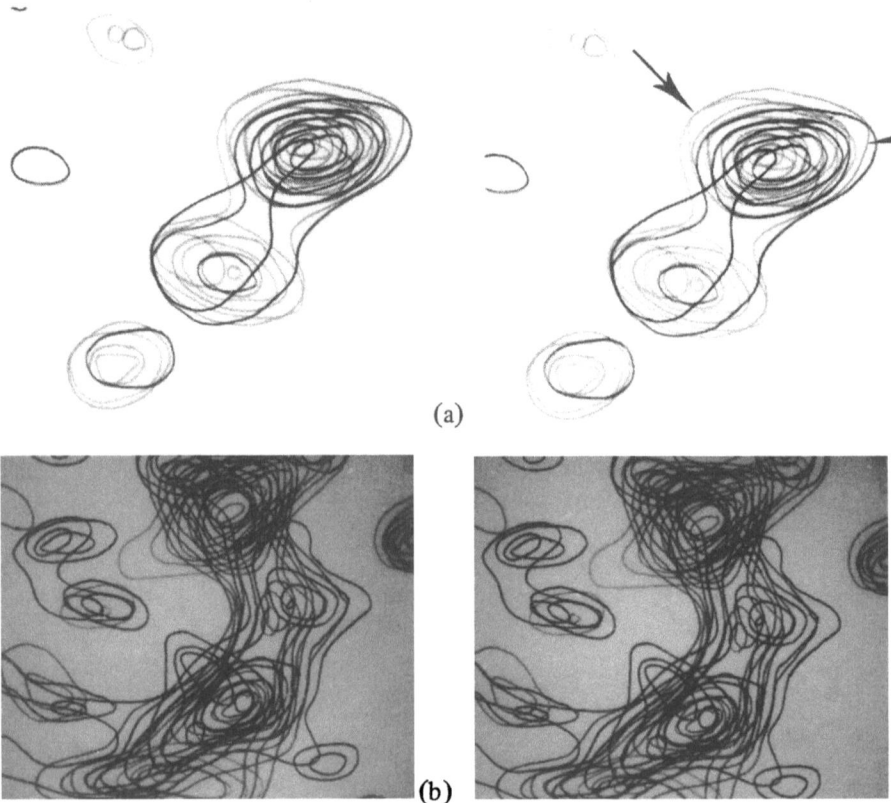

Figure 4.4 Electron density maps, in stereo, of the HCAC – acetazolamide complex (a) according to Eq. (4.2) and (b) according to Eq. (4.3). The arrow markings indicate the oxygen and nitrogen atoms of the sulphonamide group. Only the relevant part of the active site region is presented

native enzymes. One of the oxygen atoms is located near a hydrophobic pocket and is probably co-ordinated to the zinc ion as its fifth ligand.

The plane of the heterocyclic ring is located midway between the hydrophobic and hydrophilic walls of the active site with its sulphur atom in van der Waals contact with residue 121 (Ala 121 in HCAB and Val 121 in HCAC). The acetylamido moiety is in van der Waals contact with residues 91 and 131 (Leu 131 and Phe 91 in HCAB and Ile 91 and Phe 131 in HCAC). Probably no hydrogen bonds are formed from the acetylamido group to the protein.

There are some interesting differences in the binding of this inhibitor to HCAC as compared with HCAB. The sulphonamide group is slightly rotated in the HCAC - acetazolamide complex, so that the nitrogen atom which binds to the zinc ion

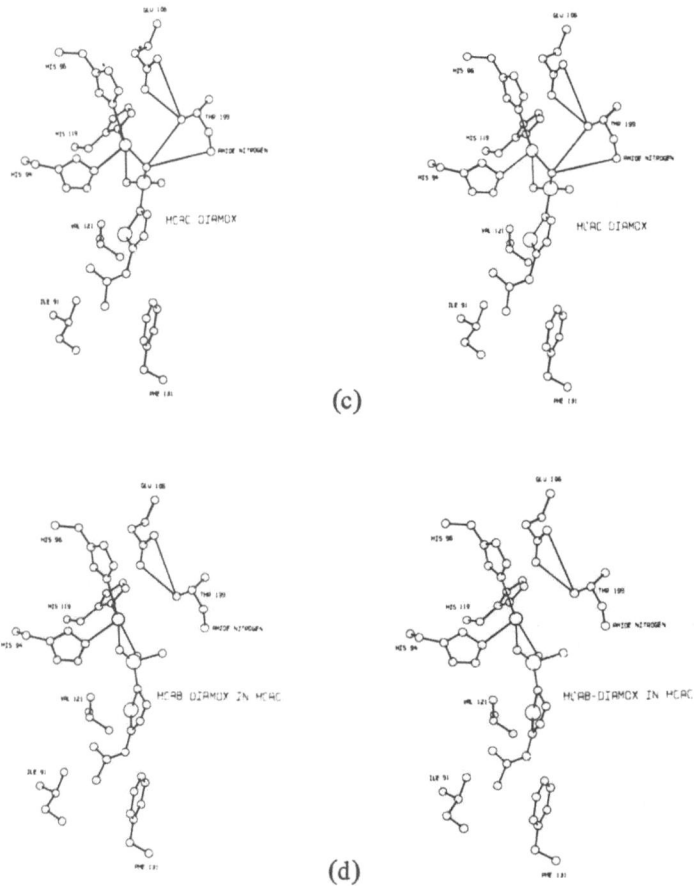

Figure 4.4(c) ORTEP drawing of acetazolamide binding to HCAC as interpreted from the electron density maps, but not in the same orientation as the maps

Figure 4.4 (d) ORTEP drawing of the acetazolamide molecule bound to HCAB drawn in the active site of HCAC. The co-ordinates of the inhibitor molecule interpreted from HCAB electron density maps were rotated and translated to the orientation of the HCAC molecule and drawn in the active site of HCAC

(replacing the solvent molecule) is hydrogen-bonded to the O^γ atom of the Thr 199 as well as to the amide nitrogen of Thr 199. The oxygen atom of the sulphonamide group that is not co-ordinated to the zinc ion is hydrogen-bonded to the amide nitrogen of Thr 199 in HCAB, whereas in HCAC this is not the case.

Acetazolamide inhibits HCAC ten times more powerfully than HCAB. An explanation for this difference should obviously lie in the differences in the molecular interactions between the inhibitor and the respective receptors. The sulphur

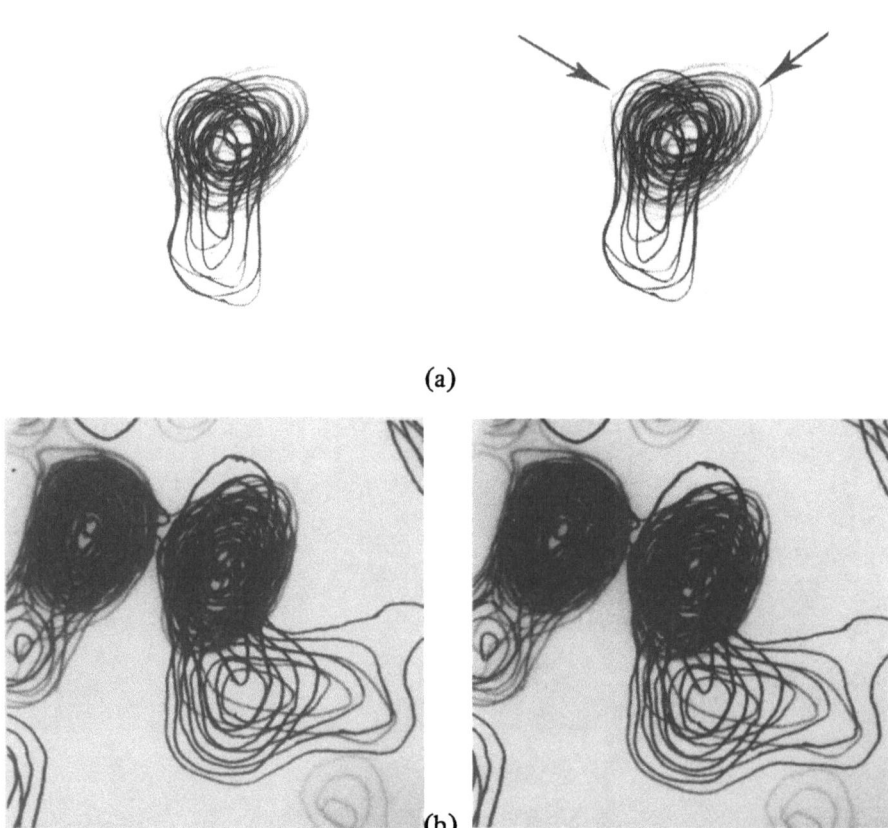

Figure 4.5 Electron density maps, in stereo, of the HCAB – AMSulph complex (a) according to Eq. (4.2) and (b) according to Eq. (4.3)

atom of the sulphonamide group is located at about the same distance from the metal ion: 3.5Å in HCAB and 3Å in HCAC. The same number of hydrogen bonds are formed in the two complexes even though the sulphonamide groups are not oriented in the same manner. The main differences in the mode of binding of acetazolamide to the isoenzymes seems, however, to be through the interaction of the heterocyclic group and the acetylamido moiety to the hydrophobic amino acids located in the active site of the respective isoenzymes. One such interaction of importance is between the sulphur atom in the ring and Val 121 in HCAC or Ala 121 in HCAB.

Sulphanilamide

Acetoxymercury sulphonamide (AMSulph), an aromatic sulphonamide, was one of the heavy atom derivatives that proved to be very useful in the structure deter-

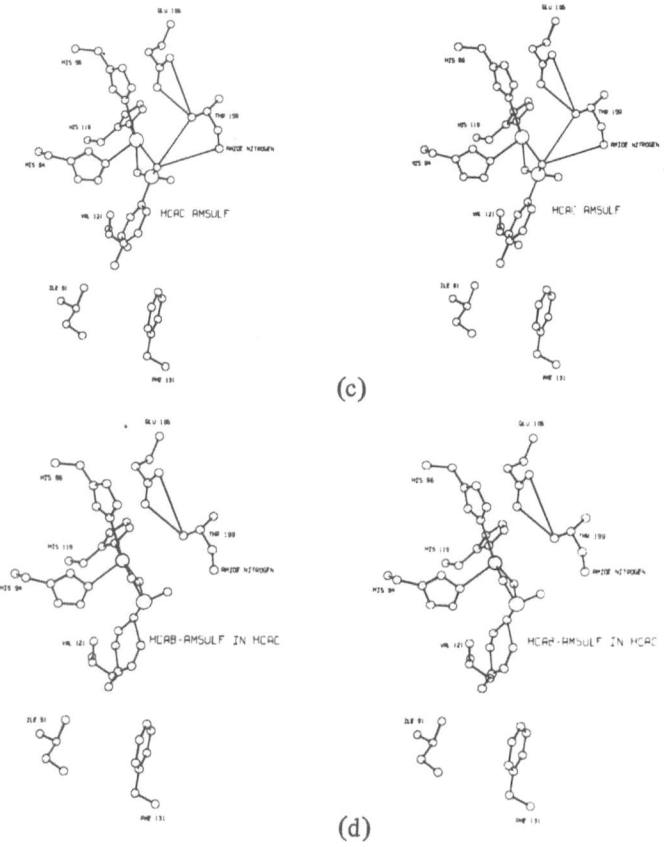

Figure 4.5 (c) ORTEP drawing of AMSulph binding to HCAB
Figure 4.5(d) ORTEP drawing of the AMSulph molecule bound to HCAC, drawn in the active site of HCAB

---

mination of HCAB (Kannan *et al.*, 1975) and HCAC (Liljas *et al.*, 1972).

The electron density maps of this inhibitor complex with HCAB (Figs. 4.5a, b) and with HCAC (Figs. 4.6a, b) clearly indicate the position of the sulphonamide group and also the most probable orientation of the ring. The interpretation of the binding of this inhibitor to HCAB is given in Fig. 4.5c and to HCAC in Fig. 4.6c. Preliminary co-ordinates of the non-hydrogen atoms of the inhibitor molecule are listed for the two isozymes in Tables 4.5 and 4.6 and the amino acids in the active site in the immediate vicinity of the inhibitor molecule in Table 4.4. The sulphur atom of the sulphonamide group could be easily located in the difference electron density maps (Figs. 4.5a and 4.6a) and the co-ordinates were improved by least squares refinement in conjunction with the isomorphous replacement method (Liljas *et al.*, 1972; Kannan *et al.*, 1975).

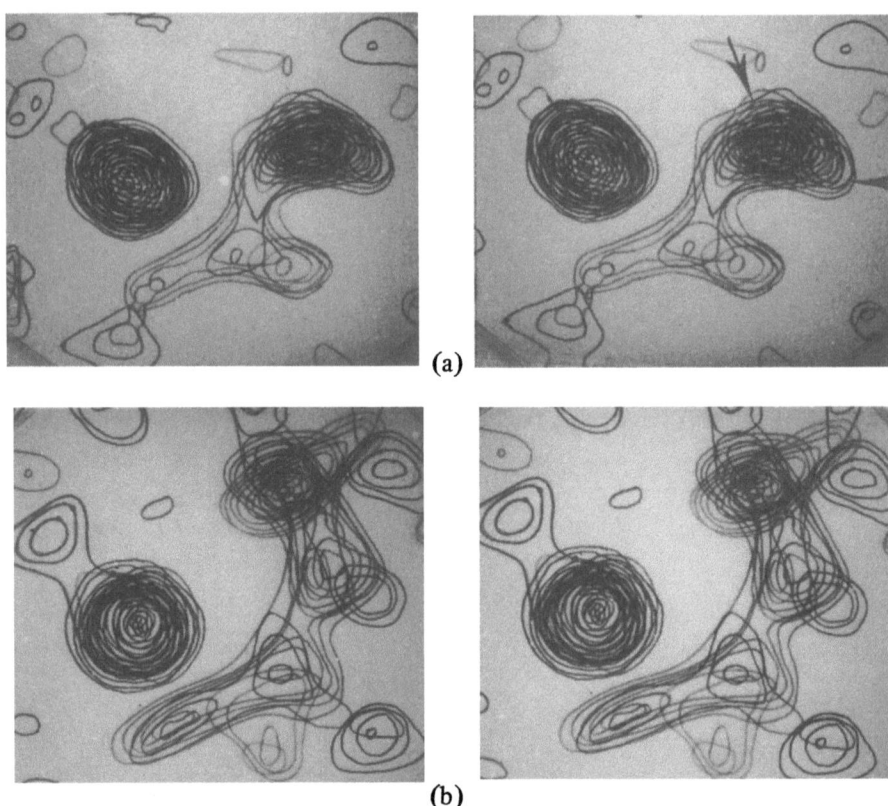

Figure 4.6 Electron density maps, in stereo, of the HCAC – AMSulph complex (a) according to Eq. (4.2) and (b) according to Eq. (4.2)

The inhibitor binds to the zinc ion via the sulphonamide group, replacing the liganded solvent molecule. The general mode of binding of the sulphonamide group to the zinc ion is very similar to that of the acetazolamide binding discussed above. The aromatic ring of the inhibitor is situated more or less midway between the hydrophobic wall and the hydrophilic wall of the active site.

Our earlier interpretation of the HCAC - AMSulph complex (Bergstén et al., 1972) was based on the assumption that the structure of the inhibitor molecule is as shown in Fig. 4.7. However, it has turned out after the structure investigation of HCAB was completed that AMSulph must be a mixture of a simple mercurial and probably sulphanilamide (Fig. 4.8) or its derivative but *not* acetoxymercury sulphanilamide, as explained below.

In HCAC one of the major mercury sites is associated with His 64 in the active site, and the other major site with Cys 206 (Liljas et al., 1972). There is no connecting density between the mercury atom at His 64 and the rest of the inhibitor electron density (Figs. 4.6a, b). It is also difficult to fit the aromatic ring to the electron density if one should account for a mercuriated inhibitor. These observa-

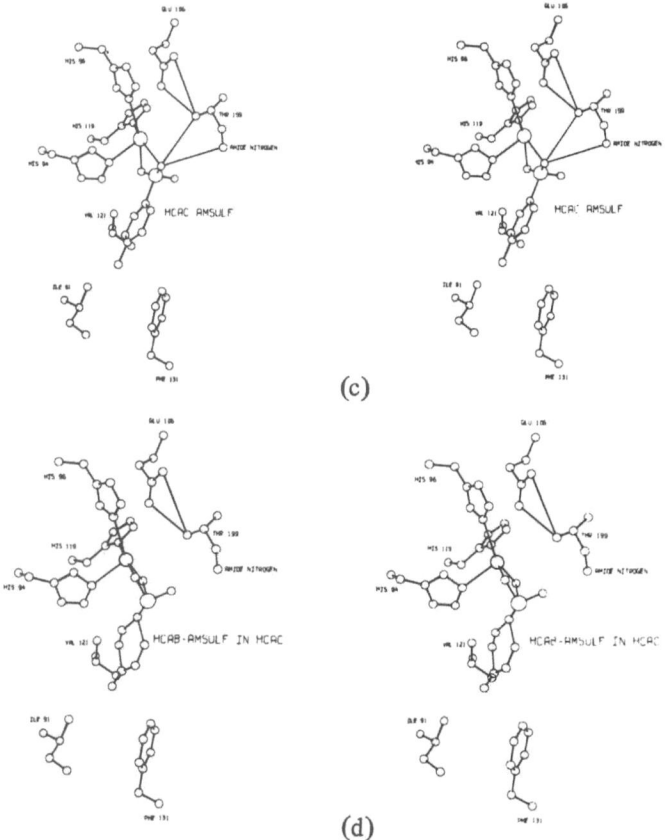

Figure 4.6(c) ORTEP drawing of AMSulph binding to HCAC
Figure 4.6(d) ORTEP drawing of the AMSulph molecule bound to HCAB, drawn in the active site of HCAC

Figure 4.7 The presumed chemical formula of AMSulph

tions, and some other evidence, point to the possibility that the inhibitor is not mercuriated. In the absence of inhibitors mercurials bind strongly only to Cys 206, but in the presence of certain inhibitors the reactivity of His 64 in HCAC is increased drastically. Thus, in the presence of inhibitors not only is Cys 206 mercuriated but also His 64 binds a mercury (Vaara *et al.*, 1972). Göthe and Nyman (1972) have shown that the modification of His 64 by bromopyruvate was accele-

Table 4.3 Atomic co-ordinates of the acetazolamide inhibitor in the HCAC–acetazolamide complex (Å)

	x	y	z
S_1	21.8	32.4	25.0
O_1	23.2	32.5	25.0
O_2	21.6	32.3	26.4
N_1	20.9	33.4	24.4
C_1	21.7	30.8	24.0
N_2	20.6	29.5	22.6
N_3	20.7	30.6	23.4
C_2	21.8	28.8	22.7
S_2	23.0	29.5	23.7
N_4	22.0	27.4	22.0
C_3	22.6	27.3	20.8
O_3	23.4	28.2	20.4
C_4	22.7	26.0	20.2
Zn ion	22.5	35.3	24.0

Matrix and translation parameters to convert HCAC co-ordinates into HCAB orientation:

M = 0.206 5   0.675 35   − 0.737 21
    − 0.862 97   0.384 36   0.327 94
      0.504 83   0.629 42   0.590 75

T = (31.21   14.14   − 63.30)

rated to a great extent by the presence of $Au(CN)_2^-$, an anionic inhibitor of carbonic anhydrase. It has also been shown by Campbell, Lindskog and White (1974, 1975) that the pK of the histidine in the active site changes on binding inhibitors. It is also known from the three-dimensional structure of HCAB that His 64 is somewhat shielded by His 67 and His 200, making it less accessible.

It is possible that the compound used in the preparation of the derivative was a mixture of two sulphonamides, one mercuriated species and one without any mercury, and that the mercuriated species binds to the C isozyme, while sulphanilamide binds to the B enzyme. It seems, however, more reasonable to believe that

Table 4.4 Active site amino acids within 5Å of the inhibitor molecule

Polar residues		Non-polar residues	
HCAB	HCAC if different	HCAB	HCAC if different
Gln 92		Phe 91	Ile
His 94		Ala 121	Val
Thr 199		Leu 131	Phe
His 200	Thr	Leu 141	
		Leu 198	
		Trp 209	

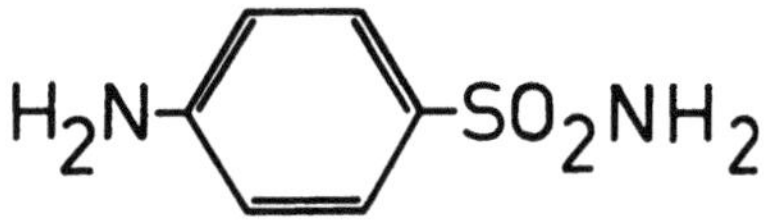

$$H_2N-\langle\bigcirc\rangle-SO_2NH_2$$

Figure 4.8 The chemical formula of sulphanilamide

the ring is not mercuriated at all and that the compound consists of a mixture of a simple mercurial such as mercuric acetate and an aromatic sulphonamide inhibitor in HCAC also. It thus seems reasonable to conclude that the inhibition of HCAC by an aromatic sulphonamide has facilitated the binding of mercury to His 64 in the active site.

Table 4.5 Atomic co-ordinates of the sulphanilamide (AMSulph) inhibitor in the HCAB – sulphanilamide complex (Å)

	x	y	z
S_1	38.4	42.1	−38.7
O_1	37.9	41.2	−36.5
O_2	37.9	43.3	−38.0
N_1	39.9	42.1	−38.0
C_1	37.8	41.1	−39.2
C_2	37.0	39.8	−39.2
C_3	36.6	39.2	−39.9
C_4	36.6	39.6	−41.9
C_5	37.1	40.9	−42.2
C_6	37.6	41.7	−41.2
N_2	36.2	38.8	−42.5
Zn ion	40.1	40.8	−36.6

Table 4.6 Atomic co-ordinates of the sulphanilamide (AMSulph) inhibitor in the HCAC – sulphanilamide complex (Å)

	x	y	z
S_1	21.8	32.4	24.8
O_1	23.2	32.7	25.2
O_2	21.4	31.9	26.3
N_1	20.8	33.2	24.3
C_1	22.1	30.8	23.8
C_2	21.0	30.5	22.9
C_3	21.2	29.3	21.9
C_4	22.5	28.7	21.9
C_5	23.2	30.0	23.8
C_6	22.6	27.6	20.9
Zn ion	22.5	35.3	24.0

DISCUSSION

A number of important features are revealed by the crystal structures of the sulphonamide complexes with the human carbonic anhydrase isoenzymes HCAB and HCAC. The sulphonamides are bound to the enzyme through the metal ion by direct co-ordination at the fourth ligand site, replacing the solvent molecule bound to the metal in the native enzyme. The metal-co-ordinated atom of the sulphonamide group is hydrogen-bonded to the O^γ atom of Thr 199 in the same way as the solvent molecule is bonded in the native enzymes. In addition, the O^γ atom of Thr 199 is hydrogen-bonded to Glu 106. These two amino acids are known to be invariant in all the carbonic anhydrases for which the sequence has so far been established. The fourth co-ordination site also coincides with the binding site of most of the anionic inhibitors investigated by X-ray diffraction methods (Bergstén *et al.*, 1972; Vaara *et al.*, 1972; Kannan, unpublished results). Thus it seems reasonable that the sulphonamides also bind to the metal ion as the anionic species, as postulated by Taylor, King and Burger (1970). Even though the oxygen and nitrogen atoms are indistinguishable at this resolution, it seems natural to assign the NH^- group of the sulphonamide to occupy the fourth ligand site.

It is interesting to note in this connection that modification of the NH_2 group of the sulphonamide moiety removes the inhibitory properties of the sulphonamide inhibitors. This is very reasonable, as their binding to the metal ion would be restricted, probably owing to change in their ionisability as well as to steric hindrance encountered with the protein molecule. Besides, the hydrogen bonding to the protein will also be limited.

One of the oxygen atoms of the sulphonamide group occupies a fifth co-ordination site of the metal ion. This site is situated near a hydrophobic pocket where imidazole is known to bind in HCAB (Kannan *et al.*, 1977). It is interesting to note that in di(histidino) zinc pentahydrate (Harding and Cole, 1963) and di(L-histidino) zinc dihydrate (Kretzinger, Cotton and Bryan, 1963) the metal has four tightly co-ordinated (2.0 Å) nearly tetrahedrally distributed ligand atoms and two distantly co-ordinated atoms (2.9 Å). The zinc ion in the carbonic anhydrase – sulphonamide complex has almost this co-ordination geometry, though the sixth co-ordination site is sterically hindered by the protein. Woolley and co-workers (1975) have shown that zinc and Co exhibit five co-ordination in some macrocyclic ligands. However, these compounds are not as efficient catalysts as the carbonic anhydrases. It seems that the microenvironment around zinc in the carbonic anhydrases is designed to allow only four more or less tightly bound ligands and a distant fifth ligand site that is utilised for fast exchange of substrates. It is also important to account for the role played by the system zinc – solvent – Thr 199 – Glu 106 in enzyme-catalysed reactions when comparing and evaluating model systems for the carbonic anhydrases. The solvent molecule, water or hydroxyl, co-ordinated at the fourth ligand site may be thought of as one of the substrates in the forward reaction (Eq. 4.1). The sulphonamides inhibit the enzyme by replacing this substrate as well as occupying the fifth co-ordination site where the other substrate, e.g. CO_2, would bind. Furthermore there is a certain similarity between the substrate HCO_3^- and the sulphonamide group. Since sulphonamides are competitive inhibitors of this substrate (Lindskog et al., 1971), it may be expected that this substrate binds in the same way as the sulphonamide group.

The potency of the heterocyclic and aromatic sulphonamides is, however, not solely derived from their binding to the metal ion. The aromatic or heterocyclic part of the inhibitor molecule is in van der Waals contact with a number of sidechains, especially those situated on the hydrophobic wall of the active site (see also Table 4.4). It may be expected that the inhibitor and substrate specificity would be dictated to some extent by the topography defined by the hydrophobic half of the active site.

It is well known (Maren, 1967; Kakeya et al., 1969) that substitution on the ring changes the inhibitory characteristics of the sulphonamides towards the two isoenzymes. Especially, *para* and *ortho* substitutions on aromatic rings have been well characterised. *Para*-substituted aromatic sulphonamides inhibit the C isozyme, in general, ten times more powerfully than the B enzyme. Taylor et al. (1970) have also shown that increasing the carbon chain length at the *para* position increases the inhibitory power. This must be due largely to increased hydrophobic bonding with more amino acids in the active site entrance. An extra ring introduced in the *para* position of the aromatic sulphonamides may be expected to improve the inhibitory effect on HCAC because of improved interaction with Phe 131. *Ortho*-substituted sulphonamides are poorer inhibitors of HCAC compared with *para*-substituted ones.

One may qualitatively identify the amino acid residues responsible for these characteristics. Three amino acid residues, 91, 121 and 131, located in the active site interact well with the ring portion of the sulphonamides. In HCAB these amino acids are Phe 91, Ala 121 and Leu 131, whereas in HCAC they are Ile 91, Val 121 and Phe 131. We have already commented on the interaction of the residue 121 (Ala/Val) with the sulphur atom in the acetazolamide ring. This residue may also be responsible for the difference in the inhibitory strength of *ortho*-substituted aromatic sulphonamides. These sulphonamides will experience significant steric hindrance from Val 121 in HCAC but less so with Ala 121 in HCAB. It is also evident from the topography of the active sites that substitution at the *ortho* and *meta* positions would have to be limited in their size owing to steric hindrance.

It is quite possible that selective carbonic anhydrase inhibitors may be designed by suitable modifications in the *meta* or *ortho* positions of the aromatic ring. However, the topography of the active sites of HCAB and HCAC should be characterised better by crystallographic refinement. It would also be necessary to investigate the interaction of a number of sulphonamides with the carbonic anhydrases at the molecular level.

ACKNOWLEDGEMENTS

We should like to thank Professor B. Strandberg and Drs A. Liljas and H. Cid-Dresdner for very useful criticism of the manuscript and valuable suggestions. We are very much indebted to Gunnel Johansson for typing the manuscript.

This work was supported by grants from the Faculty of Science, University of Uppsala, and the Swedish Natural Science Research Council.

REFERENCES

Andersson, B., Nyman, P. O. and Strid, L. (1972). *Biochem. Biophys. Res. Comm.*, **48**, 670
Armstrong, J. McD., Myers, D. V., Verpoorte, J. A. and Edsall, J. T. (1966). *J. Biol. Chem.*, **241**, 5137
Bergstén, P. C., Vaara, I., Lövgren, S., Liljas, A., Kannan, K. K. and Bengtsson, U. (1972). In *Proceedings of the Alfred Benzon Symposium IV* (ed. M. Rorth and P. Astrup), Copenhagen, Munksgaard, p. 363
Blow, D. M. and Crick, F. H. C. (1959). *Acta Cryst.*, **12**, 794
Campbell, I. D., Lindskog, S. and White, A. I. (1974). *J.Mol.Biol.*, **90**, 469
Campbell, I. D., Lindskog, S. and White, A. I. (1975). *J.Mol.Biol.*, **98**, 597
Coleman, J. E. (1971). *Progr. Bioorg. Chem.*, **1**, 159
Dickerson, R. E., Kendrew, J. S. and Strandberg, B. E. (1961). *Acta Cryst.*, **14**, 1188
Göthe, P. O. and Nyman, P. O. (1972). *FEBS Lett.*, **21**, 159
Harding, M. M. and Cole, S. J. (1963). *Acta Cryst.*, **16**, 643
Henderson, L. E., Henriksson, O. and Nyman, P. O. (1973). *Biochem. Biophys. Res. Comm.*, **52**, 1388
Henriksson, D. (1975). Dissertation, Department of Biochemistry, Gothenburg University
Järup, L., Kannan, K. K., Liljas, A. and Strandberg, B. (1970). *Computer Programs Biomed.*, **1**, 74
Johnson, C. K. (1965). Oak Ridge National Lab. Publ.
Kakeya, N., Aoki, M., Kameda, A. and Yata, N. (1969). *Chem. Pharm. Bull.*, **17**, 1010
Kannan, K. K., Fridborg, K., Bergstén, P. C., Liljas, A., Lövgren, S., Petef, M., Strandberg, B., Vaara, I., Adler, L., Falkbring, S. O., Göthe, P. O. and Nyman, P. O. (1972). *J. Mol. Biol.*, **63**, 601
Kannan, K. K., Liljas, A., Vaara, I., Bergstén, P. C., Fridborg, K., Lövgren, S., Strandberg, B., Bengtsson, U., Carlbom, U., Järup, L. and Petef, M. (1971). *Cold Spring Harbor Symposia on Quant. Biology*, **36**, 221
Kannan, K. K., Notstrand, B., Fridborg, K., Lövgren, S., Ohlsson, A. and Petef, M. (1975). *Proc. Nat. Acad. Sci. U.S.A.*, **72**, 51
Kannan, K. K., Petef, M., Fridborg, K., Cid-Dresdner, H. and Lövgren, S. (1977). *FEBS Lett.*, **73**, 115
Kretzinger, R. H., Cotton, F. A. and Bryan, R. F. (1963). *Acta Cryst.*, **16**, 651
Kuang-Tzu, D. L. and Deutsch, H. F. (1973). *J. Biol. Chem.*, **248**, 1885
Liljas, A., Kannan, K. K., Bergstén, P. C., Vaara, I., Fridborg, D., Strandberg, B., Carlbom, U., Järup, L., Lövgren, S. and Petef, M. (1972). *Nature New Biol.*, **235**, 131
Lindskog, S., Henderson, I. E., Kannan, K. K., Liljas, A., Nyman, P. O. and Strandberg, B. (1971). In *The Enzymes* (ed. P. D. Boyer), 3rd edn, Vol. 5, New York, Academic Press, p. 387
Mann, T., and Keilin, D. (1940). *Nature (London)*, **146**, 164
Maren, T. H. (1967). *Physiol. Rev.*, **47**, 595, and references therein

Marriq, C., Sciaky, M., Giraud, N., Foveau, D. and Laurent-Tabusse, G. (1973). *Biochemie*, 55, 1361
Meldrum, N. U. and Roughton, F. J. W. (1932). *J.Physiol. (London)*, 75, 4P and 15P
Notstrand, B., Vaara, I. and Kannan, K. K. (1975). In *Isoenzymes I, Molecular Structure* (ed. C. L. Markert), New York, Academic Press, p. 575
Nyman, P. O. (1961). *Biochem. Biophys. Acta*, 52, 1
Richards, F. M. (1968). *J.Mol. Biol.*, 37, 225
Strandberg, B., Tilander, B., Fridborg, K., Lindskog, S. and Nyman, P. O. (1962). *J.Mol.Biol.*, 5, 583
Tashian, R. E. (1975). In *Isoenzymes I, Molecular Structure* (ed. C. L. Markert), New York, Academic Press
Taylor, P. W., King, R. W. and Burgen, A. S. V. (1970). *Biochemistry*, 9, 3894
Vaara, I. Lövgren, S., Liljas, A., Kannan, K. K. and Bergstén, P-C. (1972). In *Second Int. Conference on Red Cell Metabolism and Function, Ann Arbor*
Woolley, P. (1975). *Nature (London)*, 258, 677, and references therein

5
Kinetic aspects of structure – activity relationships in the carbonic anhydrase – sulphonamide system

R. W. King (Division of Molecular Pharmacology, National Institute for Medical Research, Mill Hill, London, UK)

INTRODUCTION

The binding of sulphonamide inhibitors to the enzyme carbonic anhydrase (E.C.4.2.1.1) is a useful model system for the interaction of drugs with receptors. There exists a very wide range of chemically related specific inhibitors, all of those with high affinity ($K_a > 10^5$ M^{-1}) possessing the following properties. The sulphonamide group is unsubstituted on the nitrogen atom and is directly linked to an aromatic nucleus. This nucleus may be homocyclic, of the benzene or naphthalene type, or it may be heterocyclic, as in the case of the well-known drugs acetazolamide and chlorothiazide. The enzyme itself is easily purified in large quantities from mammalian blood and has the useful qualities of being extremely stable to a wide variety of storage and experimental conditions. The physical properties of the enzyme have been closely studied and an X-ray structure is available. Most of the following studies have been carried out using the C isoenzyme of human carbonic anhydrase (HCA-C).

KINETIC ANALYSIS OF SULPHONAMIDE BINDING

The advantage of the sulphonamide-carbonic anhydrase system for the measurement of equilibrium binding constants and reaction kinetics is that many of the inhibitors quench the natural tryptophan fluorescence of the enzyme when a complex is formed. The quenching can be shown to bear a linear relationship to the concentration of the complex, which simplifies experimental procedures. Equilibrium affinity constants can be measured by adding small relative volumes of the inhibitor to the enzyme solution and observing the decrease in fluorescence. A plot of fluorescence against inhibitor concentration will yield the value of K_a from the normal binding curve. Rate constants are measured using a stopped-flow apparatus adapted for fluorimetry. In the sulphonamide-carbonic anhydrase system dissociation rate constants can be measured quite simply by displacement of the bound sulphonamide by another sulphonamide of different quenching capacity. The conditions are chosen so that the dissociation of the bound inhibitor is rate-limiting, and a simple first-order plot yields the rate constant. Bimolecular association rate constants are usually measured under pseudo-first-order conditions, which, assuming a one-step reaction scheme,

$$E + I \underset{k_b}{\overset{k_f}{\rightleftharpoons}} EI \qquad (5.1)$$

yields a first-order plot from which the rate constant $k_{obs} = k_f [I] + k_b$. The values of k_b for dissociation of sulphonamide inhibitors from carbonic anhydrase are almost invariably less than 1 s^{-1}, while the values of k_f range from 10^4 to 10^7 M^{-1} s^{-1}. The concentrations of enzyme and inhibitor can easily be chosen so that the contribution of k_b to k_{obs} is negligible. The value of k_f can then be determined from $k_{obs}/[I]$.

The simple mechanism described by Eq. (5.1), when applied to the binding of small molecules to macromolecules, makes certain predictions. Alberty and

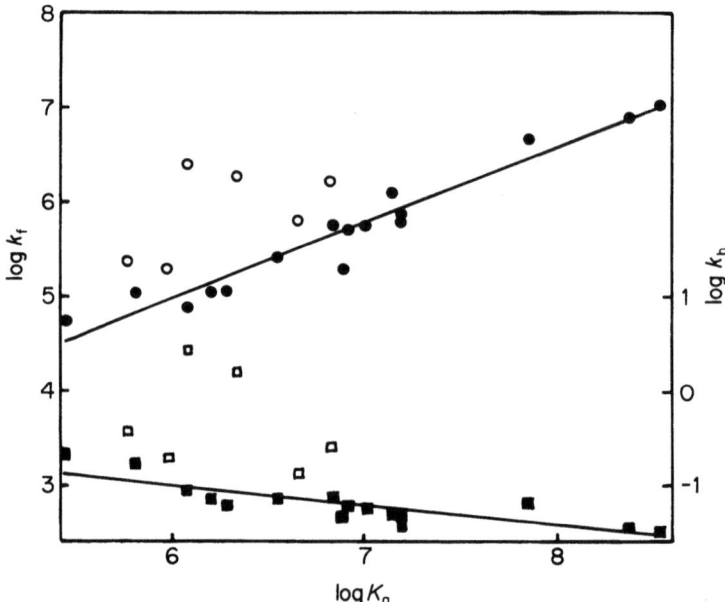

Figure 5.1 Measured kinetic constants for a variety of ring-substituted benzene sulphonamides, plotted as a function of the affinity constant. Circles are association rate constants; squares are dissociation rate constants. Filled symbols are *para*- and *meta*-substituted compounds; open symbols *ortho*-substituted compounds. Least-squares lines are drawn for filled symbols only. Data of Taylor *et al.* (1970a)

Hammes (1958) showed that the association rate constant k_f will be limited only by the rate of diffusional access to the site, as long as the site is unobstructed, and for several macromolecule - small ligand interactions k_f was calculated to be between 10^8 and 10^{10} M^{-1} s^{-1}. Other factors will also affect this rate constant, notably the charge state of the incoming ligand and the site, and to a certain extent the shape, of the ligand (Burgen, 1966). Electrostatic attractions are expected to be able to *increase* the predicted association rate constant by more than an order of magnitude only when the product of the charges exceeds 6 and the ionic strength is very low, while the effect of electrostatic repulsions on *reducing* k_f will be more pronounced. Bulky side-chains on incoming ligands, or steric restriction of the site, will decrease the effective solid angle of approach and, hence, also decrease the rate constant. For a series of very similar molecules the effects of charge and shape should be minimised. Variations in the affinity constant K_a ($= k_f/k_b$) would then be expected to be much more dependent on variation of the dissociation rate constant.

Taylor, King and Burgen (1970a) measured k_f, k_b and K_a for a group of benzene and heterocyclic sulphonamides and obtained the results shown in Fig. 5.1. Ignoring for the moment the *ortho*-substituted sulphonamides, the depen-

Table 5.1 Effect of alkyl chain extension on the binding and kinetic constants of sulphonamide inhibitors binding to human carbonic anhydrase C. F is the average multiple increase per —CH_2 group in the chain. n is the number of homologous compounds studied

Formula	n	F_{K_a}	F_{k_f}	F_{k_b}
R—⟨O⟩—SO_2NH_2	6	2.71	1.95	0.72
R—O—CO—⟨O⟩—SO_2NH_2	5	2.25	1.79	0.80
R—NH—CO—⟨O⟩—SO_2NH_2	6	2.29	1.45	0.63
R—O—CO—⟨O⟩$_S$—SO_2NH_2	5	2.57	1.82	0.70
R—CO—NH—⟨N=N/S⟩—SO_2NH_2	4	2.07	1.78	0.86

dence of affinity constant on the association rate constant is four times greater than that on the dissociation rate constant. These sulphonamides were not all closely structurally related, but the range of more than two orders of magnitude covered by the values of k_f itself suggests that the mechanism of Eq. (5.1) is too simple to explain the results. King and Burgen (1976) have extended these studies by measuring the kinetic constants of homologous series of sulphonamides under carefully controlled conditions. Some of their results are presented in Table 5.1, where they are expressed according to the relationship

$$\log Q_x = \log Q_o + x \log F$$

where x is the number of $-CH_2-$ groups in the substituent chain, Q is the measured property and F is therefore the average multiple per $-CH_2-$ group. This equation is not strictly adhered to, but it serves to illustrate the remarkable similarity of the results in the *para*-substituted benzene, 5-thiophene and 5-thiodiazole series. In each case the affinity constant increases by at least a factor of two per $-CH_2-$ group, and once again the greater part of this increase is accounted for by an increase in the association rate constant rather than by a decrease in the dissociation rate constant.

A decrease in dissociation rate constant with increasing chain length is not unexpected. There is evidence from ultra-violet difference spectroscopy (King and Burgen, 1970) and resonance Raman spectroscopy (Kumar, King and Carey, 1974, 1976) that in the equilibrium complex the sulphonamide is in its anionic state. Also, the very distinctive visible spectra exhibited by sulphonamide complexes of carbonic anhydrase in which the active-site zinc atom has been replaced by cobalt indicate the formation of a metal-sulphonamide bond (Lindskog, 1963; Lindskog and Nyman 1964). For series of sulphonamides such as these, with very similar pK_a values within the series, the strength of this bond would be expected to be roughly constant. However, an increase in the non-ionic forces stabilising the complex would increase the activation energy necessary to disrupt the complex and, hence, reduce the dissociation rate constant. Even so, the dependence of K_a on k_b is considerably less than it is on k_f, which does not fit with the theoretical predictions based on the simple one-step mechanism.

This problem can be overcome by considering the implications of a multistage mechanism. The simplest such mechanism to consider is a two-step process,

$$E + I \underset{k_{-1}}{\overset{k_1}{\rightleftharpoons}} EI_1 \underset{k_{-2}}{\overset{k_2}{\rightleftharpoons}} EI_2 \qquad (5.2)$$

where EI_1 is an intermediate form of the complex which can convert to the final form, EI_2, by a unimolecular process which may involve a simple isomerisation of EI_1 or may be more complicated. The solution of the rate equation for this mechanism will accommodate the experimental data within certain limitations. We have seen in direct determinations of the bimolecular rate constant k_f under pseudo-first-order conditions that there is no deviation from simple exponential decays. The two-step mechanism will produce this kind of result as long as the concentration of EI_1 relative to $[E] + [EI_2]$ remains small. In this case the rate constant k_f can be expressed by

$$k_f \simeq \frac{k_1 \times k_2}{k_{-1} + k_2} \qquad (5.3)$$

In the limiting case where $k_{-1} \ll k_2$ the equation becomes $k_f = k_1$, which is equivalent to the simple diffusion-limited case. However, when $k_{-1} \gg k_2$, the equation becomes

$$k_f = \frac{k_1 \times k_2}{k_{-1}} = K_1 k_2 \qquad (5.4)$$

where K_1 is the affinity constant of the intermediate species. This condition predicts that the apparent rate constants will be less than the diffusion-limited value.

The observed rate constant now contains two terms, K_1 and k_2, both of which may be structure-dependent, since there is no reason *a priori* to suppose that the structural features involved in the forces stabilising the intermediate complex are identical with those which influence the formation of the final complex.

Treating the apparent dissociation rate constant in the same way gives the relationship

$$k_b = \frac{k_{-1} \times k_{-2}}{k_{-1} + k_2} \qquad (5.5)$$

Assuming that the diffusion-limiting case $k_{-1} \ll k_2$ does not apply, then, when $k_{-1} \gg k_2$, the equation simplifies to $k_b = k_{-2}$. The dissociation rate is then primarily governed by the forces stabilising the final form of the complex. The overall affinity constant is thus composed of two terms, one of which is primarily governed by intermolecular forces involved in the intermediate form of the complex, the other by those involved in the final form.

Haselkorn *et al.* (1974), in a study of the binding of haptens to an IgA immunoglobulin produced by mouse plasma cell tumour, MOPC-315, also found that very small differences in the structure of the hapten, e.g. from a dimethylaminodinitrophenol to a diethylaminodinitrophenol, caused relatively large changes in the association rate constant. Their conclusion was similar to ours, that the diffusion-limited step led to the formation of what they called an 'encounter complex' followed by a 'transformation step' leading to the definitive complex.

Evidence for an Intermediate Complex

Evidence for the existence of an intermediate complex has not been obtained directly from stopped-flow experiments. Indeed, the kinetic analysis presented above depends on the transient existence of such a complex at low relative concentration. However, evidence for the existence of an intermediate binding site and some pointers to the forces involved in both stages of the reaction mechanism have been obtained from studies of the binding of N-acetylated sulphonamides to holoenzyme and of normal sulphonamides to metal-free apoenzyme.

Binding of N-acetylated sulphonamides

Mann and Keilin's (1940) first investigations of sulphanilamide inhibition of carbonic anhydrase showed that acetylation of the sulphonamide group caused a reduction of several orders of magnitude in the inhibitory power. Lanir and Navon (1971) found a value of 1.5×10^2 M^{-1} for the affinity constant of sulphacetamide, which compares with the normal range of $10^6 - 10^9$ M^{-1} for unsubstituted sulphonamides. Their results from NMR line-broadening experiments gave minimum values of 2×10^2 s^{-1} for the dissociation rate constant of both sulphacetamide and p-toluene sulphonamide, whereas King and Burgen (1976) and Taylor *et al.* (1970a) have made direct measurements of the dissociation rate constant of p-toluene sulphonamide by fluorescence quenching and found values of less than 0.1 s^{-1}. Lanir and Navon concluded that one species of the enzyme-inhibitor complex exchanges rapidly with its free constituents. However, they also stated that their results could not be produced by a minor fraction of a fast-exchanging complex but were consistent with a multistage mechanism.

Apart from the obvious difference in bulk around the nitrogen atom, the other property of sulphacetamide which distinguishes it from the more active sulphonamides is its low pK value of 5.0 for the sulphonamide-NH. The molecule therefore exists as an anion at neutral pH, where most measurements have been made. Several investigations (Kernohan, 1966; Lindskog and Thorslund, 1968; Taylor *et al.*, 1970b; King and Maren, 1974) of the effect of pH on binding and kinetic constants have shown bell-shaped curves of K_a or k_f against pH, while k_b is independent of pH. As can be seen from Fig. 5.2, the lower limb of these curves is controlled by the ionisation of an enzymic group with a pK near neutrality, while the other limb is controlled by the pK of the sulphonamide group. The low binding constant of sulphacetamide might therefore be due solely to the depressed pK. King and Burgen (1976) have produced evidence which indicates that the complex formed by N-acetyl-p-nitrobenzene sulphonamide (pK = 3.75), closely related to sulphacetamide, is not the same as that formed by normal sulphonamide inhibitors. The binding constant is insensitive to pH between 5.5 and 9.0; if the binding mechanism were the same as with p-nitrobenzene sulphonamide, then a 300-fold change in K_a would have been expected over this range. Furthermore, the N-acetylated sulphonamide does not produce the distinctive visible spectrum of the cobalt carbonic anhydrase complex, either at low or high pH, indicating that a metal-ligand bond is not formed. Nevertheless, the compound is an inhibitor of enzymic hydrolysis of p-nitrobenzyl acetate

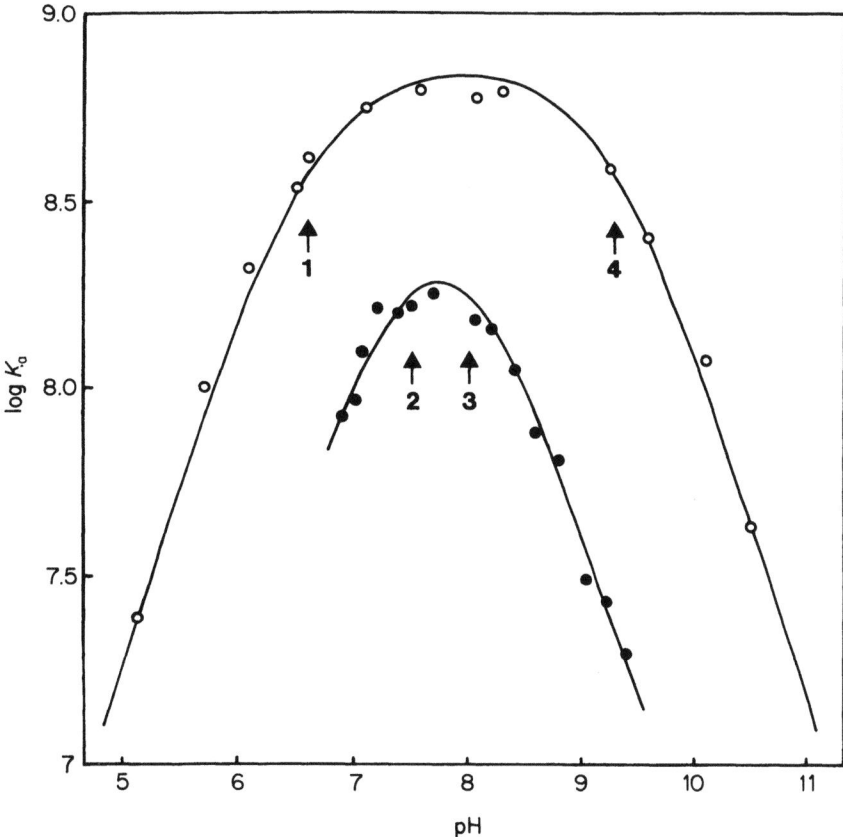

Figure 5.2 Variation of affinity constant with pH (—o—o—): HCA-C combining with salicylazobenzene sulphonamide. (—•—•—): HCA-B combining with ethoxzolamide. The pK values controlling the shape of these curves are: 1, enzymic pK of HCA-C at 6.6; 2, enzymic pK of HCA-B at 7.5; 3, pk of dissociation of ethoxzolamide sulphonamide-NH at 8.05; 4, pK of dissociation of salicylazobenzene sulphonamide-NH at 9.3. The lines are drawn according to Eq. (5.6), with the value of K_{int} being varied for best fit

and competes with p-nitrobenzene sulphonamide and dimethylaminonaphthalene sulphonamide with an affinity constant of 3×10^4 M^{-1}.

The binding site for N-acetylated sulphonamides would thus appear to overlap that for the unsubstituted ones. The N-acetyl group influences the strength of the binding by preventing the formation of the metal-ligand bond. Since there is no pH-dependence of the affinity constant, this must almost certainly be due to steric hindrance around the metal atom.

Binding experiments with apoenzyme

Further evidence for the existence of a pre-equilibrium binding site comes from experiments on binding of sulphonamides to apoenzyme. Coleman (1967) measured the binding of acetazolamide to apocarbonic anhydrase and found a reduction of approximately three orders of magnitude in the binding constant. King and Burgen (1976) have used an analytical sulphanilamide affinity column to measure the binding of a variety of ring-substituted benzene sulphonamides to apocarbonic anhydrase. They found stoicheiometric binding and similar or even greater reductions in K_a for *para*-substituted sulphonamides.

An estimate of the dissociation rate constant of sulphonamides from the apoenzyme can be obtained by assuming a diffusion-limited value (5×10^8 M^{-1} s^{-1}) for the association rate constant. The estimates of k_b then range from 1.6×10^4 s^{-1} to 6.3×10^5 s^{-1}, of the same order of magnitude as the dissociation rate constant measured by Lanir and Navon (1972) for sulphacetamide from the manganese-substituted enzyme, 5×10^4 s^{-1}, and as that calculated for N-acetyl p-nitrobenzene sulphonamide, 1.7×10^4 s^{-1}.

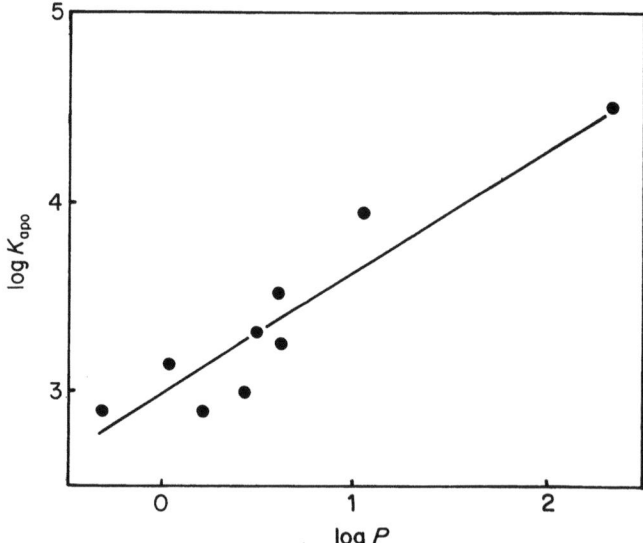

Figure 5.3 Correlation of the sulphonamide affinity constant for the apoenzyme with the octanol-water partition coefficient (P) of the sulphonamide. Data of King and Burgen (1976)

The binding site for sulphonamides on the apoenzyme thus appears to be closely related to that for N-acetylated sulphonamides on the holoenzyme, and is likely to be the same as that used in forming EI_1. Since the binding of sulphonamides to this state is pH-independent, it is probable that it is hydrophobic in nature. King and Burgen's (1976) measurements of the affinity constant for apoenzyme show a positive correlation with the octanol-water partition coefficient (P) of the sulphonamide (Fig. 5.3), which would be expected for a diffusion-controlled association reaction and a dissociation reaction which needed to overcome hydrophobic forces only.

IMPLICATIONS FOR STRUCTURE – ACTIVITY ANALYSIS

Correlations with Physical Properties

The two-step reaction scheme discussed above, in which the structure-dependent properties of the incoming ligand may have different effects at different stages of the reaction, assists an understanding of the structure-binding relationships in the combination of sulphonamides with carbonic anhydrase. In such a two-step reaction the overall affinity constant K_a is equal to the product of the affinity constants in each step, K_1 and K_2. A high value of K_1 is clearly desirable for strong binding, and since this binding appears to be hydrophobic, an increase in partition coefficient of the sulphonamide should be advantageous. Figure 5.4 contains a plot of $\log K_a$ against log partition coefficient for several series of sulphonamides and a clear correlation is present, but only within each closely structurally

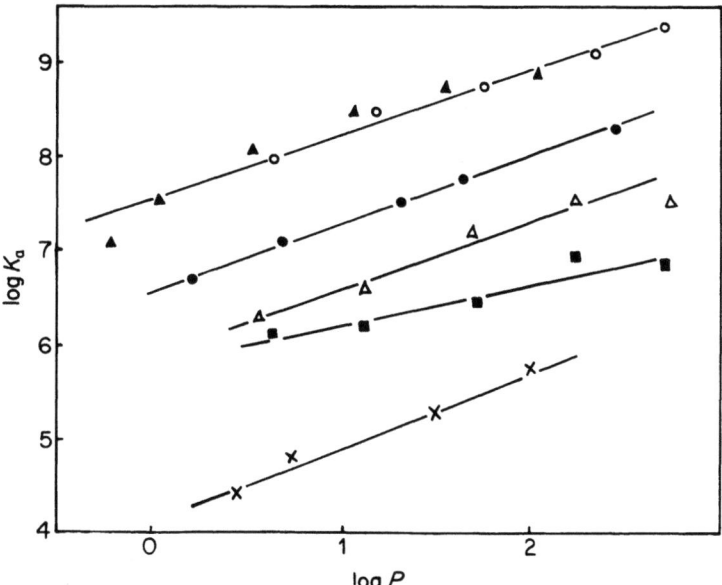

Figure 5.4 Correlation of the sulphonamide affinity constant for the holoenzyme with the octanol-water partition coefficients for several series of sulphonamides. (▲) p-amides, (○) p-esters, (●) p-alkyl, (■) m-esters, (×) o-esters, all of benzene sulphonamide; (△) 5-esters of thiophene-2-sulphonamide

related series. These results contrast with those shown in Fig. 5.3, where the correlation of K_{apo} with partition coefficient is not series-dependent, and suggests that interseries differences are more important in the second stage of the binding.

When a situation such as this occurs, the valuable properties of the first-stage binding may be counter-productive when one attempts to correlate other properties of the sulphonamide with the binding constant. This is particularly well illustrated in the case of carbonic anhydrase inhibitors by the role of the ionisation of the sulphonamide group in the binding process. The bell-shaped dependence of K_a on pH shown in Fig. 5.2 is also exhibited by k_f, since the dissociation rate constant is pH-insensitive. This has led to some disagreement in the literature concerning the interpretation of these results (Taylor et al., 1970b; Olander, Bosen and Kaiser, 1973). In a single-step reaction two reaction mechanisms will satisfy the observed dependence, combination of the anionic sulphonamide with the acidic form of the enzyme or combination of the neutral sulphonamide with the basic form of the enzyme. As we have noted above, in the final form of the complex the sulphonamide is in its anionic form, yet the exceedingly high bimolecular association rate constant required for formation of the complex from the ionised species exceeds diffusion limitation by an order of magnitude in some cases (Taylor et al., 1970b, and can be calculated for some of the higher esters in King and Burgen, 1976).

This paradoxical situation is irrelevant in a two-stage reaction scheme, when the first step, binding to form an intermediate complex, is apparently independent of the ionisation state of the inhibitor. In this case the dependence of the association rate on pH must manifest itself in the second, unimolecular step.

This presents a further problem in that two alternative pathways can exist for formation of the final complex. Either the anionic form of the sulphonamide can bind directly to the metal or the neutral species can transfer a proton to a deprotonated acceptor group on the enzyme during the transition from EI_1 to EI_2. The experimental curves of K_a against pH can be fitted by equations describing either of these mechanisms. For direct combination of the anion

$$K_{obs} = K_{int} \frac{K_I/K_E}{(1 + K_1/[H^+])(1 + [H^+]/K_E)} \quad (5.6)$$

and for the neutral species

$$K_{obs} = K_{int} \frac{1}{(1 + KI/[H^+])(1 + [H^+]/K_E)} \quad (5.7)$$

where K_{obs} is the value of K_a at any pH, K_{int} is the intrinsic affinity constant of the reactive species, K_I and K_E are the dissociation constants of the sulphonamide and enzymic groups, respectively, and $[H^+]$ is the hydrogen ion concentration.

For measurements at a fixed pH the equations can be transformed to give the following dependencies of K_{obs} on K_1. For Eq. (5.6),

$$\log K_{obs} = \text{const} - pK_I - \frac{1}{2.303}\left\{\left[\frac{K_I}{[H^+]}\right] - \frac{1}{2}\left[\frac{K_I}{[H^+]}\right]^2 + \frac{1}{3}\left[\frac{K_I}{[H^+]}\right]^3 - \ldots\right\}^n \quad (5.8)$$

and for Eq. (5.7),

$$\log K_{obs} = \text{const}' - \frac{1}{2.303}\left\{\left[\frac{K_I}{[H^+]}\right] - \frac{1}{2}\left[\frac{K_I}{[H^+]}\right]^2 + \frac{1}{3}\left[\frac{K_I}{[H^+]}\right]^3 - \ldots\right\} \quad (5.9)$$

This produces the theoretical dependence of $\log K_{obs}$ on pK_I shown in Fig. 5.5, where the pH of the measurement is taken as 8.0. Direct reaction of the anion should lead to a marked increase in K_{obs} with decreasing pK_I, whereas ionisation of the inhibitor during the $EI_1 \rightarrow EI_2$ transition should give a much less marked decrease in K_{obs} with pK_I.

Figure 5.6 shows a plot of $\log K_a$ against pK_I for some homologous series. There is no definitive trend in the results, and any apparent correlation would

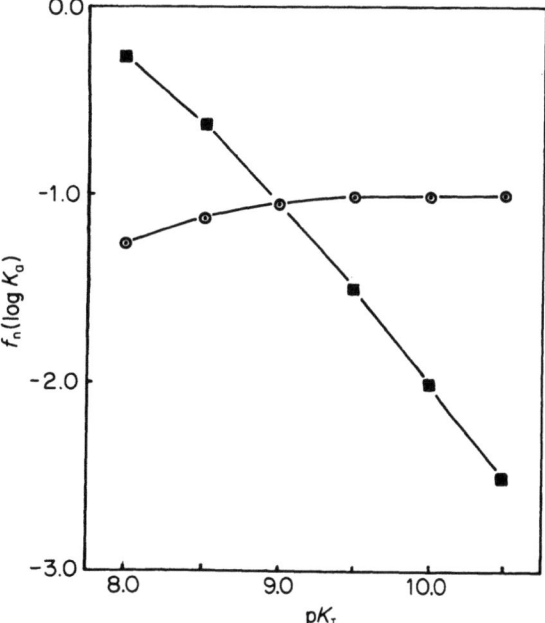

Figure 5.5 Theoretical dependence of the measured affinity constant on the pK of the sulphonamide group given by Eq. (5.8) (■) or Eq. (5.9) (○). The pH of measurement is assumed to be 8.0

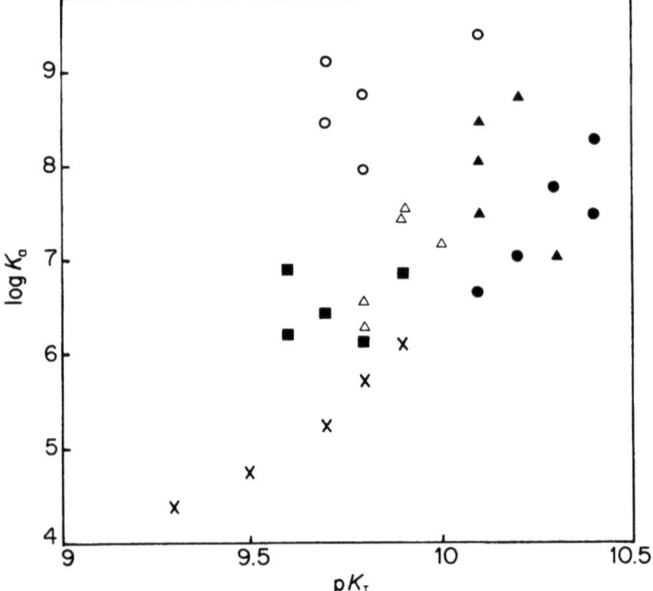

Figure 5.6 Values of log K_a measured at pH 8.0 plotted as a function of the pK of the sulphonamide. Symbols as for Fig. 5.4

suggest a large decrease in K_{obs} with pK_I, which agrees with neither prediction. This result is rather typical of the results of other workers; for example, Miller, Dessert and Roblin (1950) did find an increase in inhibiting power with decrease in pK_I for thiodiazole and thiazole sulphonamides, but there was no overlap of correlation between series, and some of the series they tested gave no correlation.

The implicit assumption in plots of K_a against pK_I that the intrinsic binding constant is the same for all sulphonamides is clearly not justified, and this is due in part at least to the varying contributions of hydrophobic interactions to the overall binding energy. Multiple regression analysis of the type used by Fujita and Hansch (1967) might provide a better indication of the reactive species.

A further complication of structure – activity relationships which has relevance to carbonic anhydrase inhibitors is the effect of positional isomers of the same sulphonamide. Kakeya et al. (1969) measured the inhibitory power of a group of benzene sulphonamides and found that for isomers of the same substituent the *ortho*-substituted compound had the least and the *para*-substituted the greatest inhibitory effect. Also, as can be seen from Fig. 5.1, *ortho*-substituted compounds did not fit the correlation of rate constants with equilibrium affinity constants obtained by Taylor et al. (1970a). These data are characterised by association and dissociation rate constants which are both too high to fit on the regression lines for the *meta*- and *para*-substituted compounds. The association rate constants measured for three of the *ortho*-substituted benzene sulphonamides were greater than for most of the *meta-* and *para*-substituted ones with higher values of K_a. This result is difficult to explain on the basis of a single-step mechanism implicating steric hindrance at the combining site, as a reduction in k_f would be expected on this model. In a two-step model involving only hydrophobic bonding as a first step the restrictions on orientation of the ligand on the initial binding may be minimal. Subsequent reorientation of the sulphonamide in the second stage of binding may be more difficult to achieve than in the case of *meta* and *para* isomers, but if the value of K_1 is sufficiently high, then a high association rate constant is achievable, since what we observe is the product of K_1 and k_2. However, if the formation of the final complex involves a reduction in the binding forces through steric strain, then an increase in the dissociation rate constant and subsequent reduction in K_a is also predicted.

King and Burgen (1976) have approached this problem by measuring binding and kinetic constants for positional isomers of series of esters of carboxyl-benzene sulphonamide. Some results are presented in Table 5.2. Binding of these

Table 5.2 Effect of positional isomerisation and alkyl chain extension on binding and kinetic constants. K_a, affinity constant for holoenzyme; K_1, affinity constant for apoenzyme; K_2, affinity constant for second-stage binding; k_2, second-stage association rate constant; k_{-2}, measured dissociation rate constant from holoenzyme

	$K_a (M^{-1})$	$K_1 (M^{-1})$	$K_2{}^a$	$k_2^b (s^{-1})$	$k_{-2} (s^{-1})$
4-Me	9.63×10^7	1.8×10^3	5.3×10^4	2.5×10^3	0.047
4-Bu	1.3×10^9	3.2×10^4	4.1×10^4	1.0×10^3	0.025
3-Me	1.43×10^6	3.3×10^3	4.2×10^2	2.6×10^2	0.61
3-Bu	8.87×10^6	3.3×10^3	2.7×10^3	2.7×10^3	1.00
2-Me	2.60×10^4	1.0×10^3	2.6×10^1	1.27×10^1	0.49
2-Bu	5.69×10^5	2.5×10^3	2.3×10^2	2.5×10^1	0.11

[a] Calculated from $K_a = K_1 \times K_2$.
[b] Calculated from $k_{app} = K_1 \times k_2$.

inhibitors to the apoenzyme does appear to be considerably less structure-dependent than binding to the holoenzyme. There is only a 32-fold variation in the measured values compared with a 50 000-fold variation in the overall binding constant. The reinforcing effects of increasing alkyl chain length on K_a seen in the *para* series are still apparent in the *meta-* and *ortho-*substituted compounds, though the kinetics involved in the production of these effects are complicated, and different in each case.

Considering first the *para* isomers, the greater part of the energy of binding arises from the second stage of the reaction, where low values of k_{-2} and relatively high values of k_2 indicate a minimal introduction of strain during the second step. Results from resonance Raman spectroscopy indicated only small deformations of *para*-substituted benzene sulphonamides in the complex with HCA-B (Kumar *et al.*, 1976). The effect of increasing chain length is to decrease both k_2 and k_{-2}. However, the overall result of these decreases is that K_2 changes very little. Very similar results were found with the amide analogues.

The situation is quite different with the *meta*-substituted compounds. Here the contribution of the second stage to the overall binding energy is less than in the first stage, but K_2 increases with chain length. This increase in K_2 is due to a tenfold increase in k_2 accompanied by a less than twofold increase in k_{-2}.

The *ortho*-substituted esters present yet another case. Once again the contribution of the second-stage binding is less than the first stage, but this is due to very low values of k_2, which increase with chain length, accompanied by fairly high values of k_{-2}, which decrease with chain length.

A detailed molecular interpretation of these effects must lie in the spatial relationship of the hydrophobic bonding areas in the enzyme-binding site to the position and direction of the co-ordinate bond formed between the active-site zinc atom and the sulphonamide group. The orientation of the sulphonamide group with respect to the zinc atom in the intermediate complex will be determined by optimisation of the hydrophobic bonding. The results from binding positional isomers to the apoenzyme suggest that steric hindrance is not a major factor in the initial binding step. If the benzene nucleus and alkyl sidechain are bound in a similar fashion in all of the positional isomers, then reorientation of the molecule will be necessary during the EI_1 to EI_2 transition in some cases. The barriers to reorientation may involve both steric hindrance and changes in hydrophobic bonding. The results for k_2 would suggest that these barriers are least in the case of *para* and *meta* substituents, yet they are subtly different in their response to chain length.

A contributory factor to the differing effects of chain length and positional isomerisation on k_2 and k_{-2} may be the asymmetry of the rest of the molecule with respect to the sulphonamide group in *meta* or *ortho* isomers. If the initial binding is optimised with respect to the aromatic nucleus and the side-chain, then the sulphonamide group can occupy a minimum of two orientations, 180° apart in the plane of the aromatic nucleus. The probability of formation of the metal-ligand bond may be much less in one orientation than another, in which case k_2 will be reduced. The effect of chain length in increasing or decreasing k_2 can then be explained in terms of steric factors at or near the side-chain binding site.

Formation of the ligand-metal bond from a preferred orientation of the sulphonamide in the initial complex will influence to some extent the energy required to rupture the bond once formed. The experiments with *para*-substituted sulphonamides demonstrated a relatively small dependence of k_{-2} on chain length, and since this rate constant is independent of pH over a very wide range, much of the energy of the final complex must arise from the metal-ligand bond.

The variation in k_{-2} with positional isomerisation is then presumably mainly due to steric strain caused by misalignment of the optimum positions for hydrophobic and co-ordinate bonding due to hindrance from the enzyme side-chains.

CONCLUSION

The results discussed above demonstrate the complex relationships which can exist in the apparently simple binding of an inhibitor to an enzyme. If the kinetic pathway of the incoming ligand involves more than a single step, then the structural features of the ligand which affect the overall association rate constant may be unrelated to those which affect the dissociation rate constant, and as such may work in concert or in opposition.

In the binding of sulphonamides to carbonic anhydrase the first step of the reaction sequence appears to be dominated by non-ionic interactions which are little affected by the overall shape of the molecule. The subsequent production of the final complex, involving the formation of a metal-ligand bond, is less sensitive to changes in hydrophobic interactions but is dependent on the ionisation state of the sulphonamide group and an enzymic group, and is subject to steric limitations.

In such circumstances attempts to correlate overall binding constants with physical properties of the drug can only meet with limited success.

REFERENCES

Alberty, R. A. and Hammes, G. G. (1958). *J. Phys. Chem.*, 62, 154
Burgen, A. S. V. (1966). *J. Pharm. Pharmacol.*, 18, 137
Coleman, J. E. (1967). *Nature (London)*, 214, 193
Fujita, T. and Hansch, C. (1967). *J. Med. Chem.*, 10, 991
Haselkorn, D., Friedman, S., Girol, D. and Pecht, I. (1974). *Biochemistry*, 13, 2210
Kakeya, N., Aoki, M., Kamada, A. and Yata, N. (1969). *Chem. Pharm. Bull.*, 17 (5), 1010
Kernohan, J. C. (1966). *Biochim. Biophys. Acta*, 118, 405
King, R. W. and Burgen, A. S. V. (1970). *Biochim. Biophys. Acta*, 207, 278
King, R. W. and Burgen, A. S. V. (1976). *Proc. R. Soc. London*, 193, 107
King, R. W. and Maren, T. H. (1974). *Mol. Pharmacol.*, 10, 344
Kumar, K., King, R. W. and Carey, P. R. (1974). *FEBS Lett.*, 48, 283
Kumar, K., King, R. W. and Carey, P. R. (1976). *Biochemistry*, 15, 2195
Lanir, A. and Navon, G. (1971). *Biochemistry*, 10, 1024
Lanir, A. and Navon, G. (1972). *Biochemistry*, 11, 3536
Lindskog, S. (1963). *J. Biol. Chem.*, 238, 945
Lindskog, S. and Nyman, P. O. (1964). *Biochim. Biophys. Acta*, 85, 462
Lindskog, S. and Thorslund, A. (1968). *Eur. J. Biochem.*, 3, 453
Mann, T. and Keilin, D. (1940). *Nature (London)*, 146, 164
Miller, W. H., Dessert, A. M. and Roblin, R. O. (1950). *J. Am. Chem. Soc.*, 72, 4893
Olander, J., Bosen, S. F. and Kaiser, E. T. (1973). *J. Am. Chem. Soc.*, 95, 1616
Taylor, P. W., King, R. W. and Burgen, A. S. V. (1970a). *Biochemistry*, 9, 2638
Taylor, P. W., King, R. W. and Burgen, A. S. V. (1970b). *Biochemistry*, 9, 3894

6
The haemoglobin molecule as a model drug receptor

P. J. Goodford (The Wellcome Research Laboratories, Beckenham, Kent, UK)

INTRODUCTION

Receptors

It is nearly a century since Langley (1878) suggested that there might be a substance in nerves or glands with which atropine and pylocarpine could combine. He was studying salivary secretion, and was attempting to interpret his observations according to the concepts of Guldberg and Waage (1864), who had recently proposed the Law of Mass Action. This Law was very attractive to Langley because it allowed him to formulate his ideas quantitatively, and many investigations of drug action have been interpreted along similar lines during the past 100 years. Such work may all be regarded as the logical extension of Langley's pioneering studies, and it is appropriate that he should be remembered at this Symposium on Drug Action at the Molecular Level.

A long time was to elapse before Langley developed his ideas about those chemical structures in living tissues which react with drugs. By 1905, however, he had inferred that an 'accessory substance' might be present which received the stimulus, and transferred it to the contractile material of muscle or the secretory material of glands. 'Since this accessory substance is the recipient of the stimuli which it transfers to the contractile material, we may speak of it as the *receptive substance* of the muscle, and we may suppose that the receptive substance is a side-chain molecule of the molecule of contractile substance. Moreover, the receptive substance affects or is capable of affecting the metabolism of the chief substance.'

With these words Langley (1905) introduced the concept of receptors, and began to consider their molecular structure. However, no significant advance was possible in this field until experimental methods had been developed for the observation of macromolecular architecture. Many such techniques have been devised in recent years, but the direct observation of structure by using the individual atoms of a crystal as a diffraction grating for X-rays was introduced by Bragg (1913) in Langley's own lifetime.

It was not possible to apply the X-ray method to biological macromolecules until electronic computers were available to carry out the extended calculations.

In 1961 Kendrew et al. established the positions of the atoms in sperm whale myoglobin. Progress was slow but steady during the succeeding decade, and by the early 1970s atomic resolution had been achieved for a number of proteins. It then seemed appropriate to consider the feasibility of designing compounds to interact in a predetermined way with receptor sites of known molecular architecture in order to produce a predetermined response. One such attempt will now be described.

The General Approach
When one chooses a drug-receptor combination for detailed structural analysis, the initial decision lies between two different ways of approaching the problem. If a pharmacological receptor were considered, it would probably be membrane-bound, and the structure of such receptors has not yet been established. Before the analysis could begin it would be necessary to isolate and purify a substantial quantity of receptor material so that the amino acid composition and protein sequence could be determined. The three-dimensional structure of the molecule would have to be observed by X-ray crystallography, and all these stages would be time-consuming and expensive. Moreover there would be no guarantee of final success, because one could not be certain of obtaining suitable crystals for X-ray work.

The alternative approach would be to study a known protein, even if it were not strictly speaking a 'pharmacological' receptor. The problems and expense of protein sequencing and X-ray analysis would then be circumvented, and one could begin immediately designing compounds to interact optimally with the site. This approach might not be directly relevant to therapy, but it was adopted for the present study in the hope that it would lead to a better understanding of some of the problems in fitting drugs to receptors.

The overall method was therefore to choose a suitable biological macromolecule whose structure and general properties were already well-established, and construct an accurate scale model. The macromolecule would have a known receptor site, and models of known interacting compounds (e.g. the natural regulator or hormone) would also be made. The nature of the bonding interactions would then be inferred, and this knowledge would be used to design new compounds which might be expected to interact more efficiently. The proposed compounds would be synthesised and their properties studied by physicochemical techniques for comparison with their biological effects.

The Choice of a Receptor for Study
In choosing the most appropriate receptor a number of criteria are relevant which may be listed under nine main headings.

(1) The molecular structure of the receptor must have been determined. However, the calculation of atomic co-ordinates is elaborate and sometimes imprecise,

and the existence of X-ray data does not necessarily imply that three-dimensional co-ordinates are available. It is also important that the structure of the crystalline receptor should be closely related to its structure in solution. In the early 1970s, when the current project was initiated, accurate atomic co-ordinates for biological macromolecules had only been published in a limited number of cases, and this imposed a severe restriction on the choice.

(2) The identical receptor must be available for biochemical, biological and physicochemical studies. Erroneous conclusions might be drawn if one receptor site were modelled and a slightly different one were used for subsequent experiments.

(3) The mode of interaction at the receptor must be defined; that is to say, it must interact with any given compound in a specific known way, and no other. If this were not so, it would be difficult to reconcile measurements of binding with measurements of biological potency. A multiple binding situation could in theory be analysed, but this might well add extra complications which would be better avoided.

(4) A range of known interacting compounds would be desirable, so that correlations could be established between biological measurements, physicochemical measurements and assessments of the goodness of fit between compound and receptor.

(5) These compounds should, ideally, fall into different pharmacological classes, e.g. agonists and antagonists.

(6) It would be helpful if similar but not identical receptors occurred in different species or tissues, and if some structural data were available concerning them. This would aid the understanding of the way in which compounds differed in their action from species to species, or from tissue to tissue.

(7) The presence of a paramagnetic transition metal atom might make possible electron spin resonance (ESR) observations on the receptor-compound complex.

(8) It would be advantageous if the properties of the chosen system could be studied simply, obviating the need to develop new and costly methods.

(9) It would be commercially advantageous if there were at least a remote chance of this preliminary exercise yielding a clinically useful drug.

The first three criteria in the above list are essential, and must apply to the chosen receptor if meaningful results are to be obtained. Criteria (4)-(6) are highly desirable, since they should give further clues about the way in which interactions take place, and might be expected therefore to facilitate the design of other compounds. Criteria (7) and (8) are practical points which make it easier to test hypotheses concerning the interactions. Criterion (9) is the most daunting, but it is a commercial one and is not relevant to the exercise of determining whether the method may or may not be viable.

It was therefore decided to ignore criterion (9) initially, and to perform the present exercise solely in order to establish the feasibility of the method. The aim would be to gain a better understanding of receptors, in preparation for the time when the structure of a therapeutically relevant receptor might become available.

The Selection of Haemoglobin for Investigation

When the present project was initiated, there were only a few biological macromolecules whose atomic structure had been established. These included the enzymes carbonic anhydrase, carboxypeptidase, chymotrypsin, lysozyme, papain, ribonuclease and subtilisin; the oxygen carriers myoglobin and haemoglobin; the hormone insulin; and the structural proteins collagen and keratin. It was clear from the outset that haemoglobin was a strong contender, and in fact haemoglobin was the only protein which satisfied the first eight criteria on the above list. Its amino acid composition and sequence (Matsuda, Gehring-Müller and Braunitzer, 1963) were known, and the high-resolution X-ray structure had been determined (Perutz *et al.*, 1968). Dr Perutz at Cambridge kindly agreed to make the atomic co-ordinates available on magnetic computer tape, and without his advice and collaboration the present project would have been impossible. Blood is readily available, and reasonably straightforward procedures have been established for the preparation of pure haemoglobin (Drabkin, 1946; Benesch, Benesch and Yu, 1967; Williams and Tsay, 1973). Furthermore, there exists a small naturally occurring sugar phosphate (2,3-diphosphoglycerate; DPG), which combines with a known site on the haemoglobin tetramer, and the DPG-haemoglobin interaction has been investigated in some detail. A range of other compounds was also known to interact, which might allow a correlation between biological and physicochemical measurements and goodness of fit to be determined. In addition, a wide range of different haemoglobins was available for study, both from different animal species and from human mutants (Stamatoyannopoulos, 1972). The haem groups also contain iron atoms which should facilitate ESR observations, and the biological properties of haemoglobin can be simply observed by measuring the dissociation curve (Barcroft and Haldane, 1902; van Slyke and Neill, 1924; Allen, Guthe and Wyman, 1950).

A possible disadvantage was the large size of the haemoglobin molecule, which occurs as a tetramer, containing nearly 600 amino acid residues. Accurate molecular modelling was therefore a daunting task, and it was necessary to devise special methods (Norrington, 1974) in order to proceed at a reasonable speed. Another problem was the complex nature of the stepwise reaction

$$4Hb + 4O_2 = Hb_4(O_2)_4$$

since the kinetics and conformational changes which accompany the intermediate steps have not been fully investigated. However, a very large body of general knowledge is available concerning the haemoglobin-oxygen relationship, and it soon became clear that haemoglobin would be the macromolecule of choice for the new project.

The Haemoglobin Molecule as a Model Drug Receptor

HAEMOGLOBIN

Physiology

The primary function of haemoglobin is to carry oxygen from the lungs to the body tissues, where it is used by the enzyme cytochrome oxidase to initiate the series of reactions which constitute the respiratory chain. Haemoglobin must therefore take up oxygen at its partial pressure in air in the lungs, and must release it at the partial pressure of the capillary bed where the oxygen is needed in the body. The reaction is necessarily reversible, and the equilibrium is determined by the partial pressure of oxygen, as shown by the dissociation curves in Fig. 6.1. By the early twentieth century it was well established that the curve for whole blood was sigmoidal in shape (Fig. 6.1).

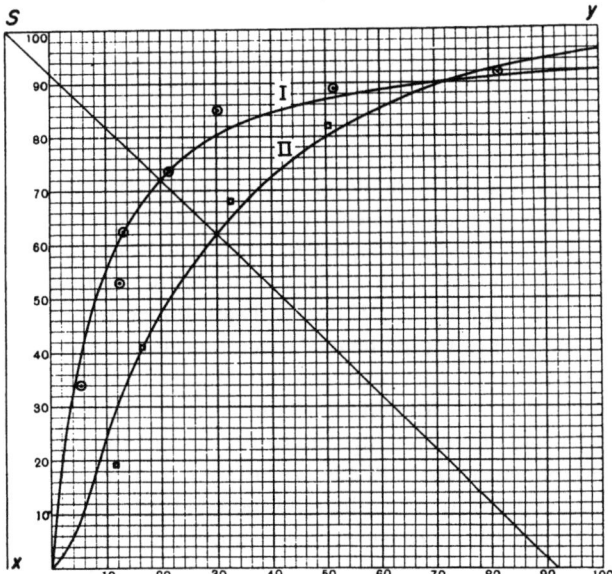

Fig. 1. Ordinates = Percentage saturation of hæmoglobin with oxygen. Abscissæ = tension of oxygen in mm. of mercury. Curve I = rectangular hyperbola. $xy = 800$. Curve II = Bohr's dissociation curve of hæmoglobin.
⊙ Points determined from dialysed solution.
□ Points determined from undialysed solution.

Figure 6.1 The haemoglobin dissociation curves observed by Barcroft and Roberts (1909). The left-hand curve, which does not deviate appreciably from a rectangular hyperbola, was measured on the sample of haemoglobin which these authors purified. The right-hand signoid curve is more characteristic of whole blood

The early workers recognised that the Law of Mass Action should result in a rectangular hyperbola when applied to the simple reaction

$$Hb + O_2 = Hb\, O_2$$

and they realised that a hyperbola would not deliver oxygen as efficiently as the observed sigmoid. Many ingenious suggestions were put forward to explain the sigmoidicity, but no agreement was reached. Ostwald (1908) suggested that oxygen uptake was not a chemical reaction at all, but merely physical absorption. Bohr (1909) made the bizarre proposal that haemoglobin dissociated into its separate haem and globin components. Another ingenious idea was based on the finding that lowering the pH diminished the affinity of haemoglobin for oxygen. If deoxyhaemoglobin were a strong acid, it would be expected to diminish its own oxygen affinity. Oxygen would therefore be liberated more easily as deoxygenation proceeded, which would lead to a sigmoid curve. However, this elegant hypothesis had to be abandoned because deoxyhaemoglobin is in fact a weaker acid than oxyhaemoglobin itself.

Barcroft and Roberts (1909) separated the haemoglobin from erythrocytes, and as far as they could tell the dissociation curve of salt-free haemoglobin solution was the rectangular hyperbola which would be expected for simple chemical reaction. This finding led Douglas, Haldane and Haldane (1912) to attribute the sigmoidal curve observed in whole blood to the presence of salts in the erythrocytes, and their interpretation has been fully confirmed by later findings. For a long time, however, no-one could repeat Barcroft and Roberts, observations and at last, reluctantly, even Barcroft came to accept that he might have been mistaken (Adair, Barcroft and Bock, 1921). He always hoped to unravel the matter, and in the very last year of his life he exclaimed on one occasion, 'If only I could find out why Roberts and I got rectangular hyperbolas in 1909, I would cheerfully order my coffin tomorrow' (Roughton, 1949).

In 1925 Greenwald discovered high concentrations of the intermediary metabolite 2,3-diphosphoglycerate (DPG) in erythrocytes, and by the early 1940s this sugar phosphate had been found in the red blood cells of many animal species (Rapoport and Guest, 1941). However, it was not until 1963 that Sugita and Chanutin observed electrophoretically that adenosine triphosphate (ATP) and DPG both form reversible complexes with haemoglobin. Other phosphates also complex, but relatively weakly.

Four more years elapsed before Chanutin and Curnish (1967) discovered that the oxygen dissociation curve of haemoglobin solutions is modified in the presence of ATP or DPG. It is now known that the shape is always sigmoidal, but it is still not easy to differentiate between the hyperbola and the sigmoid when pure haemoglobin is studied, unless accurate measurements are available at the lowest oxygen pressures. In the presence of DPG, however, the right-shifted dissociation curve is clearly sigmoidal. Other phosphates have a similar but smaller effect, although the potency of ATP in red blood cells is reduced because it complexes with the high concentrations of magnesium in the erythrocyte. Chanutin and Curnish therefore concluded that a primary physiological function of DPG is to diminish the oxygen affinity of haemoglobin and to shift its dissociation curve to the right, so that oxygen is liberated more readily in the tissues. Thus DPG was finally identified as the salt whose presence in red blood cells was predicted some 50 years earlier by Douglas *et al.* (1912), and the observations of Barcroft and Roberts (1909) were finally confirmed.

The Molecular Structure of Haemoglobin
The haemoglobin molecule, as it occurs in the red blood cell, is an aggregate of four separate protein chains. Two of these (the two alpha chains) are chemically identical, and are folded into the same globular structure round their respective haem groups and iron atoms. Moreover, they are held in a symmetrical relationship to each other about a perfect diad axis of symmetry. The other two protein chains (the beta chains) are also identical with each other but show many small differences from the alpha chains, although there is a strong superficial resemblance. In particular, the haem groups and iron atoms are held similarly by both alpha and beta chains, and the beta chains are also disposed about the *same* axis of symmetry as the alpha chains. The overall arrangement is roughly tetrahedral, so that each chain has contacts with the other three, forming a tetramer.

Haemoglobin is therefore an aggregate of several separate molecules, but the spatial relationships between these constituents are not rigidly fixed. If, for example, the pH of the surrounding environment be changed, this affects the charge distribution over the entire macromolecule, leading to widespread small structural alterations. It is not possible to consider any one of these in isolation, because an effect at one part of the haemoglobin tetramer is immediately relayed throughout the molecule and causes changes elsewhere. Similarly, an alteration in the partial pressure of oxygen may add or remove an oxygen molecule from one of the iron atoms, thereby changing its electronic properties and modifying its interaction with the protein. Once again the effects are relayed throughout the

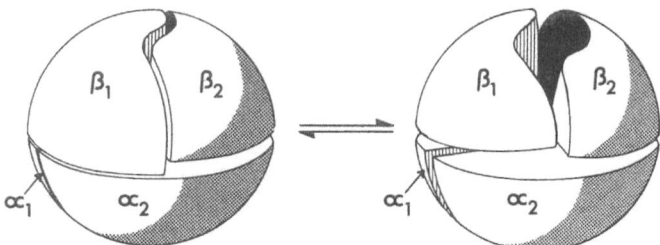

Figure 6.2 Haemoglobin consists of four protein chains which pack tightly together (left) in the presence of oxygen. The chains rearrange (right) when oxygen is removed, and a crevice appears between the beta subunits. This is the DPG receptor site

haemoglobin molecule, causing generalised structural alterations. Each iron atom is liganded to an oxygen molecule at high oxygen partial pressures, and the four protein chains then pack tightly together to form a stable conformation. On the other hand, the oxygen is removed as the partial pressure falls to zero, and under these circumstances crevices appear between some of the subunits and the molecular structure becomes less stable (Fig. 6.2).

The DPG – Haemoglobin Interaction

As the X-ray crystallographic analysis of haemoglobin was progressively refined, it became clear that one particular crevice between the subunits opened wider, after deoxygenation, than any other. This wide gap appeared between the two beta chains (Fig. 6.2), and there was evidence suggesting that a small molecule might enter this gap. Arnone (1972) therefore decided, in view of the observations on DPG binding, to crystallise deoxyhaemoglobin in the presence of DPG, and his X-ray analysis of the DPG-haemoglobin complex revealed the mode of binding in some detail.

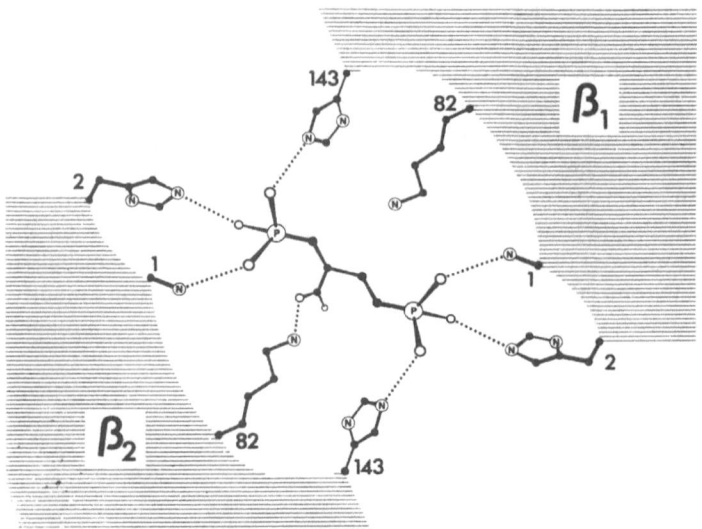

Figure 6.3 A schematic representation (Arnone, 1972) of the mode of binding of DPG in the crevice between the beta subunits of deoxyhaemoglobin. See text

The DPG receptor site is a basic region of the protein tetramer, and *each* beta chain contributes one terminal amino group, two histidines and one lysine residue, giving a total of eight basic functions symmetrically arranged at the receptor

(Fig. 6.3). DPG is an acid containing a carboxyl and two phosphate functions which present eight oxygen atoms for interaction with the protein:

$$\begin{array}{c} O O^- \\ \diagdown\!\!\diagup \\ O^-HCO^- \\ \diagdown||\diagup \\ O=P-O-C-C-O-P=O \\ \diagup||\diagdown \\ {}^-OHHO^- \end{array}$$

Arnone found that seven of these eight atoms are associated with seven of the eight basic groups on the receptor (Fig. 6.3), but the eighth potential interaction does not take place. Nevertheless the DPG - haemoglobin relationship must be regarded as a fair example of a natural process, and it is interesting to note that one functional group is apparently superfluous. This suggests that attempts to design drugs by modelling natural compounds may, in some respects, be misconceived.

It is not immediately obvious why DPG shifts the dissociation curve of haemoglobin to the right, thereby diminishing oxygen affinity, and this question may be considered at different levels of complexity. At its simplest the chemical equilibria

$$Hb \cdot O_2 \rightleftharpoons O_2 + Hb$$

$$Hb + DPG \rightleftharpoons Hb \cdot DPG$$

would move to the right when the DPG concentration was increased, promoting the breakdown of $Hb \cdot O_2$ and causing the liberation of oxygen, and this interpretation is not totally inaccurate, although it is oversimplified. In particular, the equations demonstrate that DPG interacts primarily with the deoxy protein (Hb), and it may be seen by inspection that a different situation would exist if the reaction

$$DPG \cdot Hb \cdot O_2 \rightleftharpoons DPG + Hb \cdot O_2$$

could also take place. The overall effect of DPG would then depend on the chemical equilibrium constants of the different equations. On the other hand, an increase of [DPG] would always promote the breakdown of $Hb \cdot O_2$ if the first two reactions occurred but not the last, and this appears to happen in practice.

The significance of the widely opening crevice between the beta chains of deoxyhaemoglobin is now apparent. As oxygenation proceeds, there are major structural changes in this region of the protein, and the crevice closes up (Fig. 6.2).

In the deoxy form there is a receptor for DPG which no longer exists after oxygenation and so the $DPG \cdot Hb \cdot O_2$ interaction may be largely neglected. As a result the effect of increasing [DPG] is to diminish oxygen affinity, and the DPG receptor site is ideally situated to produce this effect because of the extensive structural changes in this part of the macromolecule.

DESIGNING COMPOUNDS

The Method of Receptor Fit
The specific experimental approach to be adopted is now clear. Compounds would be designed to interact with the deoxyhaemoglobin conformation of the DPG site, care being taken that they could not also react with the changed conformation after oxygenation. Such compounds should shift the dissociation curve of haemoglobin to the right, diminishing the oxygen affinity and promoting the liberation of oxygen. Any of these effects could be measured in order to obtain a quantitative index of the biological potency of the compounds.

The briefest inspection of the DPG site shows that it contains two relatively uncommon features in the two terminal amino groups of the beta chains. Their rarity is apparent because the haemoglobin tetramer contains over 500 amino acid residues, yet there are only four terminal amino functions overall. Moreover, they are directly joined to the main protein chain, in contrast to the primary amino groups of lysine residues, and may therefore be better placed to influence the overall conformation of the protein. In attempting to design compounds to fit the deoxyhaemoglobin site for DPG, attention was first directed to the beta terminal amino groups.

In the normal course of events drugs are often designed by consideration of known active compounds, and this imposes certain constraints on the design process. It has already been mentioned that such a procedure can be misleading if the known compounds contain redundant information, but there is no need to adopt the approach at all when the structure of the receptor is known. One can then ignore earlier chemical types and design completely different compounds, subject only to the requirement that they should react appropriately with the receptor. In the present instance one would no longer be restricted to sugar phosphates but could search for any molecules which reacted with primary amines, and this idea led directly to an investigation of the aldehyde group which would react to form a Schiff base:

$$R-CHO + H_2N-R' \rightleftharpoons R-CH{=}N-R' + H_2O$$

The terminal amino groups of the beta chains move several hundred picometers relative to each other during the oxy - deoxy transition, and this observation suggested that dialdehydes might interact specifically with the deoxy form if they were designed so that the distance between the aldehyde groups matched deoxyhaemoglobin, but did not match the oxy protein. Thus the general type of compound would be

$$OHC \frown CHO$$

with a carefully tailored distance between the functional groups.

The PAR Method

In attempting to design a successful drug, it is not sufficient to find a compound which reacts optimally with the appropriate receptor. The compound must also satisfy a number of other criteria and must, for example, reach the receptor in an adequate concentration after the administration of a reasonable dose by an acceptable route. It might need to ionise appropriately in the gastrointestinal tract for optimal absorption, and in the present case it should have the right lipophilicity for passage through the red cell membrane. Hence, it is necessary to give some consideration to the physiocochemical properties of compounds which were, in the first case, designed to fit a specific receptor.

The method of Physicochemical-Activity Relationships (the PAR method) is an empirical technique for comparing different compounds in a congeneric series, in order to find the particular member which has the best overall combination of physicochemical properties. Although the approach can be applied to any type of compound, it has been developed with particular relevance to substituted benzenes (Goodford, 1973), and so there is a clear advantage to be gained by incorporating benzene rings when compounds are designed. For example, the chemical reactivity of the —CHO group in benzaldehydes can be modified in a predictable fashion by introducing appropriate benzenoid substituents, and so the compound type for interaction with the DPG site of deoxyhaemoglobin can be narrowed down to

$$OHC-\bigcirc\!\!\!-\!\!\frown\!\!-\!\!\bigcirc\!\!\!-CHO$$

The Unified Method

It was now necessary to combine the method of Receptor Fit with the PAR method, in order to design specific compounds for synthesis. Modelling studies and simple geometrical calculations showed that two methylene groups between the benzene rings would give a structure of optimal length to react with the two terminal groups of deoxyhaemoglobin, if the compound were in an extended conformation:

$$OHC-\bigcirc\!\!\!-CH_2-CH_2-\bigcirc\!\!\!-CHO$$

Other conformations could occur but this is preferred in the solid state (Robertson, 1934), although crystal packing forces may exert a significant influence in that environment (Jeffrey, 1946). Moreover, the conformational flexibility of the bibenzyl molecule may allow it to accommodate minor perturbations of the receptor structure, while the rigidity provided by the benzene rings limits the number of conformations which have to be considered and may not be greatly disadvantageous. Thus the molecule is neither completely rigid nor completely flexible, and it might have about the optimal degree of flexibility. Finally one may note that the compound is not long enough to reach both the beta terminal amino groups of the undistorted oxyhaemoglobin structure and should therefore favour the deoxy conformation.

Compound 1 was synthesised by Dr S. Wilkinson as the simplest example of the bibenzyl dialdehyde type designed to interact with the beta terminal amino groups of deoxyhaemoglobin, but not surprisingly it was almost insoluble in water and so could not be tested on haemoglobin. It was therefore necessary to consider ways of increasing its solubility without inhibiting its fit to the receptor. Aqueous solubility is not the easiest physicochemical property to predict for a novel compound, but a plausible approach was the addition of extra atoms that might form hydrogen bonds to water. The question then arose whether these extra atoms could be disposed around the molecule so that they would also interact favourably with the receptor and perhaps improve the fit, and this concept led to a study of the aldehyde - bisulphite addition complex:

$$HO-S(=O)(=O)-CH(OH)-C_6H_4-CH_2-CH_2-C_6H_4-CH(OH)-S(=O)(=O)-OH$$
$$\mathbf{2}$$

Three separate lines of argument pointed to this compound. On the one hand, it might be in equilibrium in water with enough of the free dialdehyde (compound 1) for that to react with haemoglobin by Schiff base formation as originally postulated. On the other hand, the oxygen atoms attached to the sulphur might interact with the basic groups of the DPG site, much as the phosphate functions of DPG itself. Finally it might react as an α-hydroxysulphonic acid:

$$R-CH(SO_3H)-OH + H_2N-R' \rightleftharpoons R-CH(SO_3H)-NH-R' + H_2O$$

forming a covalent bond but still leaving the oxygen atoms free for interaction.

In order to assess these possibilities it was necessary to know the structure of compound 2, and there has been much disagreement in the scientific literature on the nature of aldehyde - bisulphite complexes, although the balance of the evidence (Sheppard and Bourns, 1954) is in favour of an α-hydroxysulphonic acid as shown above. We are indebted to Mr A. G. Ferrige, who studied compound 2 by nuclear magnetic resonance, and conclusively demonstrated the direct sulphur-carbon bond which must be present if this structure is indeed correct. It therefore seemed not unreasonable to hope that compound 2 would be more soluble than compound 1 and that it would also interact more favourably with the DPG site, since covalent bonds, hydrogen bonds and salt bridges might all be formed.

The Assessment of Biological Potency

It was hoped that the designed compounds would shift the dissociation curve of haemoglobin to the right. However, in order to define their activity fully it would be necessary to study a range of drug concentrations and oxygen partial pressures, at different temperatures and pH values and varied carbon dioxide concentrations. This would be a substantial undertaking, and it was decided that a single measurement should be chosen to give a rough comparative assessment of the potency of each compound.

Dilute solutions of human haemoglobin of low phosphate and low methaemoglobin content were prepared as described by Paterson *et al.* (1976), and were mixed with a large excess (100 mmol dm^{-3}) of Hepes buffer (Good *et al.*, 1966) in order to ensure accurate pH control. The solution was equilibrated with oxygen-free nitrogen at 37°C in a special tonometer, and small measured aliquots of air were then admitted at intervals. After each admission and equilibration the proportion of oxyhaemoglobin in the solution was determined spectroscopically by a modification of the method of Allen *et al.* (1950), and the dissociation curve was calculated after applying appropriate corrections (Beddell *et al.*, 1976). The experiment was repeated in the presence of a 2.5 mmol dm^{-3} concentration of each compound, and the right shift of the dissociation curve was measured at the half-way point where the haemoglobin was half saturated with oxygen. This value (expressed in kilopascals) was termed the 'right shift of the p50' and was taken as a measure of potency, DPG itself giving a right shift of about 1.7 ± 0.1 kPa. The experiments were all carried out by Dr F. E. Norrington.

One other factor should be mentioned. Compound 2 was soluble in water as expected, but after some time it hydrolysed, forming a precipitate of compound 1. This could be prevented by the addition of a low concentration of sodium metabisulphite to the solution, and control experiments showed that this substance had little effect on the p50 value by itself. Nevertheless a consistent procedure was adopted, and sodium metabisulphite at a concentration of 5 mmol dm^{-3} was always included in control samples whenever it was added to stabilise a drug.

The Activity of the Compounds

Compound 2 at the standard concentration of 2.5 mmol dm^{-3} gave a right shift of about 1.2 ± 0.1 kPa relative to the appropriate control, and was therefore judged to be showing the expected type of behaviour, although it was less potent than DPG. This was an exciting finding which was repeated many times (Beddell et al., 1976), although any interpretation of the result was complicated by the need to include sodium metabisulphite in the solution. Another line of approach was therefore adopted simultaneously in order to obtain a soluble analogue of compound 1 which should also fit the receptor site.

Compound 1 has a diad axis of symmetry, but the perfect symmetry of DPG is broken by the carboxyl group which interacts with residue $Lys^{\beta}{}_{82}$ of the receptor. It was decided to copy this feature, and Dr Wilkinson therefore synthesised compound 3:

$$OHC-\langle\bigcirc\rangle-CH_2-CH_2-\langle\bigcirc\rangle-CHO$$
$$O-CH_2\cdot COOH$$
3

in which it was reasonable to hope that the carboxyl group might be able to react with $Lys^{\beta}{}_{82}$, while the additional oxygen atoms might render the compound sufficiently soluble for testing at 2.5 mmol dm^{-3} without the need for conversion to the bisulphite complex. It was successfully studied in the absence of sodium metabisulphite and also displayed the expected type of activity, giving a right shift of 0.7 ± 0.1 kPa, which was again confirmed in a number of experiments. Compound 3 was significantly less potent than compound 2, which suggested that the latter might not interact solely after conversion to the dialdehyde 1, but rather that the sulphonate functions might also participate in the process.

In order to follow up this idea further, compound 4 was also prepared by Dr Wilkinson:

4

and was tested in the presence of metabisulphite relative to the appropriate control. At a concentration of 2.5 mmol dm^{-3} it caused a right shift of 2.5 ± 0.2 kPa and was therefore significantly more potent than either of the other compounds or, indeed, than DPG itself. The most straightforward way of accounting for this behaviour is to assume that the sulphonate function does indeed participate, because it is not easy to explain why compound 4 should be more potent than compound 3 if it works only by formation of the latter compound.

In summary, therefore, at this stage of the work, a general type of compound has been designed to fit the DPG site. Its structure has been modified to promote solubility and improve receptor interaction, leading to compound 3, which can form Schiff bases at two points and has a side-chain available to form salt bridges or hydrogen bonds to the receptor. This is active but less so than compound 2, which can also interact covalently at the same two sites, but has a greater capacity for salt bridges and hydrogen bond formation. Finally compound 4 combines all the chemical functions and, as might be expected, this is the most potent oxygen-liberating compound of those described.

CONCLUSIONS

The ultimate objective of the present study was to devise and implement a rational procedure for designing drugs, and the general approach has been to combine different methods into a unified strategy. I have been extremely fortunate to work with a group of colleagues whose range of skills has facilitated interdisciplinary liaison, and I am particularly indebted to those who are acknowledged below. The work would not have been possible without their joint contribution, and any credit will be theirs if the final outcome is at all successful.

It must be borne in mind that society today is setting very high standards before it is prepared to accept any new therapeutic agent. Compounds such as aspirin or digoxin, which have relieved the pain or prolonged the life of millions of people in the past, would no longer be acceptable if they were recent discoveries, because much higher safety margins would now be required. The rate of discovery of acceptable new drugs has inevitably fallen, and it may be many years before the present approach leads to a significant therapeutic advance, if it ever does. Nevertheless it is my belief that a combination of rational and traditional methods into a unified strategy offers the best hope of satisfying today's stringent requirements. Four general aspects need to be considered.

First, it is necessary to choose a physiologically important process, and interpret its properties in order to establish how they may be exploited therapeutically. In the present case we have chosen to study the delivery of oxygen to the tissues, and have focused attention on the haemoglobin molecule. It is plausible to suggest that an ability to control the oxygen affinity of haemoglobin might well yield therapeutic benefits in one situation or another. Moreover, the physiology and biochemistry of haemoglobin have been extensively studied, and provide a background to the central problem of designing new drugs. The importance of this background is well demonstrated by the emphasis of the present chapter, in which one of the main sections is devoted entirely to the normal physiology, structure and function of haemoglobin. The final objective is to cure disease, but the emphasis is placed originally on understanding the normal healthy state.

Second, it is necessary to find a compound which acts on the chosen process to produce the desired effect. A traditional way of doing this has been to study as many compounds as possible, using a cheap, simple biological test. Another traditional method has been to study compounds which are structurally related to a natural hormone or regulator. However, neither of these approaches has been used in the present work. Instead we have adopted the novel method of receptor fit which yielded a compound having the desired properties.

Third, we have used a mixture of methods in order to devise related compounds for testing. This stage could be described as a logical extension of the receptor fit approach, or an empirical application of PAR methodology, or a use of traditional screening. It is in fact a combination of methods into a unified strategy, and I believe that this is the most worthwhile policy to adopt after finding the starting compound.

It must be emphasised that none of the observations so far prove that the present approach has worked as intended. Nevertheless the results have been sufficiently encouraging for us to proceed to the fourth stage of the strategy, in which a new generation of compounds are to be designed. The initial bibenzyl compounds were chosen to fit a receptor site as it exists in solid haemoglobin crystals, and this is therefore the most appropriate environment for testing the accuracy of the forecasts. We have already succeeded in crystallising deoxyhaemoglobin from a solution containing one of the bibenzyl compounds, and low-resolution X-ray photographs show differences from the native crystals which suggest that the compound is indeed binding to the protein. We intend to carry out a full structural analysis as soon as facilities for high-resolution X-ray crystallography are available, and this should enable us to design better second-generation compounds.

Attention must now be drawn to the fact that the method becomes self-correcting at this stage. It is of course highly improbable that the forecast modes of binding are correct in every respect. Some functional groups on the compound may not take part in the binding process at all. The receptor may also be distorted by the compound so that it takes up a different conformation from that of the native protein, but as long as one of the first-generation compounds can be studied at its site by X-ray crystallography, any error in the original forecasts can be observed. The second-generation compounds can then be designed to take account of this, each functional group being tailored to the receptor site after allowing for any receptor-distortion which may be revealed by the first-generation compounds.

The role of nuclear magnetic resonance (NMR) in the drug design process should now be considered briefly. Once an active compound has been found, then NMR methods should throw light on the drug-receptor interaction. This will be of value at stage three of the strategy, when a small group of compounds are being designed around the first active molecule. It will also provide a check on any differences between binding to the solid protein crystal and binding in solution, and will therefore complement the X-ray studies. However, it is not yet easy to envisage how the NMR technique could be used to design the starting compound in a series without prior information about the structure of potential receptor sites.

One other aspect of the stage-four strategy should be mentioned. Different compounds may produce qualitatively different results. In the case of the DPG – haemoglobin interaction this is shown by studying the shape of the dissociation curves, which show less sigmoidicity in the presence of some bibenzyl compounds. It is both desirable and feasible at stage four to relate these qualitative differences in biological effect to differences in the mode of binding, and this also provides information for designing second-generation compounds.

There is a natural temptation to withhold publication of the present study until the details of binding have been fully established. However, the work on haemoglobin should be regarded as a trial run, and although some of the present arguments may eventually be justified, others will certainly have been misconceived. The main interest will then lie in comparing the different lines of approach. For instance, it is tacitly assumed in the present work that the receptor site is undistorted by the bibenzyl compounds from its conformation in native deoxyhaemoglobin. On the other hand, Arnone (1972) has evidence suggesting that DPG does in fact distort the site, and it is not unlikely that we might have found more potent compounds by modelling to the distorted structure. In order to prevent any possible confusion at a later date as to the exact way in which the first-generation compounds were designed, it is essential at the start of the exercise to write out a full description of all the logical steps. This is not difficult in the present case, because we have always chosen the simplest and most straightforward option whenever a decision had to be made. It will be interesting to find out how often we were justified in doing so, if at all.

ACKNOWLEDGEMENTS

I am deeply indebted to my colleagues at the Wellcome Research Laboratories, including C. R. Beddell, P. A. M. Eagles, A. Ferrige, G. C. Lees, S. Mahmood, M. Norman, F. E. Norrington, K. D. Patel, R. A. Paterson, E. Rahr, V. S. Rose, G. C. Sheppey, C. Vaughan, S. Wilkinson, R. Wootton, R. Wrigglesworth and D. A. B. Young, and also to Dr F. Brown, Professor R. D. Cohen and Dr M. F. Perutz.

REFERENCES

Adair, G. S., Barcroft, J. and Bock, A. V. (1921). *J. Physiol.*, **55**, 332
Allen, D. W., Guthe, K. F. and Wyman, J. Jr. (1950). *J. Biol. Chem.*, **187**, 393
Arnone, A. (1972). *Nature (London)*, **237**, 146
Barcroft, J. and Haldane, J. S. (1902). *J. Physiol.*, **28**, 232
Barcroft, J. and Roberts, Ff. (1909). *J. Physiol.*, **39**, 143
Beddell, C. R., Goodford, P. J., Norrington, F. E., Wilkinson, S. and Wootton, R. (1976). *Br. J. Pharmacol.*, **57**, 201
Benesch, R., Benesch, R. E. and Yu, C. I. (1968). *Proc. Nat. Acad. Sci. U.S.A.*, **59**, 526
Bohr, C. (1909). *Nagels Handbuch*, Vol. 1, p. 73
Bragg, W. L. (1913). *Proc. R. Soc. London A*, **89**, 248
Chanutin, A. and Curnish, R. R. (1967). *Arch. Biochem. Biophys.*, **121**, 96

Douglas, C. G., Haldane, J. S. and Haldane, J. B. S. (1912). *J. Physiol.*, **44**, 275
Drabkin, D. L. (1946). *J. Biol. Chem.*, **164**, 703
Good, N. E., Winget, G. D., Winter, W., Connolly, T. N., Izawa, S. and Singh, R. M. M. (1966). *Biochemistry*, **5**, 467
Goodford, P. J. (1973). *Adv. Pharmacol. Chemother.*, **11**, 51
Greenwald, I. (1925). *J. Biol. Chem.*, **63**, 339
Guldberg, C. M. and Waage, P. (1864). *Les Mondes*, **5**, 107
Jeffrey, G. A. (1946). *Proc. R. Soc. London A*, 1946-47, **188**, 222
Kendrew, J. C., Watson, H. C., Strandberg, B. E., Dickerson, R. E., Phillips, D. C. and Shore, V. C. (1961). *Nature (London)*, **190**, 666
Langley, J. N. (1878). *J. Physiol.*, **1**, 339
Langley, J. N. (1905). *J. Physiol.*, **33**, 374
Matsuda, G., Gehring-Müller, R. and Braunitzer, G. (1963). *Biochem. Z.*, **338**, 669
Norrington, F. E. (1974). *Lab. Pract.*, April, 191
Ostwald, W. (1908). *Z. Chem. Ind. Koll.*, **11**, 264
Paterson, R. A., Eagles, P. A. M., Young, D. A. B. and Beddell, C. R. (1976). *Int. J. Biochem.*, **7**, 117
Perutz, M. F., Muirhead, H., Cox, J. M. Goaman, L. C. G., Mathews, F. S., McGandy, E. L. and Webb, L. E. (1968). *Nature (London)*, **219**, 29
Rapoport, S. and Guest, G. M. (1941). *J. Biol. Chem.*, **138**, 269
Robertson, J. M. (1934). *Proc. R. Soc. London A*, **146**, 473
Roughton, F. J. W. (1949). *Obituary Notices of Fellows of the Royal Society*, **6**, 315
Sheppard, W. A. and Bourns, A. N. (1954). *Can. J. Chem.*, **32**, 4
van Slyke, D. D. and Neill, J. M. (1924). *J. Biol. Chem.*, **61**, 523
Stamatoyannopoulos, G. (1972). *Ann. Rev. Genet.*, **6**, 47
Sugita, Y. and Chanutin, A. (1963). *Proc. Soc. Exp. Biol. Med.*, **112**, 72
Williams, R. C. Jr. and Tsay, K-Y. (1973). *Anal. Biochem.*, **54**, 137

7
Substrate and inhibitor binding to dihydrofolate reductase

G. C. K. Roberts (Division of Molecular Pharmacology, National Institute for Medical Research, Mill Hill, London, UK)

INTRODUCTION

Dihydrofolate reductase (5, 6, 7, 8-tetrahydrofolate:NADP⁺ oxidoreductase, E.C.1.5.1.3), an enzyme found in the vast majority of both prokaryotic and eukaryotic organisms, catalyses the reduction of dihydrofolate to tetrahydrofolate, using NADPH as coenzyme:

7, 8-dihydrofolate + NADPH + H⁺ ⇌ 5, 6, 7, 8-tetrahydrofolate + NADP⁺

The product of this reaction, tetrahydrofolate, plays a vital role in intermediary metabolism, acting as a 'carrier' of one-carbon fragments in the biosynthesis of a number of amino acids, thymidylate and purines (for a review, see Blakley, 1969). In most of these one-carbon transfer reactions, the folate coenzyme remains at the tetrahydro oxidation level, but in the reaction catalysed by thymidylate synthetase,

dUMP + 5, 10-methylene-tetrahydrofolate ⇌ dTMP + dihydrofolate

the product is dihydrofolate. This must then be reduced by dihydrofolate reductase in order to maintain the cellular pool of tetrahydrofolate derivatives (Fig. 7.1). In the absence of a functional dihydrofolate reductase, this pool will rapidly

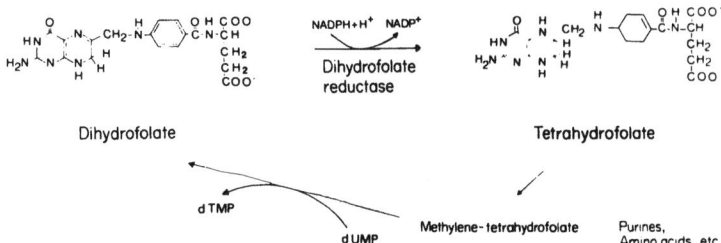

Figure 7.1 The reaction catalysed by dihydrofolate reductase, and its metabolic relationship to that catalysed by thymidylate synthetase

become depleted, leading to a deficiency of purines and of thymidylate and thus to a disruption of nucleic acid synthesis.

The first drug which acts by inhibiting dihydrofolate reductase, aminopterin, was synthesised 30 years ago (Seeger, Smith and Hultquist, 1947) as an antimetabolite of folic acid, whose structure had recently been established, and was soon found to be beneficial in some cases of leukaemia (Farber *et al.*, 1948). Shortly thereafter, Nichol and Welch (1950) showed that aminopterin inhibited the conversion of folic acid to 'citrovorum factor' (5-formyltetrahydrofolate), and on the identification and partial purification of dihydrofolate reductase, aminopterin and related compounds were found to be powerful inhibitors of this enzyme (Futterman, 1957; Osborn, Freeman and Huennekens, 1958; Zakrzewski and Nichol, 1958). Since that time, a vast number of inhibitors of dihydrofolate reductase have been synthesised, and a number of them have found clinical application, notably in the treatment of malaria (pyrimethamine), bacterial infections (trimethoprim) and some neoplastic diseases (methotrexate). The available evidence indicates that in all cases the major effect of these 'anti-folate' drugs is to inhibit dihydrofolate reductase (see Blakley, 1969; Bertino, 1971).

This therefore represents one of the simplest kinds of drug action, in which the drugs are relatively straightforward structural analogues of the natural substrate, and appear to act by simple competitive inhibition. Since dihydrofolate reductase is a soluble enzyme, and the bacterial and mammalian enzymes are monomeric proteins of moderate molecular weight (16 000 – 40 000), this is a system in which one might expect to be able, with presently available techniques, to obtain a good deal of information on the binding of substrates and inhibitors. Although the inhibition of the enzyme by the 'anti-folate' drugs has been studied extensively for many years, it is only in the last five years or so that pure dihydrofolate reductase has become available in sufficient quantity to permit the kind of systematic structural and spectroscopic studies which are capable of providing a description of ligand binding in molecular detail. At this point it is useful to survey briefly the salient features of the structure – activity relationships in this system, to bring out those questions for which we seek answers in molecular terms.

Structure – Activity Relationships

The central role of 2,4-diamino substitution

The natural substrate of the enzyme dihydrofolate is a 2-amino-4-keto-substituted pteridine. Known inhibitors of dihydrofolate reductase include, as well as close structural analogues of the substrate such as methotrexate and aminopterin, pteridines (triamterine), quinazolines (methasquin), pyridopyrimidines, triazines (cycloguanil triazine, the active metabolite of paludrine) and pyrimidines (pyrimethamine, trimethoprim); these structures are illustrated in Fig. 7.2. The essential structural fragment is apparently a 2,4-diaminopyrimidine ring (in which the 5- or, more rarely, the 6-carbon can be replaced by a nitrogen; Fig. 7.3). The vital role of 2,4-diamino substitution is dramatically illustrated by

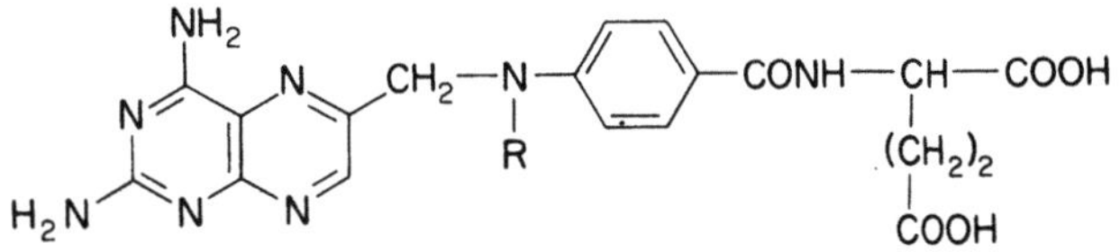

R = H aminopterin
R = CH_3 methotrexate

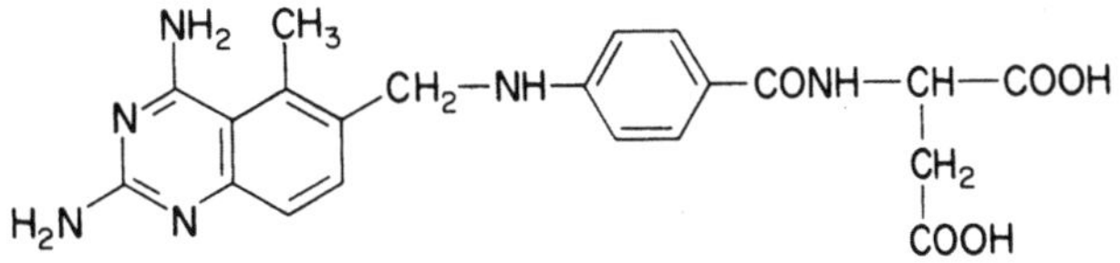

methasquin

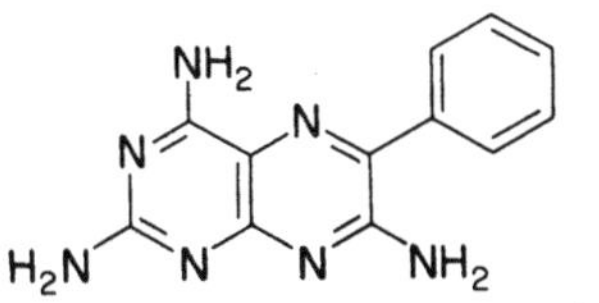

triamterine

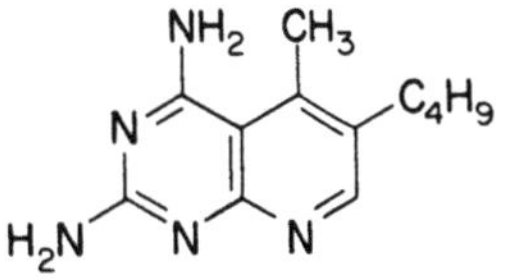

2,4-diamino-5-methyl-6-butyl-pyrido[2,3-*d*]pyrimidine

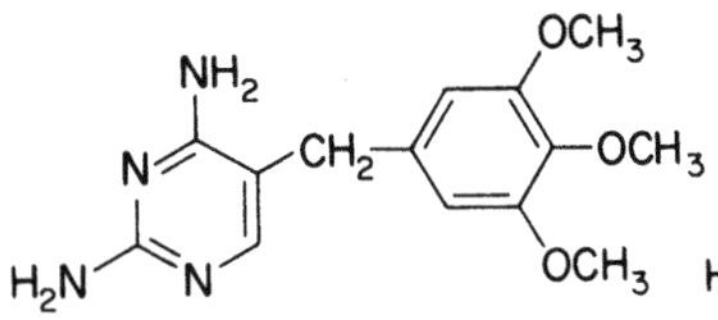

trimethoprim

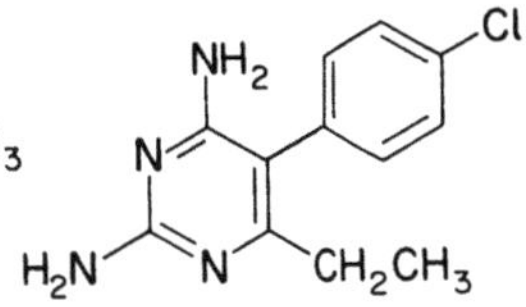

pyrimethamine

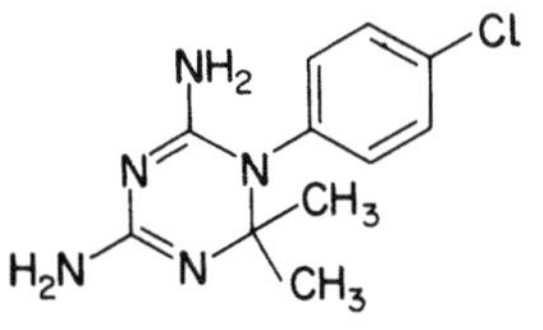

chlorguanide triazine

Figure 7.2 The structures of some powerful inhibitors of dihydrofolate reductase

a comparison of folate and aminopterin. The latter differs from folate, a substrate, only in the replacement of the 4-keto group by a 4-amino group, yet it is not a substrate, and binds to dihydrofolate reductase from various sources some 10 000 - 50 000-fold (6 - 8 kcal/mol) more tightly than does folate (cf. Blakley, 1969).

Two contrasting hypotheses have been advanced to explain this substantial effect of the 4-amino group on binding to the enzyme. Zakrzewski (1963) has proposed that folate and related compounds, which exist in solution as the 4-keto (imido) tautomer, bind to the enzyme in the enol form, the 4-hydroxy group acting as hydrogen-bond donor. The weaker binding of these compounds simply reflects, on this hypothesis, the low population in solution of that form of the ligand which binds to the enzyme, while compounds such as aminopterin always have a hydrogen-bond donor at the 4-position. Though this hypothesis can perhaps be questioned on evolutionary grounds, there is at present no evidence concerning the tautomeric form of folate when bound to the enzyme. Baker (1959, 1967) and Pullman (Perault and Pullman, 1961; Collin and Pullman, 1964) have drawn attention to the marked increase in basicity at N_1 which accompanies the replacement of the 4-keto group by an amino group. Baker (1959, 1967) has further proposed that the 2,4-diamino compounds bind to the enzyme in the protonated form and that their tighter binding can be explained by an additional coulombic interaction which is not possible for folate. The ultraviolet difference spectrum generated on the binding of methotrexate to the enzyme bears a general similarity to that generated by protonation of free methotrexate (Erickson and Mathews, 1972; Poe et al., 1974, 1975; K. Hood, G. C. K. Roberts and A. S. V. Burgen, unpublished work), and a detailed analysis

Table 7.1 Effects of 5 and 6-substitution on the activity of 2,4-diamino- and 2-amino-4-keto-pyrimidines as inhibitors of pigeon liver dihydrofolate reductase

R_1	R_2	K_i^a (μM) X = O	K_i^a (μM) X = NH_2	$\dfrac{K_i(X = O)}{K_i(X = NH_2)}$
CH_3	H	3 800	220	17.3
CH_3	n-C_4H_9	52	0.4	130
CH_3	C_4-ϕ	6	0.005	1 200
CH_3	C_3-$NH\phi$	63	0.024	2 625
NH_2	H	2 600	240	10.8
NH_2	n-C_4H_9	8	4.6	1.7
NH_2	C_4-ϕ	1.7	0.7	2.4
CH_2-ϕ	C_4-ϕ	10	0.03	333
n-C_3H_7	C_4-ϕ	150	0.003	50 000

[a]Approximate K_i values, calculated from data reviewed by Baker (1967).

of the difference spectra confirms that methotrexate and trimethoprim do bind to the enzyme preferentially in the protonated form (K. Hood, G. C. K. Roberts, A. S. V. Burgen, unpublished work). As yet, however, no quantitative estimate of the difference in binding energy between the protonated and unprotonated forms of the inhibitors is available. It would be surprising if a single additional coulombic interaction alone could account for the 6 - 8 kcal/mol difference in binding energy between methotrexate and folate.

Both these hypotheses are essentially 'static' ones, in that they envisage the substrates and inhibitors fitting, with varying affinities, in the same orientation into a rigid binding site. However, a detailed examination of the structure - activity relationships, notably in the large series of pyrimidines and triazines studied by Baker and his colleagues (reviewed by Baker, 1967), suggests that the real situation is more complex. As shown in Table 7.1, alkyl and aralkyl substitution at the 5- and/or 6-positions of the pyrimidine ring not only radically affects the affinity of these compounds for the enzyme, but also leads to a variation of several hundredfold in the *relative* affinities of the 4-amino and 4-keto compounds. This clearly implies that the alkyl or aralkyl substituents interact with the enzyme in a significantly different way in the two series of compounds, indicating, in turn, a difference in orientation within the binding site or a difference in conformation of the complex. It is clear that, as yet, there is no wholly satisfactory explanation of the origin of the tight binding of the 2,4-diamino-substituted compounds.

Selectivity

Since a functional dihydrofolate reductase is apparently essential for all cells, the therapeutic effectiveness of inhibitors of the enzyme must depend on their ability to distinguish in their effects between different cell types. This selectivity, and the related phenomenon of acquired resistance, which is also of considerable therapeutic importance, can arise in a number of ways, many of which are reviewed in Mihich (1973). Sensitive and resistant cells may differ in the rate and/or extent of uptake of the drug (see, for example, Goldman, 1971; Harrap *et al.*, 1971; Hutchison, 1971), in its metabolism (Johns *et al.*, 1966; Johns and Valerino, 1971), in the level of dihydrofolate reductase in the cell (Hakala, Zakrzewski and Nichol, 1961; Ferone, O'Shea and Yoeli, 1970; Huchison, 1971) or in the inhibitor-binding characteristics of the enzyme.

It is this last finding, that therapeutically exploitable differences in inhibitor binding to dihydrofolate reductase from different species do exist, which has led to much of the success of 'anti-folate' drugs in chemotherapy. The classic example of this is trimethoprim, whose usefulness as an antibacterial agent arises from its substantially (30 000-fold) greater affinity for bacterial than for mammalian dihydrofolate reductase. A comparison of the effects of a number of inhibitors on the bacterial and mammalian enzymes (Burchall and Hitchings, 1965; Burchall, 1971) is presented in Table 7.2. The effectiveness of pyrimethamine as an anti-malarial similarly depends on the fact that it is some four orders of magnitude more powerful an inhibitor of *Plasmodium berghei* dihydrofolate

Table 7.2 Effects of dihydrofolate reductase inhibitors on the mammalian and bacterial enzymes. (Data from Burchall and Hitchings, 1965, and Burchall, 1971)

Compound number	Concentration (10^{-8} M) for 50% inhibition of enzyme from				
	Human liver	Rat liver	E. coli	S. aureus	P. vulgaris
1	9	9	0.6	0.1	0.5
2	30 000	26 000	0.5	1.5	0.4
3	180	70	2500	300	1500
4	55	14	65 000	50 000	100 000
5	95	46	50	4	50
6	24	26	2	7	1

Compounds
1: Methotrexate
2: Trimethoprim
3: Pyrimethamine (I_{50} for *Plasmodium berghei* enzyme = 5 × 10^{-10} M; Ferone *et al.*, 1969)
4: 1-(*p*-butylphenyl)-2,2-dihydro-2,2-dimethyl-4,6-diamino-s-triazine
5: 2,4-diamino-6-butylpyrido (2,3-*d*) pyrimidine
6: 2,4-diamino-5-methyl-6-butylpyrido (2,3-*d*) pyrimidine

reductase than of the human enzyme (Ferone *et al.*, 1969).

As can be seen from Table 7.2, methotrexate (compound 1) shows considerably less selectivity than do the pyrimidine and other 'small molecule' inhibitors. Close structural analogues of the substrate would be expected to have less discriminatory power than compounds which can exploit small differences in the topography of the protein immediately outside the essential substrate site (Hitchings *et al.*, 1952; Hitchings and Burchall, 1965; Baker, 1967). An indication of the relative positions of the ligand groupings conferring selectivity, as deduced from the extensive studies of Hitchings and his colleagues, is given in Fig. 7.3. All the information we have at present on the structural basis of selectivity has come from 'classical' structure-activity studies, but this is clearly an area in which a detailed knowledge of the protein structure around the binding site could be exploited in the design of new compounds.

Lactobacillus casei Dihydrofolate Reductase

A complete understanding at the molecular level of the action of the 'anti-folate' drugs will clearly require studies of the enzyme from a number of species. We chose to begin by making a detailed examination of the enzyme from a single source, and since the methods, such as X-ray crystallography and nuclear magnetic resonance (NMR) spectroscopy, which have the power to give information in the necessary kind of molecular detail require relatively large amounts of material, a bacterial source was indicated. In common with many other resistant cell lines (see Blakley, 1969; Mihich, 1973), the methotrexate-resistant strain of *Lactobacillus casei* we have used has greatly elevated levels of dihydrofolate reductase, so that the enzyme is available in gram quantities. The dihydrofolate reductase of

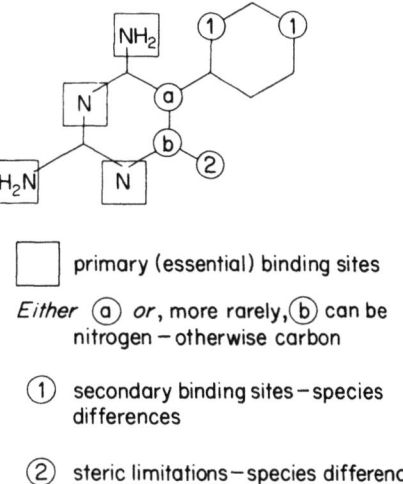

Figure 7.3 A schematic indication of the essential (primary) and species-specific (secondary) binding groups on dihydrofolate reductase inhibitors. Redrawn from Hitchings and Burchall (1965)

L. casei consists of a single polypeptide chain, of molecular weight 18 000, with no disulphide bonds (Dann *et al.*, 1976). The study of this enzyme is still at an early stage; the amino acid sequence is being determined by H. R. Morris and K. Batley (London), while crystallographic studies have been begun by W. D. Mercer and A. C. T. North (Leeds). In the present paper, which is essentially a progress report, we shall consider first some of the general features of substrate and inhibitor binding, and then attempt to relate these to the structural information obtained by NMR spectroscopy. Coenzyme binding is discussed elsewhere (Roberts *et al.*, 1974; Way *et al.*, 1975; Feeney *et al.*, 1975; Birdsall *et al.*, 1977a).

CO-OPERATIVE BINDING OF LIGANDS TO DIHYDROFOLATE REDUCTASE

The equilibrium constants for the formation of the binary complexes between *L. casei* dihydrofolate reductase and some substrates and inhibitors are listed in Table 7.3. Methotrexate binds some 20 000-fold (5.8 kcal/mol) more tightly to the enzyme than does folate — indeed even trimethoprim binds a hundredfold more tightly.

As a part of any detailed analysis of the structure – activity relationships (which in this simple system amount to structure – binding constant relationships), we need to assess the contributions of the various parts of the ligand molecules to the overall binding energy. The importance of the 2,4-diaminopyrimidine moiety has been discussed in general terms above; a number of experiments have indicated that the *p*-aminobenzoyl-L-glutamate moiety also contributes signifi-

Table 7.3 Equilibrium constants for the formation of binary complexes between *L. casei* dihydrofolate reductase and substrates, inhibitors and coenzymes (Dann et al., 1976)

	$K_a (M^{-1})$
Dihydrofolate	2×10^6
Folate	5×10^4
Methotrexate	$\sim 10^9$
Trimethoprim	3×10^6
NADPH	1×10^8
NADP$^+$	2×10^5

cantly to methotrexate binding (Baker et al., 1964, 1966; Greenberg et al., 1966; Plante, Crawford and Friedkin, 1967; Chaykovsky et al., 1974) while the pyrazine ring *probably* makes only a minor contribution (Baker, 1967). We have therefore studied the binding of 2,4-diaminopyrimidine and *p*-aminobenzoyl-L-glutamate (Fig. 7.4) to *L. casei* dihydrofolate reductase. Under conditions where the binding constant of methotrexate is approximately 10^9 M^{-1} ($\Delta F = -11.6$ kcal/mol), the binding constant of 2,4-diaminopyrimidine is 8×10^3 M^{-1} (-5.0 kcal/mol) and that of *p*-aminobenzoyl-L-glutamate is 1×10^3 M^{-1} (-3.9 kcal/mol) (Roberts et al., 1974, Birdsall et al., 1977b). It is clear that simple addition of the binding energies of these two 'fragments' does not reproduce the total binding energy of the methotrexate molecule. A number of difficulties in attempts of this sort to 'partition' the binding energy of a ligand to a protein are well known. First, the comparison is clearly *only* valid if the 'fragments' bind to the enzyme in the same way as the corresponding parts of the whole ligand; this can *not* be judged from

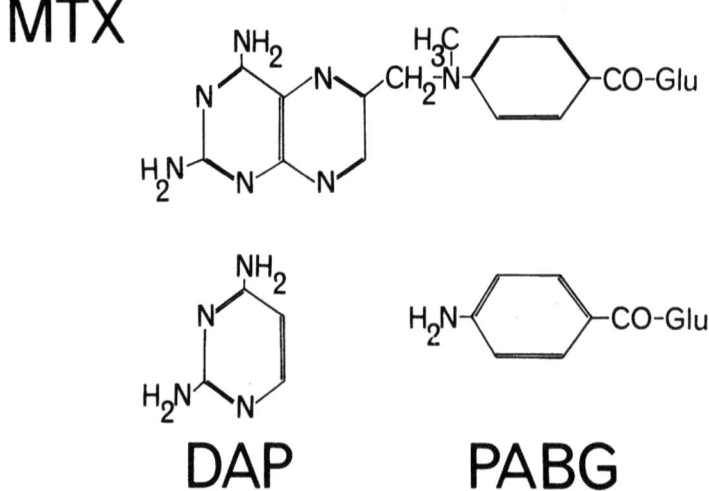

Figure 7.4 The structures of methotrexate (MTX) and its 'fragments' 2,4-diaminopyrimidine (DAP) and *p*-aminobenzoyl-L-glutamate (PABG)

the binding constants alone, but in the present case the NMR evidence, discussed below, suggests that it is probably true. Second, the entropic contributions (both translational and internal) to the binding energies are clearly not the same for the binding of two 'fragments' as for the binding of the whole ligand, and a complete accounting of the different entropic contributions is usually extremely difficult (as discussed by, for example, Jencks, 1975).

In the present case, however, a major contribution to the apparent non-additivity of free energies comes from an effect which is less usually considered. Not only can 2,4-diaminopyrimidine and p-aminobenzoyl-L-glutamate bind simultaneously to the enzyme, as would be expected, but they also bind *co-operatively*, in the sense that p-aminobenzoyl-L-glutamate binds some 25-fold more tightly to the enzyme – 2,4-diaminopyrimidine complex than to the enzyme alone. The binding scheme and equilibrium constants are shown in Fig. 7.5. These binding constants were obtained by NMR and are of limited precision; experiments designed to obtain the more precise values required for a proper thermodynamic analysis are in progress (J. F. Rodriguez de Miranda, B. Birdsall, A. S. V. Burgen and G. C. K. Roberts, unpublished work). Preliminary results

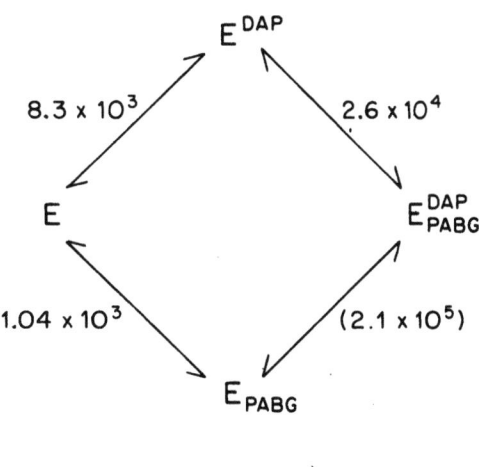

Figure 7.5 Binding constants (M^{-1}) for 2,4-diaminopyrimidine (DAP) and p-aminobenzoyl-L-glutamate(PABG) binding – separately and together – to *L. casei* dihydrofolate reductase. The 'free energy of cooperativity', ΔF_{xy} (cf. Weber, 1975) is defined by

$$\Delta F_{xy} = \Delta F(E \rightarrow E^{DAP}) - \Delta F(E_{PABG} \rightarrow E^{DAP}_{PABG})$$

$$= \Delta F(E \rightarrow E_{PABG}) - \Delta F(E^{DAP} \rightarrow E^{DAP}_{PABG})$$

The binding constant given in parentheses could not be measured directly, but was calculated from the other three values

indicate that co-operative binding can be observed for a number of ligands related to the 'fragments' shown in Fig. 7.4, but that the *degree* of co-operativity is a rather sensitive function of the structure of the ligands.

The equilibrium constants given in Fig. 7.5 show that the additional free energy change associated with the co-operative binding of p-aminobenzoyl-L-glutamate and 2,4-diaminopyrimidine is approximately -1.8 kcal/mol. That is, the overall free energy change accompanying the formation of the ternary enzyme - 2,4-diaminopyrimidine - p-aminobenzoyl-L-glutamate complex is more negative by 1.8 kcal/mol than the sum of the free energies of formation of the two binary complexes. While this energy difference is relatively small, it is comparable to those observed in other, better known, co-operative systems (such as oxygen and diphosphoglycerate binding to haemoglobin; for a discussion of the magnitudes of these free energy differences, see Weber, 1975). The degree of co-operativity which it implies can be illustrated by the fact that, at ligand concentrations sufficient to saturate 50 per cent of the enzyme molecules with each ligand, 80 per cent of the enzyme molecules which have *any* ligand bound will have *both* ligands bound.

If we now compare the *overall* free energy change for the formation of the enzyme - 2,4-diaminopyrimidine - p-aminobenzoyl-L-glutamate complex (-10.7 kcal/mol) with that for the formation of the enzyme - methotrexate complex (~ -11.6 kcal/mol), we see that they are within 1 kcal/mol of each other — though once again uncertainties in the treatment of the entropic contributions prevent a rigorous comparison. What is the origin of this co-operativity in binding? The two obvious possibilities are a direct interaction between the two bound ligands, or an effect transmitted by a conformational change in the protein. At present we cannot distinguish unequivocally between these two explanations, though the NMR evidence clearly favours the conformational one. While the existence of this co-operativity makes it more difficult to 'partition' the ligand binding energy, it does provide a valuable approach to the understanding of the molecular mechanism of methotrexate binding.

In addition to the co-operativity between parts of the methotrexate molecule, a similar co-operativity in binding between substrates or inhibitors and coenzyme has been noted for dihydrofolate reductase from a number of sources (Perkins and Bertino, 1966; Poe *et al.*, 1974; Greenfield, 1975; Way *et al.*, 1975). With the *L. casei* enzyme the presence of NADPH leads to increases in binding constant ranging from threefold for p-aminobenzoyl-L-glutamate to approximately 100-fold for methotrexate (Roberts *et al.*, 1974; A. S. V. Burgen and G. C. K. Roberts, unpublished work).

^{1}H NUCLEAR MAGNETIC RESONANCE STUDIES

The power of NMR spectroscopy as a tool for the study of protein - ligand interactions arises first from the fact that the spectrum contains at least one signal from each amino acid residue in the protein, and secondly from the considerable sensitivity of the spectral parameters such as chemical shift (resonance position) to molecular interactions and conformation. These two important advantages of the method bring with them corresponding disadvantages. The very richness of the spectrum means that it is usually difficult to resolve the resonances of more than a small fraction of the amino acid residues, though this problem can be partially overcome by various methods of spectral simplification, notably selective deuteration. The chemical shift of a resonance is sensitive to many features of the environment of the proton(s) from which it arises — including its proximity to charges or aromatic rings, the polarisability of its surroundings, hydrogen bonding, and so on — and consequently an *a priori* interpretation of a particular chemical shift change is rarely possible. One must rely on empirical arguments, often based on a comparison of related ligands or on extrinsic perturbations of the system (such as studies of pH-dependence).

It is useful to distinguish two general classes of effects on the NMR spectrum of the protein which can accompany ligand binding — direct effects, due to the proximity of the ligand molecule to the proton whose resonance is being observed, and effects on residues more distant from the binding site whose environment is altered as a result of a ligand-induced conformational change in the protein. In special cases one can distinguish between these effects by the use of paramagnetic ligands, or by intermolecular nuclear Overhauser effects, but no *general* method for making the distinction exists. In the present work we have relied on a comparison of the effects of related ligands for a tentative identification of 'direct' effects.

Thus, in the absence of a crystal structure for the protein, there are considerable limitations on the kind of structural information which can be obtained by NMR spectroscopy. However, valuable *comparative* information is more readily available. Thus, in the case of dihydrofolate reductase (1) studies of different ligands and of 'fragments' of the ligands should allow us to establish which residue is affected by which structural feature of the ligand, and to say tentatively whether this is a direct effect; (2) in examining the binding of 'fragments' of the inhibitors, we can look for structural counterparts of the co-operative binding discussed above; and (3) a particularly important comparison is clearly that of 2,4-diamino- and 2-amino-4-keto-substituted compounds, i.e. of substrates and inhibitors.

To be meaningful, such comparisons must be based on studies of the resonances of individual amino acid residues. At present, we have been able to resolve individual resonances for approximately 20 residues; the present discussion will be limited to those we have studied in most detail, the six histidine and five tyrosine residues.

Histidine Residues

The resonances of the C2 protons of the imidazole ring of histidine residues can usually be resolved in the ^{1}H NMR spectra of proteins. The chemical shifts of these resonances are dependent on the charge state of the imidazole ring, and thus provide a convenient method for determining the pK of *individual* histidine residues

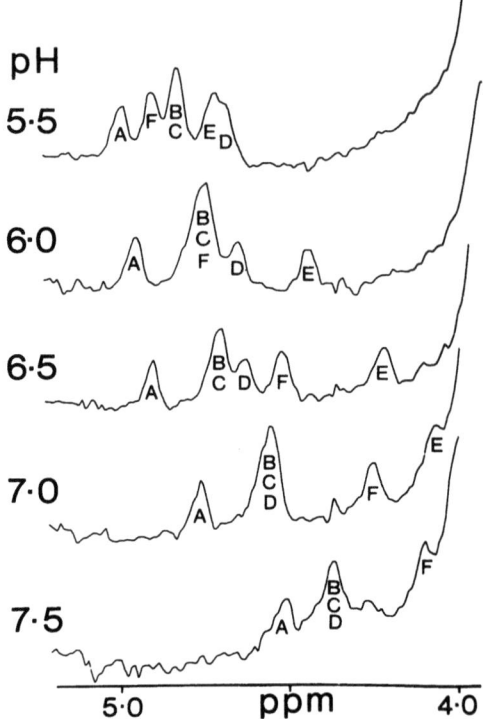

Figure 7.6 The histidine C2-H resonances in the 100 MHz ^{1}H NMR spectra of the *L. casei* dihydrofolate reductase – trimethoprim complex at various pH* values. Chemical shifts in p.p.m. from dioxan

in proteins and their complexes with ligands. As an example, Fig. 7.6 shows the histidine C2-H resonances in the dihydrofolate reductase – trimethoprim complex at various pH* values. (pH* = pH meter reading in D_2O without correction for the isotope effect on the glass electrode.) The six histidine residues give rise to five separate C2-H resonances, whose pH-dependence allows us to construct titration curves for the six histidine residues (Fig. 7.7). (In the absence of assignments to particular residues in the sequence, the six histidine residues are labelled $H_A - H_F$.)

In the absence of ligands, the six histidines of dihydrofolate reductase give rise to only three distinct titration curves, corresponding to residues $H_A + H_B + H_C$ (pK† ~ 7.5), residue H_D (pK† ~ 7.7) and residues $H_E + H_F$ (pK = 6.54). A comparison of the titration curves of the free enzyme and of the enzyme – trimethoprim complex (Roberts *et al.*, 1974; Birdsall *et al.*, 1977b) shows that two of the six histidine residues are affected by trimethoprim binding. In order to establish

†As the enzyme is unstable at pH > 7.5, complete titration curves cannot be obtained for these residues, and these pK values are estimates, subject to an error of up to ± 0.2 units.

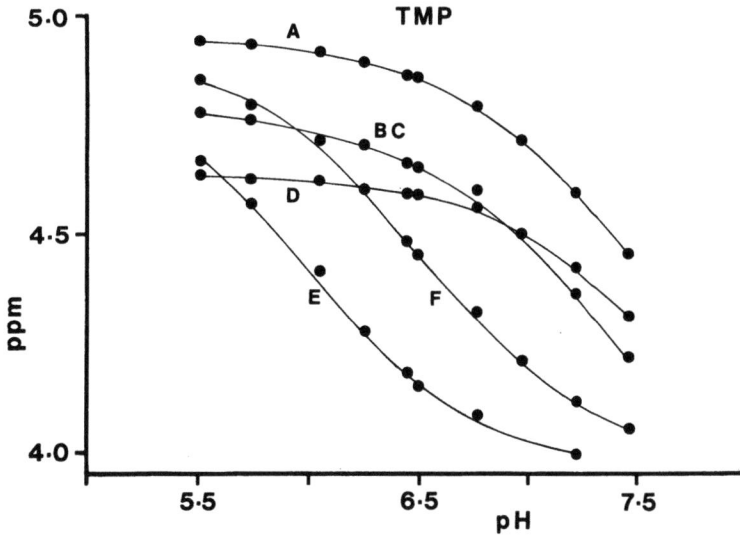

Figure 7.7 Titration curves for the six histidine residues of *L. casei* dihydrofolate reductase in its complex with trimethoprim

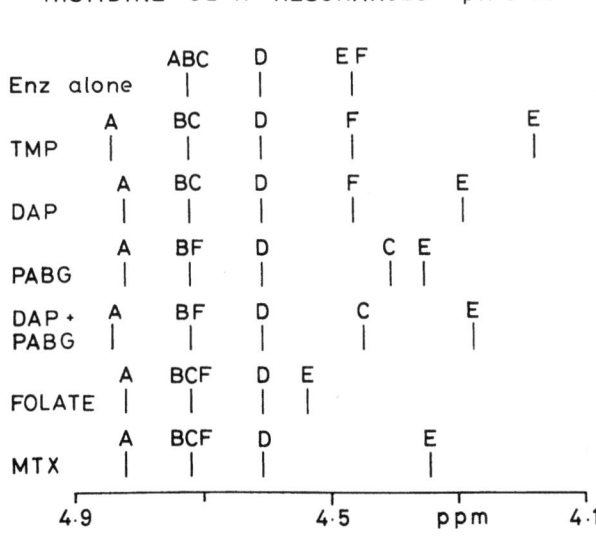

Figure 7.8 A schematic indication of the positions (at pH* 6.50) of the six histidine C2-H resonances of *L. casei* dihydrofolate reductase, alone and in its complexes with substrates and inhibitors. (TMP = trimethoprim; MTX = methotrexate; DAP = 2,4-diaminopyrimidine; PAGB = p-aminobenzoyl-L-glutamate)

which two residues these are, it is necessary to connect the resonances in the spectrum of the free enzyme with those in the spectrum of the complex. Since trimethoprim binds tightly to the enzyme ($K_a = 3 \times 10^6$ M^{-1}; Dann et al., 1976), exchange between the bound and free states is slow on the NMR time scale, and the connection cannot be made directly. However, for 2,4-diaminopyrimidine, a 'fragment' of trimethoprim which binds more weakly, the connection can readily be made, and since the effects of trimethoprim and 2,4-diaminopyrimidine on the histidine residues are closely similar (see below), we can conclude that the resonance assignments in the two complexes are the same. By similar procedures, we have analysed the histidine titration curves of dihydrofolate reductase in its complexes with a variety of substrates and inhibitors. The results of these experiments are summarised in Fig. 7.8 (which shows diagrammatically the resonance positions in the various complexes at pH*6.50) and in Table 7.4; details are given by Birdsall et al. (1977b).

Two (H_B and H_D) of the six histidine residues are entirely unaffected by ligand binding, though another (H_C) is affected only by p-aminobenzoyl-L-glutamate — this is discussed further below. The three 4-keto compounds examined, the substrates folate and dihydrofolate and the product analogue folinic acid, have identical effects on the histidine residues, producing a substantial increase in the pK of residue H_F, a smaller increase in that of H_E and a downfield shift of the

Table 7.4 The effects of ligands on the pK and C2-H chemical shift of the histidine residues of L. casei dihydrofolate reductase (Birdsall et al., 1976b).

Ligand	Histidine residue[a]			
	H_A $\Delta\delta$[b]	H_C $\Delta\delta$[b]	H_E ΔpK[c]	H_F ΔpK[c]
Folate Dihydrofolate Folinic acid	+0.12	0	+0.20–0.25	+ ~0.7
Methotrexate Aminopterin	+0.11	0	−0.27–0.33	+ ~0.7
Trimethoprim	+0.16	0	−0.62	0
2,4-diaminopyrimidine	+0.11	0	−0.40	0
p-aminobenzoyl-L-glutamate	+0.10	−0.60[d]	−0.26	+ ~0.7
2,4-diaminopyrimidine + p-aminobenzoyl-L-glutamate	+0.14	−0.59[d]	−0.39	+ ~0.7

[a] Residues H_B and H_D are not affected by ligand binding.
[b] Change in chemical shift of C2-H resonance of the protonated form (p.p.m.); positive shifts downfield.
[c] Increase in pK indicated by positive number.
[d] Effect due to p-aminobenzoyl-L-glutamate binding to its second site (see text)

C2-H resonance of residue H_A. Since these three compounds have the same effect on the histidine residues, it is unlikely that there is a histidine residue in close proximity to the pyrazine ring of these ligands, since a change in the reduction state of this ring would be expected to influence neighbouring residues (if only by the change in ring-current effects). Methotrexate and aminopterin affect the same three histidine residues as do the substrates, and for two of them, H_A and H_F, the effect is the same. For residue H_E, in contrast, the inhibitors produce a *decrease* in pK. Trimethoprim affects only two histidines, H_A and H_E; its effects on these two residues are similar to those of methotrexate on the one hand, and to those of 2,4-diaminopyrimidine on the other (though trimethoprim causes a rather larger decrease in the pK of H_E than do the other ligands).

In attempting to go beyond these rather general comparisons, we must first attempt to distinguish between direct and indirect effects of ligand binding on the histidine residues; this is most easily done by considering each histidine in turn. Histidine H_E shows an increase in pK of about 0.7 units on the binding of folate, dihydrofolate, folinic acid, methotrexate and aminopterin, but not with trimethoprim or 2,4-diaminopyrimidine. This suggests that the p-aminobenzoyl-L-glutamate moiety of the ligands might be responsible for this effect, and indeed p-aminobenzoyl-L-glutamate itself leads to an identical increase in pK. An increase in pK would be expected if histidine H_F interacted directly with one of the carboxylate groups of p-aminobenzoyl-L-glutamate, and the results of preliminary studies of the pH-dependence of p-aminobenzoyl-L-glutamate binding (J. F. Rodriguez de Miranda, B. Birdsall, G. C. K. Roberts, J. Feeney and A. S. V. Burgen, unpublished work) are in agreement with this idea. The effects of ligand binding on histidine H_F can thus readily be explained as a direct effect; if this explanation is correct, then the glutamate moieties of both substrates and inhibitors (as well as p-aminobenzoyl-L-glutamate itself) must bind to the enzyme in the same way.

The C2-H resonance of histidine H_A is shifted downfield by 0.10-0.16 p.p.m. on the binding of any of the ligands listed in Table 7.4. This effect can thus not be associated with any particular structural feature of the ligand — indeed coenzyme binding produces a very similar shift in this resonance (Birdsall *et al.*, 1977a). It is very difficult to explain these observations in terms of a direct effect of some group on the ligand, and an indirect effect, mediated by a conformational change common to all ligands, seems more likely.

Histidine H_E is the only one of the six histidine residues which shows a clear distinction between substrates, which cause an increase in its pK, and inhibitors, which cause a decrease. This, of course, focuses attention on the pyrimidine ring as a possible source of these effects. However, the observation that p-aminobenzoyl-L-glutamate also produces a decrease in the pK of residue H_E indicates that the effects of ligand binding on this residue are more complicated than this simple picture would suggest, and a proper understanding of the role of this histidine will require studies of a wider range of ligands. To the extent that a simple

Table 7.5 Comparison of the two binding sites for p-aminobenzoyl-L-glutamate on *L. casei* dihydrofolate reductase (data from Roberts *et al.*, 1974 and Birdsall *et al.*, 1977b)

	Site I	Site II
Binding constant (M^{-1})	1.0×10^3	34
Histidine residues affected	H_A, H_E, H_F	H_C
Change in chemical shift of aromatic protons of ligand	-0.4, -0.58	0
Competitive with methotrexate?	Yes	No
Co-operativity with 2,4-diaminopyrimidine?	Yes	No

suggest the possibility that the conformational changes induced by ligand binding may differ, in some respects, for substrates and inhibitors.

Of the ligands examined, only p-aminobenzoyl-L-glutamate has any effect on histidine H_C. This effect is in fact due to the binding of p-aminobenzoyl-L-glutamate to a second, weaker binding site, distinct from that occupied by the corresponding moiety of substrates or inhibitors such as methotrexate. The two binding sites for p-aminobenzoyl-L-glutamate are compared in Table 7.5. The finding that the aromatic protons of p-aminobenzoyl-L-glutamate show no change in chemical shift on binding to the second site suggests that the glutamate moiety is of primary importance for this interaction. Since it is known that the folate enzymes in *L. casei* exist primarily as polyglutamates (Baugh, Braverman and Nair, 1974; Brown *et al.*, 1974; Buehring, Tamura and Stokstad, 1974), it is tempting to suggest that the weak binding site for p-aminobenzoyl-L-glutamate corresponds to the binding site for one of the 'extra' glutamate residues. Experiments to test this are in progress.

The usefulness of the 'fragments' 2,4-diaminopyrimidine and p-aminobenzoyl-L-glutamate as an aid in understanding the binding of substrates and inhibitors depends, as noted above, on their binding to the enzyme in the same way. As far as the histidine residues are concerned, this seems to be true: 2,4-diaminopyrimidine and trimethoprim have very similar effects, as do 2,4-diaminopyrimidine + p-aminobenzoyl-L-glutamate and methotrexate (discounting the effects due to the binding of p-aminobenzoyl-L-glutamate to site II). A comparison of the effects of 2,4-diaminopyrimidine and p-aminobenzoyl-L-glutamate binding separately and in combination is of interest in view of the co-operativity in their binding. The increase in the pK of histidine H_F produced by p-aminobenzoyl-L-glutamate is unaffected by the simultaneous binding of 2,4-diaminopyrimidine, but the effects of the two ligands on histidines H_A and H_E are distinctly non-additive. Indeed, in both cases the effects of binding *both* 'fragments' are very similar to those of binding 2,4-diaminopyrimidine *alone*. While it is not impossible to explain this non-additivity in terms of direct effects, the other comparisons discussed above suggested a conformational contribution to the effects of ligand binding on these two histidines, and it seems likely that the non-additivity of the effects of the two 'fragments' reflects the structural basis for the co-operativity in their binding.

Tyrosine Residues

While the individual histidine C2-H resonances are readily resolved in the spectrum of the enzyme, this is not the case for the resonances of the other aromatic amino acids. The aromatic region of the ^{1}H NMR spectrum of dihydrofolate reductase (Fig. 7.9) contains resonances from the aromatic protons of eight phenylalanine, five tyrosine and five tryptophan residues, and from the C4 protons of the six histidines — a total of 91 protons. As a result, only an ill-resolved envelope of overlapping resonances is observed, and although the binding of methotrexate or trimethoprim clearly has substantial effects on this part of the spectrum (Fig. 7.9), no *individual* resonances can be resolved, so that a detailed description of these effects is not possible. To overcome this problem, a substantial simplification of the spectrum is required, and this can be achieved by selective deuteration. Figure 7.10 shows the aromatic region of the ^{1}H NMR spectrum of a selectively deuterated dihydrofolate reductase, in which all the aromatic protons of histidine, phenylalanine and tryptophan have been replaced by deuterium, as have the 3',5'-protons of tyrosine. The only remaining resonances are those of the 2,6-protons of the five tyrosine residues, and the effects of ligand binding on the tyrosine residues can thus be followed in detail (Feeney et al., 1977).

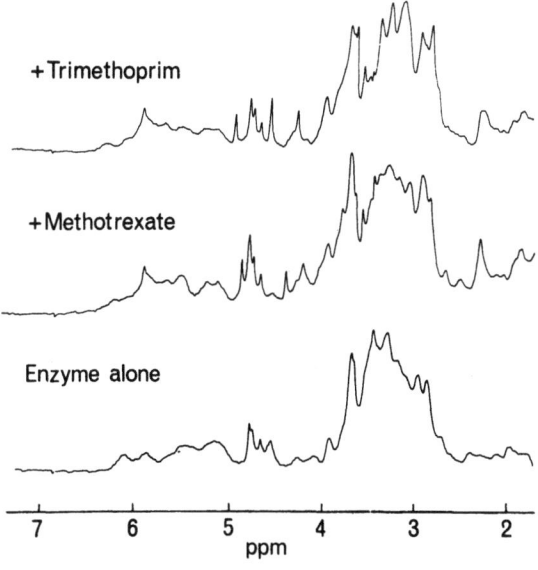

Figure 7.9 The aromatic region of the 270 MHz ^{1}H NMR spectra of *L. casei* dihydrofolate reductase and its complexes with methotrexate and trimethoprim

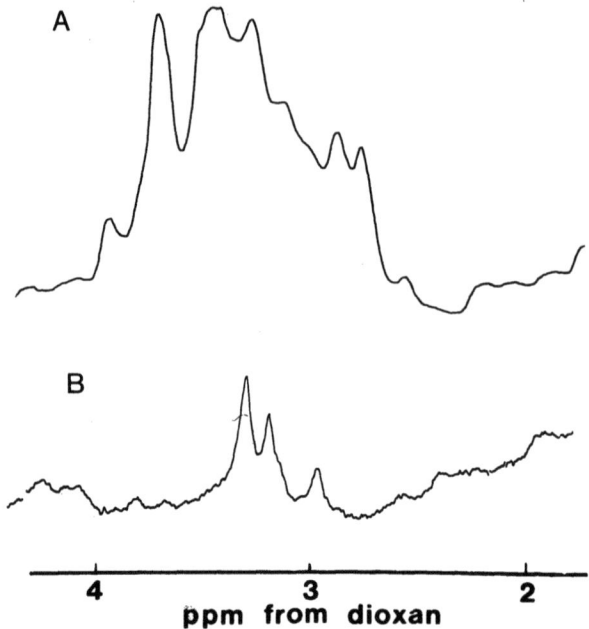

Figure 7.10 A comparison of the aromatic region of the 270 MHz ^{1}H NMR spectrum of *L. casei* dihydrofolate reductase (A) with that of a selectively deuterated analogue (B) in which only the 2,6-proton resonances of the tyrosine residues remain

Spectra of the complexes of the enzyme with inhibitors and substrates are shown in Fig. 7.11, and the chemical shifts of the tyrosine resonances (identified as tyrosines Y_A-Y_E) are summarised in Table 7.6. As was noted for the histidine C2-H resonances, the tyrosine resonances of the free enzyme are incompletely resolved, appearing as three absorption bands ($Y_A + Y_B$, $Y_C + Y_D$ and Y_E, respectively), while addition of inhibitors spreads out the resonances and also sharpens them, so that in the methotrexate complex, for example, five separate resonances can be observed. This improved resolution on addition of ligands, particularly inhibitors, appears to be a general phenomenon; it may reflect a decrease in conformational flexibility on ligand binding.

Two of the tyrosine residues, Y_B and Y_C, appear to be unaffected by ligand binding (a small shift of the resonance of Y_B on addition of *p*-nitrobenzoyl-L-glutamate† is most probably only apparent, due to overlap with the resonance of Y_A). The 4-keto compounds, folate and folinic acid, affect only a single tyrosine residue, Y_E, folate causing a slightly smaller shift in its resonance than does folinic

†In this experiment we have used *p*-nitro- rather than *p*-aminobenzoyl-L-glutamate, since the aromatic resonances of the latter overlap those of the tyrosines. The two compounds appear to bind in a closely similar way (Roberts *et al.*, 1974; Feeney *et al.*, 1977).

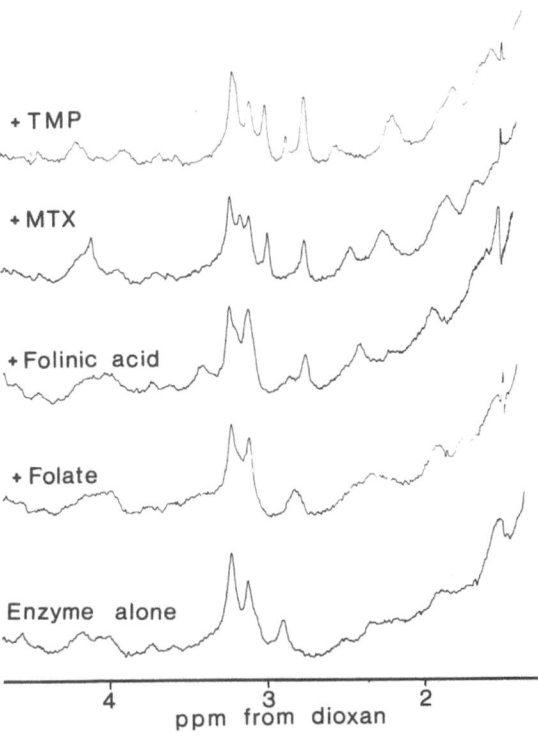

Figure 7.11 The aromatic region of the 270 MHz ^{1}H NMR spectra of selectively deuterated *L. casei* dihydrofolate reductase alone and in its complexes with substrates and inhibitors. (TMP = trimethoprim; MTX = methotrexate)

acid. This tyrosine is affected in the same way by methotrexate binding, which, however, also leads to changes in the chemical shift of two other tyrosine resonances, those of Y_A and Y_D. There is thus a clear distinction between the effects of substrates and of inhibitors.

None of these three tyrosine residues show the simple kind of behaviour which would suggest a direct effect of ligand binding (as was observed with histidine H_E) — indeed all three of them are also affected by coenzyme binding (see below). An upfield shift of the resonance of tyrosine Y_E is seen on the binding of all the substrates and inhibitors examined, and, with the exception of folate, the magnitude of the shift observed is essentially identical in each case. In particular, the shift produced by 2,4-diaminopyrimidine *and* p-nitrobenzoyl-L-glutamate is the same as that produced by *either* fragment alone. The behaviour of tyrosine Y_E is thus analogous to that of histidine H_A. Tyrosine Y_A is affected by methotrexate, 2,4-diaminopyrimidine and p-nitrobenzoyl-L-glutamate but only slightly by trimethoprim. The effect of p-nitrobenzoyl-L-glutamate is similar to that of methotrexate, but since folate has no effect, a straightforward direct interaction

Table 7.6 Chemical shifts of the tyrosine 2,6-proton resonances of dihydrofolate reductase alone and in its binary complexes with substrates and inhibitors (Birdsall et al., 1976b)

Ligand	Chemical shift[a]				
	Y_A	Y_B	Y_C	Y_D	Y_E
None	−0.16	−0.16	−0.26	−0.26	−0.48
Folate	−0.15	−0.15	−0.27	−0.27	−0.57
Folinic acid	−0.15	−0.15	−0.27	−0.27	−0.63
Methotrexate	−0.22	−0.15	−0.27	−0.39	−0.63
Trimethoprim	−0.18	−0.15	−0.27	−0.38	−0.63
2,4-diaminopyrimidine	−0.12	−0.16	−0.27	−0.32	−0.63
p-nitrobenzoyl-L-glutamate	−0.22	(−0.22)	−0.26	−0.26	−0.60
2,3-diaminopyrimidine + p-nitrobenzoyl-L-glutamate	−0.28	−0.17	−0.28	−0.40	−0.63

[a] p.p.m. (± 0.02) from the 2,6-proton resonance of N-acetyl tyrosine amide; negative numbers denote upfield shifts.

is unlikely; further experiments will be needed to clarify the behaviour of this residue. The resonance of tyrosine Y_D is shifted upfield on the addition of methotrexate, trimethoprim or 2,4-diaminopyrimidine, but is unaffected by folate. This suggests that a direct effect of the diaminopyrimidine ring may be involved. However, while p-nitrobenzoyl-L-glutamate alone has no effect on this resonance, it doubles the shift produced by 2,4-diaminopyrimidine (bringing it much closer to the effect of methotrexate). Therefore, *if* the effect on tyrosine Y_D is due to a direct interaction with the 2,4-diaminopyrimidine ring, the relative orientation of the tyrosine and pyrimidine rings must be altered in the presence of p-nitrobenzoyl-L-glutamate. Alternatively, the presence of the diaminopyrimidine ring may alter the conformation of the enzyme in such a way that p-nitrobenzoyl-L-glutamate now also has a direct effect on tyrosine Y_D. In either event, a conformational change accompanying the binding of the fragments must be postulated. Since the spectrum of the complex with the two fragments is again very similar to that of the methotrexate complex (Table 7.6), and this is also true in the presence of the coenzyme NADPH (Fig. 7.12), we must conclude that the conformational change(s) accompanying fragment binding also occur when methotrexate binds.

The spectra of the selectively deuterated enzyme in its complexes with coenzyme and in its ternary complexes with coenzyme and substrates or inhibitors are discussed in detail by Feeney et al. (1977), but two points arising from them are of interest here. Both NADPH and NADP+ produce shifts in the resonances of tyrosines Y_A, $Y_C + Y_D$ and Y_E (Table 7.7). Residues Y_A and $Y_C + Y_D$ are

Substrate and Inhibitor Binding to Dihydrofolate Reductase   147

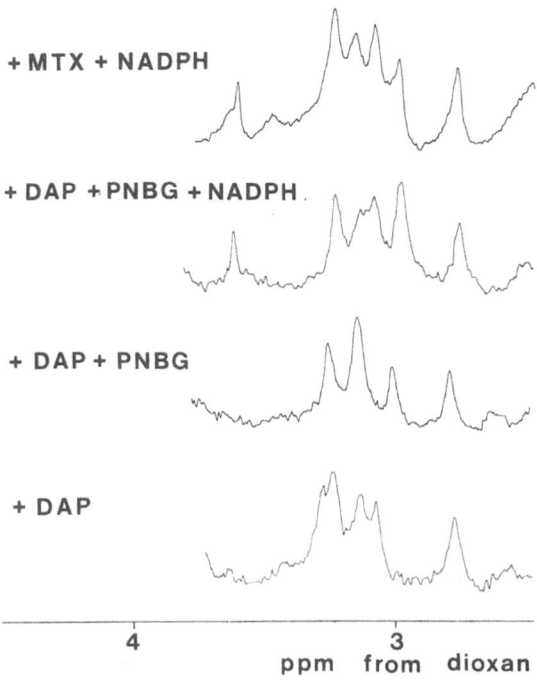

Figure 7.12 The aromatic region of the 270 MHz ^{1}H NMR spectra of selectively deuterated *L. casei* dihydrofolate reductase in its binary and ternary complexes with various inhibitors. (DAP = 2,4-diaminopyrimidine; PNBG = *p*-nitrobenzoyl-L-glutamate; MTX = methotrexate)

Table 7.7 Chemical shift of the 2,6-proton resonances of *L. casei* dihydrofolate reductase in some of its binary and ternary complexes

Ligands	Chemical shift[a]				
	Y_A	Y_B	Y_C	Y_D	Y_E
NADPH	−0.10	−0.17	−0.30	−0.30	−0.41
NADP$^+$	−0.07	−0.17	−0.28	−0.28	−0.54
Methotrexate	−0.22	−0.15	−0.27	−0.39	−0.63
Methotrexate + NADPH	−0.24	−0.16	−0.32	−0.39	−0.64
Methotrexate + NADP$^+$	−0.16	−0.16	−0.31	−0.36	−0.63
Folate + NADP$^+$	−0.15	−0.16	−0.31	−0.34	−0.60

[a] As for Table 7.6.

affected in the same way by both oxidised and reduced coenzyme, and this effect is associated with the 2′-phosphoadenosine-5′-diphosphoribose 'backbone' of the coenzymes, while tyrosine Y_E (whose resonance is shifted in opposite directions by NADP$^+$ and NADPH) is influenced only by the nicotinamide ring (Birdsall et al., 1976a). Although NADPH binding thus affects the same tyrosine residues as does methotrexate binding, the spectra of the enzyme - methotrexate complex and the enzyme - methotrexate - NADPH complex are closely similar (Table 7.7; Figs. 7.11 and 7.12). In contrast, the enzyme - methotrexate - NADP$^+$ complex gives a spectrum which is distinct from that of the binary complex (Table 7.7) as far as the chemical shift of the resonance of tyrosine Y_A is concerned. Furthermore, although, as noted above, the spectra of the binary complexes with folate and methotrexate are quite different, the spectra of the enzyme - folate - NADP$^+$ and enzyme - methotrexate - NADP$^+$ complexes are very similar (Table 7.7). In the presence of NADP$^+$, folate is able to shift the resonances of Y_A and Y_D, on which, by itself, it has no effect. It is apparent that the coenzyme can have a profound influence on the way in which the substrates and inhibitors interact with the enzyme; again the effects seen in the NMR spectra probably reflect the structural basis of the co-operativity in binding.

CONCLUSIONS

In the absence of a crystal structure for the enzyme, the experiments described here can not be interpreted to give a geometric picture of the binding site of dihydrofolate reductase. However, the rather fragmentary information presently available clearly shows that even the simplest type of drug - receptor interaction — inhibition of an enzyme by substrate analogues — can be a complex process. There is clear evidence from stopped-flow kinetic experiments (R. W. King, J. G. Batchelor, S. Dunn, A. S. V. Burgen and G. C. K. Roberts, unpublished work) that conformational changes accompany substrate, coenzyme and inhibitor binding to L. casei dihydrofolate reductase, and the NMR experiments described here do allow us to make some general comments on the nature of these changes. Substrate and/or inhibitor binding affects four of the six histidine residues and three of the five tyrosine residues. These residues can be divided into two classes (omitting for the moment histidine H_C, which is affected by p-aminobenzoyl-L-glutamate binding to its second site). Histidines H_A and H_F and tyrosine Y_E are affected in a very *similar* way by both folate and methotrexate. Histidine H_F probably interacts directly with the glutamate moiety of the ligands, but the effects on residues H_A and Y_E can not be correlated with any particular structural feature of the ligand. If, as argued above, the effects on these two residues are conformational in origin, then the very similar behaviour of H_A and Y_E reflects a conformational change which occurs on the binding of *both* substrates and inhibitors. The second group of residues, comprising histidine H_E and tyrosines Y_A and Y_D, are those which are affected *differently* by folate and methotrexate.

The pK of histidine H$_E$ is altered in opposite directions by folate and methotrexate, while Y$_A$ and Y$_D$ are affected only by methotrexate. The behaviour of these residues is difficult to explain solely in terms of direct effects, and it seems likely that it reflects some difference in the conformational changes produced by substrates and inhibitors.

The task of unravelling this complex series of conformational changes will be made significantly easier by the observation of co-operative binding of 'fragments' of methotrexate, and its structural counterparts as manifest in the NMR spectrum. Since the spectrum of the complex of the two 'fragments' with the enzyme is closely similar to that of the 'complete' ligand, we can conclude that the conformational changes which accompany the binding of the fragments, and which are responsible for their co-operative binding, also occur when methotrexate binds. Thus studies of 'fragment' binding may well allow us to examine 'partial' conformational changes and to build up gradually a structural, kinetic and thermodynamic picture of the overall binding process. To this end, we must clearly study a wide range of ligands and, particularly, as many amino acid residues in the enzyme as possible; experiments along these lines are in progress.

ACKNOWLEDGEMENTS

The work described here was carried out in collaboration with a number of past and present members of the Division of Molecular Pharmacology: A. S. V. Burgen, J. Feeney, R. W. King, B. Birdsall, D. V. Griffiths, J. G. Batchelor, J. G. Dann, R. A. Bjur, V. Yuferov, J. P. Rodriguez de Miranda, S. Dunn, B. J. Kimber, G. Ostler, P. Scudder and P. Turner.

REFERENCES

Baker, B. R. (1959). *Cancer Chemother. Rep.*, 4, 1
Baker, B. R. (1967). *Design of Active-site-directed Irreversible Enzyme Inhibitors*, New York, Wiley
Baker, B. R., Santi, D. V., Almaula, P. I. and Werkheiser, W. C. (1964). *J. Med. Chem.*, 7, 24
Baker, B. R., Schwan, T. J., Novotny, J. and Ho, B. T. (1966). *J. Pharm. Sci.*, 55, 295
Baugh, C. M., Braverman, E. and Nair, M. G. (1974). *Biochemistry*, 13, 4952
Bertino, J. R. (Ed.) (1971). Folate antagonists as chemotherapeutic agents. *Ann. N. Y. Acad. Sci.*, 186
Birdsall, B., Feeney, J., Roberts, G. C. K. and Burgen, A. S. V. (1977a). Manuscript in preparation
Birdsall, B., Griffiths, D. V., Roberts, G. C. K., Feeney, J. and Burgen, A. S. V. (1977b). *Proc. R. Soc. London*, in press.
Blakley, R. L. (1969). *The Biochemistry of Folic Acid and Related Pteridines*. Amsterdam, North-Holland
Brown, J. P., Dobbs, F., Davidson, G. E. and Scott, J. M. (1974). *J. Gen. Microbiol.*, 84, 163
Buehring, K. U., Tamura, T. and Stokstad, E. L. R. (1974). *J. Biol. Chem.*, 249, 1081
Burchall, J. J. (1971). *Ann. N. Y. Acad. Sci.*, 186, 143
Burchall, J. J. and Hitchings, G. H. (1965). *Mol. Pharmacol.*, 1, 126

Chaykovsky, M., Rosowsky, A., Papathanasopoulos, N., Chen, K. K. N., Modest, E. J., Kisliuk, R. L. and Gaumont, Y. (1974) *J. Med. Chem.*, **17**, 1212
Collin, R., and Pullman, B. (1964). *Biochim. Biophys. Acta*, **89**, 232
Dann, J. G., Ostler, G., Bjur, R. A., King, R. W., Scudder, P., Turner, P. C., Roberts, G. C. K., Burgen, A. S. V. and Harding, N. G. L. (1976). *Biochem. J.*, **157**, 559
Erickson, J. S. and Mathews, C. K. (1972). *J. Biol. Chem.*, **247**, 5661
Farber, S., Diamond, L. K., Mercer, R. D., Sylvester, R. J. Jr. and Wolff, J. A. (1948). *New Engl. J. Med.*, **238**, 787
Feeney, J., Birdsall, B., Roberts, G. C. K. and Burgen, A. S. V. (1975). *Nature (London)*, **257**, 564
Feeney, J., Roberts, G. C. K., Birdsall, B., Griffiths, D. V., King, R. W., Scudder, P. and Burgen, A. S. V. (1977). *Proc. R. Soc. London*, in press
Ferone, R., Burchall, J. J. and Hitchings, G. H. (1969). *Mol. Pharmacol.*, **5**, 49
Ferone, R., O'Shea, M. and Yoeli, M. (1970). *Science, N. Y.*, **167**, 1263
Futterman, S. (1957). *J. Biol. Chem.*, **228**, 1031
Goldman, I. D. (1971). *Ann. N. Y. Acad. Sci.*, **186**, 400
Greenberg, D. M., Tam, B. D., Jenny, E. and Payes, B. (1966). *Biochim. Biophys. Acta*, **122**, 423
Greenfield, N. J. (1975). *Biochim. Biophys. Acta*, **403**, 32
Hakala, M. T., Zakrzewski, S. F. and Nichol, C. A. (1961). *J. Biol. Chem.*, **236**, 952
Harrap, K. R., Hill, B. T., Furness, M. E. and Hart, L. I. (1971). *Ann. N. Y. Acad. Sci.*, **186**, 312
Hitchings, G. H. and Burchall, J. J. (1965). *Adv. Enzymol.*, **27**, 417
Hitchings, G. H., Falco, E. A., Vanderwerff, H., Russell, P. B. and Elion, G. B. (1952). *J. Biol. Chem.*, **199**, 43
Hutchison, D. J. (1971). *Ann. N. Y. Acad. Sci.*, **186**, 172
Jencks, W. P. (1975). *Adv. Enzymol.*, **43**, 219
Johns, D. G., Ianotti, A. T., Sartorelli, A. C. and Bertino, J. R. (1966). *Biochem. Pharm.*, **15**, 555
Johns, D. G., and Valerino, D. M. (1971). *Ann. N. Y. Acad. Sci.*, **186**, 378
Mihich, E. (Ed.) (1973). *Drug Resistance and Sensitivity: Biochemical and Cellular Basis*, New York, Academic Press
Nichol, C. A. and Welch, A. D. (1950). *Proc. Soc. Exp. Biol. Med.*, **74**, 403
Osborn, M. J., Freeman, M. and Huennekens, F. M. (1958). *Proc. Soc. Exp. Biol. Med.*, **97**, 429
Perault, A. M. and Pullman, B. (1961). *Biochim. Biophys. Acta*, **52**, 266
Perkins, J. R. and Bertino, J. R. (1966). *Biochemistry*, **5**, 1005
Plante, L. T., Crawford, E. J. and Friedkin, M. (1967). *J. Biol. Chem.*, **242**, 1466
Poe, M., Bennett, C. D., Donoghue, D., Hirshfield, J. M., Williams, M. N. and Hoogsteen, K. (1975). In *Chemistry and Biology of Pteridines (Proc. 5th Int. Symp.)* (ed. W. Pfleiderer), p. 51
Poe, M., Greenfield, N. J., Hirshfield, J. M. and Hoogsteen, K. (1974). *Cancer Biochem. Biophys.*, **1**, 7
Roberts, G. C. K., Feeney, J., Burgen, A. S. V., Yuferov, V., Dann, J. G. and Bjur, R. A. (1974). *Biochemistry*, **13**, 5351
Seeger, D. R., Smith, J. M. Jr. and Hultquist, M. E. (1947). *J. Am. Chem. Soc.*, **69**, 2567
Way, J. L., Birdsall, B., Feeney, J., Roberts, G. C. K. and Burgen, A. S. V. (1975). *Biochemistry*, **14**, 3470
Weber, G. (1975). *Adv. Protein Chem.*, **29**, 1
Zakrzewski, S. F. (1963). *J. Biol. Chem.*, **238**, 1485
Zakrzewski, S. F. and Nichol, C. A. (1958). *Biochim. Biophys. Acta*, **27**, 425

8
The molecular basis for the inhibitory action of 6-(arylhydrazino)-pyrimidines on the replication-specific DNA polymerase III of Gram-positive bacteria

Neal C. Brown and George E. Wright (Department of Pharmacology, University of Massachusetts Medical School, Worcester, Mass., USA)

INTRODUCTION

6-(*p*-Hydroxyphenylazo) uracil (HPUra, Fig. 8.1), 6-(*p*-hydroxyphenylazo)-2-amino 4 oxo pyrimidine (HPIsocytosine, Fig. 8.1) and several related 6 (arylazo)pyrimidines were conceived and synthesised by Bernard Langley of Imperial Chemical Industries, Ltd in the early 1960s. Langley and his colleagues, in their initial studies of biological activity of the arylazopyrimidines, observed that they were potent inhibitors of the growth of Gram-positive bacteria and that they possessed little or no toxicity for Gram-negative organisms or for animal cells.

The selective toxicity of the arylazopyrimidines prompted Brown and Handschumacher to investigate their mechanism in the drug-sensitive, Gram-positive bacterium, *Streptococcus faecalis*, using HPUra and HPIsocytosine as model inhibitors. The results of Brown and Handschumacher's studies (Brown,

6-(p-HYDROXYPHENYLAZO)-PYRIMIDINES

HPUra　　　　HPIsocytosine

Figure 8.1 Model arylazopyrimidines. Left, 6- (*p*-hydroxyphenylazo)uracil (HPUra); right, 6-(*p*-hydroxyphenylazo)-2-amino-4-oxo-pyrimidine (HPIsocytosine)

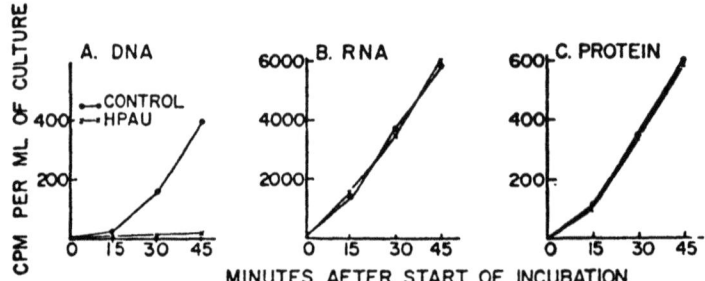

Figure 8.2 Effects of HPUra on the incorporation of radioactivity into DNA, RNA and protein in *S. faecalis*. At zero time radioisotopes and HPUra (or drug diluent as a control) were added to identical cultures of *S. faecalis* in the exponential phase of growth. Culture samples were removed for determination of incorporation into RNA, DNA and protein fractions. [^{14}C] adenine was used in A and B; [^{14}C]-L-lysine was used in C. HPUra, when present, was at a concentration of 150 µM. (Reproduced with permission from Brown and Handschumacher, 1966)

1966; Brown and Handschumacher, 1966) clearly indicated that these arylazopyrimidines inhibited the replicative synthesis of DNA and, further, that they achieved their effect selectively, without inhibiting the formation of RNA, protein or cell wall material, and without affecting the operation of pathways involved in the anabolism of 2'-deoxyribonucleoside 5'-triphosphates, the putative immediate precursors of DNA. The selectivity of the azopyrimidine inhibition in sensitive bacteria is shown by the experiment of Fig. 8.2, which depicts the effects of HPUra on the synthesis of DNA, RNA and protein in *S. faecalis*.

Brown and Handschumacher also determined that the drug-induced inhibition of DNA synthesis was effected essentially instantaneously upon addition to susceptible cultures and readily reversed by removal of drug from inhibited cells. Brown (1970, 1971) extended the investigation of azopyrimidine action to *Bacillus subtilis*, examining the effects of the drug on the non-semi-conservative synthesis of DNA associated with dark repair (Boyce and Howard-Flanders, 1964) of damage induced by ultra-violet light. Brown observed that repair synthesis, *unlike* replicative synthesis, was completely resistant to azopyrimidines.

The critical clues to the identification of the site and mechanism of azopyrimidine action on replicative DNA synthesis were derived from the examination of drug effects on an *in vitro* DNA-synthesising system derived from toluene-treated *B. subtilis*. This permeable cell system (Matsushita, White and Sueoka, 1971), like its counterpart derived from *Escherichia coli* (Moses and Richardson, 1970), utilises ATP and 2'-deoxyribonucleoside 5'-triphosphates to replicate DNA with considerable fidelity. It revealed two important facts regarding drug action (Brown, 1972; Brown, Wissemann and Matsushita 1972). First, it revealed that *azo*pyrimidines *per se* are inactive and require reduction to the *hydrazino* form; i.e.

$$-N=N- \quad \xrightarrow{[H]} \quad -\underset{H}{\underset{|}{N}}-\underset{H}{\underset{|}{N}}-$$

Second, it indicated that these active hydrazino ($H_2 \cdot$) forms act in part by mimicking specific *purine* $2'$-deoxyribonucleoside $5'$-triphosphates; dATP in the case of HPIsocytosine and dGTP in the case of HPUra; the actions of the two drugs were competitively reversed, *specifically* by the appropriate purine deoxyribonucleotide.

DNA Polymerase III as the Site of Drug Action

The observation that the arylhydrazinopyrimidines mimicked specific purine deoxyribonucleoside triphosphates strongly suggested a specific DNA polymerase as the target of drug action *in vivo*. The independent efforts of three laboratories — ours and those of Cozzarelli and of Bazill and Gross — confirmed this suggestion (Bazill and Gross, 1972; Neville and Brown, 1972; Gass, Low and Cozzarelli, 1973; Mackenzie *et al.*, 1973), by identifying in extracts of *B. subtilis* a discrete polymerase specifically sensitive to the arylhydrazinopyrimidines. The drug-sensitive polymerase, DNA polymerase III (pol III), is one of three DNA polymerases (pol I, pol II and pol III), typically found in bacteria; at present the DNA polymerases III of *B. subtilis* and *E. coli* are the only bacterial DNA polymerases with an established role in replicative DNA synthesis (Gefter *et al.*, 1971; Bazill and Gross, 1973; Cozzarelli and Low, 1973). The *B. subtilis* pol III, which forms the basis for all studies on the molecular mechanism of arylhydrazinopyrimidines, has been purified several thousand-fold by Low, Rashbaum and Cozzarelli (1976) and by Clements, D'Ambrosio and Brown (1975); it consists of a single, 167 000 dalton polypeptide, which possesses — in addition to its polymerase activity — a $3'$ exonuclease activity (Low *et al.*, 1976) with a distinct preference for single-stranded DNA.

Mutations in the structural gene for polymerase III readily occur, yielding functional enzymes, which upon isolation display increased levels of resistance to the arylhydrazinopyrimidines (Cozzarelli and Low, 1973; Gass and Cozzarelli, 1973; Clements *et al.*, 1975). The *azp-12* enzyme, derived from a *B. subtilis* mutant selected for spontaneous resistance to both HPUra and HPIsocytosine (Clements *et al.*, 1975), has been purified extensively, and its properties are described in considerable detail below.

Interest in the arylhydrazinopyrimidines has prompted considerable investigation of the effects of these drugs on a variety of prokaryotic and eukaryotic DNA polymerases. The results, many of which are unpublished, warrant the following summary. The arylylhydrazinopyrimidines do not inhibit significantly the activity of pol I and pol II of *B. subtilis* (Gass and Cozzarelli, 1973; Mackenzie *et al.*, 1973). The drugs also *do not inhibit* significantly the activity of: (1) any of the *E. coli*

DNA polymerases — including pol III (N. Brown, unpublished results); (2) the α, β and γ polymerases of mammalian cells (E. Baril, personal communication); (3) the coliphage T4-specific DNA polymerase; or (4) *B. subtilis* RNA polymerase (T. Leighton, personal communication). Thus the arylhydrazinopyrimidines presently enjoy the status of reagent inhibitors, essentially specific for replication-specific DNA polymerases of Gram-positive bacteria.

MECHANISM OF POL III INHIBITION — A TWO-COMPONENT MECHANISM

Hydrogen Bonding with Template Pyrimidines

The capacity of specific purine deoxyribonucleoside triphosphates to antagonise the inhibitory effect of the arylhydrazinopyrimidines — observed initially in toluene-treated cells (Brown, 1972) and confirmed with the isolated *B. subtilis* pol III (Neville and Brown, 1972; Gass *et al.*, 1973; Mackenzie *et al.*, 1973) — suggested that the inhibitory properties of the drugs resided, in part, in a capacity to pair with specific template pyrimidines — cytosine in the case of H_2·HPUra and thymine in the case of H_2·HPIsocytosine. Two experimental approaches (Gass *et al.*, 1973; Mackenzie *et al.*, 1973; Clements *et al.*, 1975) confirmed this suggestion. The first, summarised in Table 8.1, involved the examination of drug effects on the activity of pol III in the presence of the synthetic template-primers, poly (dC) : oligo (dG), poly (dT) : oligo (dA) and poly (dA) : oligo (dT). H_2·HPUra inhibited specifically the poly (dC)-directed synthesis of oligo (dG); H_2·HPIsocytocine inhibited specifically the poly (dT)-directed synthesis of oligo (dA); and *neither* drug affected the poly (dA)-directed formation of oligo (dT). Thus the presence of specific *template* pyrimidines was absolutely required for expression of arylhydrazinopyrimidine-induced inhibition.

The second approach to the dissection of template pyrimidine function in drug mechanism was direct, employing nuclear magnetic resonance analysis in an attempt to specify the manner in which the arylhydrazinopyrimidines and tem-

Table 8.1 Template composition as a determinant of inhibitor specificity[a]

	Nucleotide incorporation		
Substrates	Control	H_2·HPUra (100 μM)	H_2·HPIso cytosine (100 μM)
		pmol	
[^{3}H] dGTP + (dG)$_{12-18}$ – poly(dC)	27.4	1.7	27.1
[^{3}H] dATP + (dA)$_{12-18}$ – poly(dT)	5.4	5.8	0.6
[^{3}H] TTP + (dT)$_{10}$ – poly(dA)	18.1	18.0	18.4

[a]From Clements *et al.* (1975).

plate pyrimidines interact (Mackenzie *et al.*, 1973). The results of NMR analysis demonstrated the formation of novel, specific hydrogen-bonded complexes between H_2·HPUra and cytosine and H_2·HPIsocytosine and thymine. The structures, which we have proposed for these pairs on the basis of the NMR analysis, are depicted in Fig. 8.3. The parts of the molecules which participate in pairing are the 2, 3 and 4 moieties of the thymine and cytosine and the 6, 1 and 2 moieties of the inhibitors. These pairing models, which have withstood considerable testing,

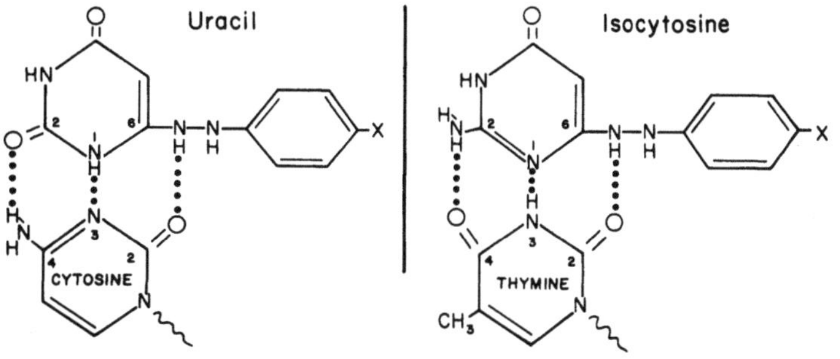

Figure 8.3 Proposed mechanism of arylhydrazinopyrimidine – pyrimidine pairing. Left, arylhydrazino uracil – cytosine; right, arylhydrazinoisocytosine – thymine.

clearly explain the purine-like character of the inhibitors, the respective capacities of H_2·HPUra and H_2·HPIsocytosine to mimic dGTP and dATP, and the generation of the active inhibitory forms of the compounds via reduction of the azo group.

Sequestration of Enzyme in a Drug-induced Complex with DNA – the Actual Basis for Inhibition

During the course of investigation of the mechanism of drug–enzyme interaction it soon became clear that arylhydrazinopyrimidine action did not depend *solely* on the capacity of these drugs to compete with purine deoxyribonucleotides for hydrogen-bonding sites on template pyrimidines. The clearest indication of a more complicated mechanism came from the observation that the arylhydrazinopyrimidines, in the presence of a natural, pyrimidine-containing template: primer DNA, strongly inhibited the *residual* synthesis catalysed by pol III when the competing purine deoxyribonucleoside triphosphate was deleted. This effect of drugs on the purine *independent* catalytic activity of pol III clearly suggested that the inhibitor, given a pyrimidine-containing template, somehow induced a sequestration of pol III, impeding its catalytic activity; more simply stated, the drug appeared to induce the formation of a relatively inactive DNA – enzyme complex.

The first clear evidence for complex formation was obtained by Gass *et al.* (1973) in an experiment exploiting pol III, H_2·HPUra and the synthetic template:primer poly(dA); oligo(dT), which promotes the H_2·HPUra-resistant formation of poly(dT). Gass *et al.* observed that addition of a small amount of a suitable template primer (i.e. calf thymus DNA), in amounts which, alone, produced no obvious effect on dTMP incorporation, caused the homopolymer – oligomer system to become drug-sensitive. The interpretation of the latter experiment was clear: the cytosine-containing DNA, in the presence of drug, sequestered pol III in a relatively stable, inactive complex.

The homopolymer experiments were confirmed in our laboratory and in Cozzarelli's laboratory by a direct demonstration of the complex (Low, Rashbaum and Cozzarelli, 1974; Clements *et al.*, 1975). The direct approach involved the examination of the effect of the drug on the elution behaviour of pol III, DNA and pol III – DNA mixtures on small columns of agarose gel capable of separating DNA and free enzyme. The results of a typical experiment performed in our laboratory (Clements *et al.*, 1975) are depicted in Fig. 8.4. Parts A and D

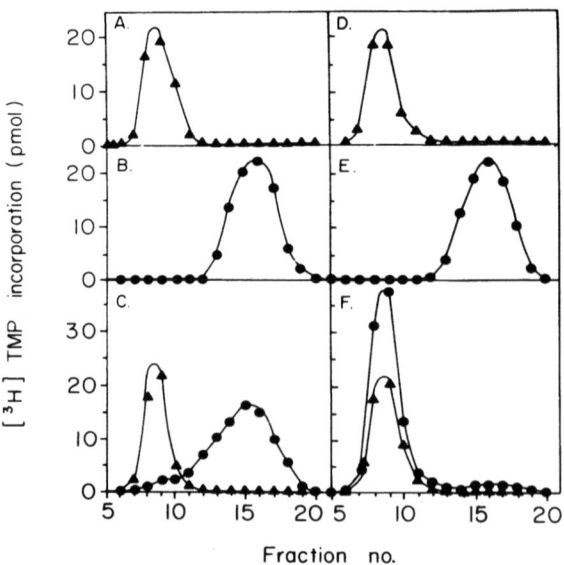

Figure 8.4 Demonstration of the drug-induced formation of a pol III – DNA complex by agarose gel filtration. Pol III and calf thymus template – primer DNA were incubated either separately or in combination in a small volume (0.125 ml) of a DNA polymerase assay buffer devoid of deoxyribonucleoside-5'-triphosphates and containing H_2·HPUra or a suitable diluent. Each mixture was filtered at 4°C through a 2 ml column of a Bio-gel A5M agarose equilibrated with assay buffer devoid of DNA and enzyme, but, otherwise, of a composition identical with that of the input mixture. Fractions (0.1 ml) were collected and 25 µl portions were assayed for pol III activity (●) or template activity (DNA, ▲). dGTP was included in high concentration in all assays to allow the expression of enzyme activity in the presence of H_2·HPUra. A, D, DNA only; B, E, enzyme only; C, F, DNA – enzyme mixture. Left panels, controls; right panels, plus 50 µM H_2·HPUra. (Reproduced with permission from Clements *et al.*, 1975)

Action of 6-(Arylhydrazino)pyrimidines on DNA Polymerase III

depict the profile of template - primer DNA incubated and filtered in the absence and presence of 50 μM H_2·HPUra; the drug had no effect on the elution pattern. Parts B and E depict the elution profile of pol III, which migrated well behind the position of DNA; H_2·HPUra also did not affect the elution profile of the enzyme. Parts C and F show the elution profile of DNA-enzyme mixtures. In the absence of the drug (C), the peak of the enzyme activity skewed slightly towards the DNA peak, and a small amount of activity (<10 per cent) co-eluted with DNA, suggesting a rather weak polymerase - DNA interaction. The presence of H_2·HPUra (Part F) promoted a much stronger interaction; indeed, under these conditions more than 90 per cent of the enzyme activity co-eluted with DNA, indicating the formation of a surprisingly stable enzyme - DNA complex.

We exploited the column approach to compare the conditions modulating complex formation with those which modulate arylhydrazinopyrimidine-induced inhibition; several observations clearly demonstrated that enzyme inhibition was the direct result of complex formation (Clements et al., 1975). First, the induction of complex required the inhibitory, hydrazino, form of the drug; the azo forms were inactive. Second, the concentration dependence of drug-induced inhibition and that of complex formation were essentially identical; the respective inhibitor constants (K_is) of wild-type and drug-resistant pol III (0.8 μM and 20-30 μM, respectively) were essentially identical with the respective values of K_{cx}, the drug concentration required for half-maximal complex induction. Third, specific purine deoxyribonucleoside 5'-triphosphates, which selectively antagonise and reverse drug-induced inhibition, antagonised with the same absolute specificity the capacity of the appropriate inhibitor to induce complex formation.

The primer - template requirements of complex formation also were studied with the gel filtration method (Low et al., 1974; Clements et al., 1975); the results indicated that complex formation does not occur in the presence of single-stranded DNA, or double-stranded DNA devoid of nicks, gaps and 3'-hydroxyl termini; complexation absolutely required a template - primer suitable as a substrate for pol III and containing a base-paired 3'-OH primer terminus and a distal,

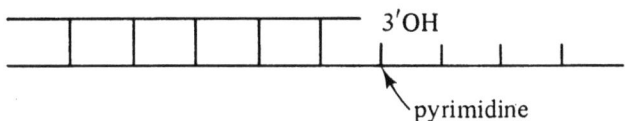

unapposed template pyrimidine, i.e. The requirement that the 3'-hydroxyl group be base-paired to template in order to provide part of the site of drug-induced inhibition was demonstrated further by Low et al. (1974). who showed that H_2·HPUra did not inhibit the capacity of pol III to catalyse the exonucleolytic degradation of *single-stranded,* cystosine-containing DNA.

THE MOLECULAR DETAIL OF THE DRUG-INDUCED DNA – ENZYME COMPLEX

The Model

The drug-induced complex, as it is currently envisioned (Low et al., 1974; Clements et al., 1975), is depicted schematically in Fig. 8.5. The complex is ternary, composed of DNA, enzyme and a base-paired primer/terminus in 1:1:1 stoicheiometry. The drug acts as a bridge between pol III and DNA, hydrogen-bonding to an unapposed, specific template pyrimidine immediately distal to the 3'-OH primer terminus and reacting, via its aryl moiety, with an enzyme site close to the deoxyribonucleoside triphosphate binding site. Another important site of enzyme – DNA interaction implied in the model is the 3'-hydroxyl terminus, which is absolutely necessary for complex formation, probably lending it considerable stability; the enzyme site involved in binding of the hydroxyl terminus is likely to be identical with that normally involved in primer extension.

Other sites of DNA – enzyme or DNA – drug interaction which may be implied by the nature of the figure are not specifically proposed and, therefore, are unintentional.

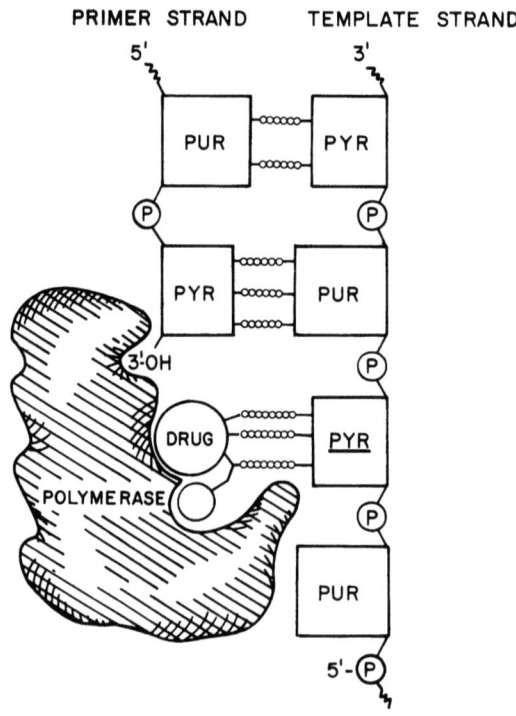

Figure 8.5 Proposed model of the arylhydrazinopyrimidine – DNA – polymerase III complex

The experimental basis for the model
The certainty of several features of the model varies considerably; each feature and the evidence for its assignment in the model are summarised below.

Stoicheiometry
The 1:1:1 relationship of drug, enzyme and primer-template, although likely, is not established; discerning the exact stoicheiometry will require the preparation of considerable amounts of pure pol III and the synthesis of radioactively labelled arylhydrazinopyrimidines — either of the conventional type or in a novel form capable of covalently attaching to DNA and/or enzyme. Both approaches are currently being explored in our laboratory.

Hydrogen-bonding mechanism
The formation of hydrogen bonds between the 2, 3 and 4 moieties of template pyrimidines and the 6, 1 and 2 moieties of the inhibitors, a feature which specifies the purine-like character of the drugs, is perhaps the most firmly established feature of the model. The hydrogen bonding has been elucidated directly by NMR analysis (Mackenzie et al., 1973) and its plausibility enhanced by examination of the structure of drug in the crystalline state (Coulter and Cozzarelli, 1975). The proposed mechanism of hydrogen bonding also is strengthened by the observation that modification of moieties critical to base pairing, i.e. methylation of

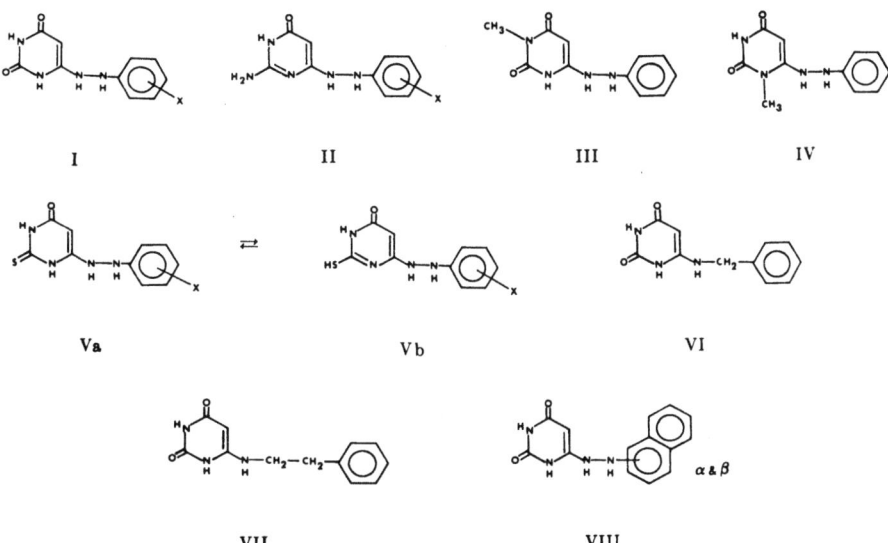

Figure 8.6 Structures of active arylhydrazinopyrimidines and related compounds. (I), 6-(arylhydrazino)uracil; (II), 6-(arylhydrazino)isocytosine; (III), 3-methyl-6-(phenylhydrazino)uracil; (IV), 1-methyl-6-(phenylhydrazino)uracil; (V), 2-thio-4-oxo-6-(arylhydrazino)pyrimidine (a, thiolactam tautomer; b, thiolactim tautomer); (VI), 6-(benzylamino)uracil; (VII), 6-(phenylethylamino)uracil; (VIII), 6-(α- and β-naphthylhydrazino)uracil

the N-1 moiety (IV, Fig. 8.6) simultaneously destroys inhibitory activity of the drug and its ability to pair with the appropriate pyrimidine (Wright, 1976).

The importance of the base-pairing mechanism in determining the adenine/guanine character of inhibitors has been supported by examination of structure – activity relationships involving ring-substituted uracil and isocytosine derivatives (Wright and Brown, 1974, 1976, and results to be published). A variety of substitutions can be made in the aryl and hydrazino groups of the uracil and isocytosine derivatives without changing the respective guanine- and adenine-like character of these compounds. The only substitutions which have changed the specific character have been the substitution of sulphur for oxygen at C2 in the pyrimidine ring; these 2-thio compounds (cf. Va, Vb, Fig. 8.6), which are relatively weak inhibitors (K_i, approximately 50 μM), require *both* dATP and dGTP to effect complete reversal of their inhibitory and complex-forming activity. We have proposed that thiolactam – thiolactim tautomerism (cf. Va, Vb, Fig. 8.6) is responsible for their ability to mimic both dATP and dGTP; the proposed mechanism (Wright and Brown, 1976) is depicted in Fig. 8.7.

The 6-NH moiety of the inhibitors is absolutely essential to bonding; its essential nature, which was implied by the requirement for azo-reduction (Mackenzie *et al.*, 1973), has been demonstrated unequivocally by the demonstration that alkylation of this moiety destroys inhibitory activity (G. E. Wright and N. C. Brown, unpublished results).

The NH group *distal* to the pyrimidine ring, as implied by the model, is clearly not involved in base pairing, nor is it required for inhibitor activity. The evidence for the latter conclusion is derived from our observation (G. E. Wright and N. Brown, results to be published) that this N may be *alkylated* or even *replaced* by a—CH$_2$—group without destroying activity; the latter compound, 6-(benzylamino) uracil (cf. VI, Fig. 8.6) is an excellent dGTP-specific inhibitor ($K_i = 2 - 3$ μM). In

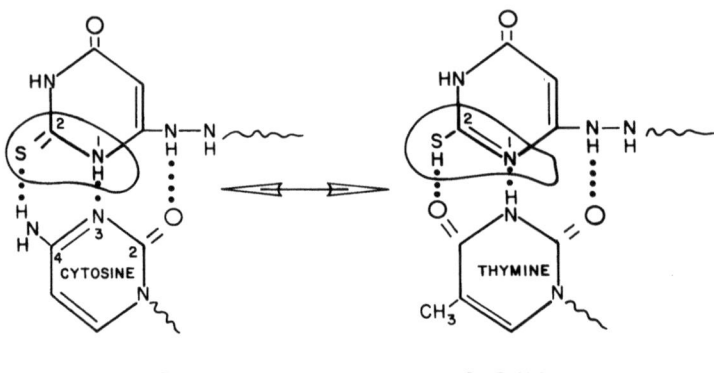

Figure 8.7 Proposed mechanism of interaction of 6-(arylhydrazino)-2-thiouracil tautomers with template pyrimidines. Left, thioketone – cytosine interaction; right, thiol – thymine interaction. (Reproduced with permission from Wright and Brown, 1976)

the context of the observed activity of the benzylamino compounds, it is appropriate to indicate that 6-(phenylethylamino)uracil (VII, Fig. 8.6) is also an active, dGTP-specific inhibitor, albeit somewhat weaker (K_i, 30 μM) than the benzyl analogue. Therefore the three bonds separating the aryl and pyrimidine moieties of the drugs can be replaced with four.

The aryl moiety as the major site of drug-enzyme interaction
A planar, unsaturated aryl moiety, either unsubstituted (i.e. a phenyl group) or substituted with a variety of substituents (*para* or *meta* CH_3, OH, Cl, Br, F, C_2H_5, etc.; cf. Wright and Brown, 1974) is absolutely required for inhibitory activity and complex formation. Removal of the aryl moiety or replacement of it with simple alkyl substituents destroys inhibitory activity.

The most convincing evidence for a primary role of the aryl moiety in complex formation and, conversely, for the presence of a specific aryl binding site in pol III is derived from our recent experiments, summarised in Table 8.2, with the mutant polymerase purified from *B. subtilis azp-12*; this enzyme is *specifically* resistant to the *p*-hydroxy compounds (K_i approximately 40 times that of wild-type pol III), and it is surprisingly nearly normally sensitive to the phenylhydrazino analogues and somewhat *hypersensitive* to compounds (i.e. *p*-CH_3) in which the *m*- or the *p*-position of the aryl moiety is occupied by a distinctly hydrophobic group.

Table 8.2 Properties of wild-type compared with those of HPUra/HPIsocytosine-resistant enzyme

— X	$K_i(\mu M)^a$	
	Wild-type enzyme[b]	'Resistant' enzyme[b,c]
— OH	0.6	>20.0
— H	1.4	2.2
— CH_3	0.5	0.4
dGTP K_m =	~0.5	~0.5

[a]Concentration of inhibitor required for half-maximal inhibition.
[b]Fraction VII (Clements *et al.*, 1975).
[c]From HPUra/HPIsocytosine-resistant mutant *B. subtilis azp-12* (Clements *et al.*, 1975).

Important details of the nature of aryl-enzyme reaction have also been derived from examination of the effects of aryl modification; the major findings can be summarized as follows.

(1) Activity is retained when the phenyl ring is replaced by other unsaturated aromatic ring systems, i.e. 6-(α, β-naphthylhydrazino)-uracils (cf. VIII, Fig. 8.6) are active dGTP-specific inhibitors.

(2) Substitutions on the phenyl moiety of phenylhydrazino-uracils allow three major generalisations. First, placement of halogens or alkyl groups *para* or *meta* to the hydrazino group has only a limited effect on the inhibitory potency. The *para* and *meta* Cl, Br and CH_3 inhibitors and the phenyl derivative are essentially equal in potency to their p-OH analogues; the weakest of the latter series is the m-Cl analogue with a K_i of approximately 4 μM. The second generalisation concerns the striking effect of the substitution of strongly electron-attracting groups, i.e. p-NO_2, p-SO_2CH_3, p-COOH, which essentially *abolish* inhibitor activity; we believe that the negative effects of these substituents derive from their capacity to render the phenyl ring and the attached NH coplanar, thus reducing the mobility of the aryl group and, therefore, its ability to conform to the enzyme's aryl binding site (cf. Fig 8.8). Thirdly, substitution *ortho* to the hydrazino moiety (i.e. o-C_2H_5 or o-CH_3) *weakens* the inhibitory activity profoundly by at least 100-fold. The basis for the effect of *ortho* substitution is not clear, although we suspect that it is primarily steric in nature.

(3) Substitutions in the p-OH series of inhibitors demonstrate a marked negative effect on inhibitory potency; the effects of substitution, which are summarised in Table 8.3, suggest strongly that substitution profoundly affects a critical interaction of the p-OH group and the aryl binding site of the enzyme (cf. discussion below).

Table 8.3 Effect of substitution on the potency of p-hydroxy derivatives

X	Y	K_i (μM)
H	H	0.8
Cl	H	8.8
Br	H	24.2
Me	H	51.2
Me	Me	124.0

Action of 6-(Arylhydrazino)pyrimidines on DNA Polymerase III 163

Enzyme sites required for drug action

Two sites are specified in the model of Fig. 8.5 – a $3'$-hydroxyl terminus binding site and an aryl binding site. The evidence for the existence and requirement of the former site has been discussed above; therefore we limit the following discussion to the *aryl* site.

(i) *Evidence for the presence of aryl binding site.* The specific response of the mutant, resistant polymerase of *B. subtilis azp-12* to alterations of the aryl group (cf. Table 8.2 and relevant discussion, above) has clearly demonstrated the presence of a distinct mutable site of reaction with the aryl group.

(ii) *Characteristics of the aryl site.* The aryl binding site has two reasonably well-defined characteristics: it is very close to the site of binding of deoxyribonucleoside triphosphates, and it is apparently hydrophobic in character. The proximity of the aryl and nucleotide binding sites is strongly suggested by the ability of the purine substrates to reverse drug-induced inhibition. The observation that mutant, drug-resistant enzymes can be altered profoundly with respect to K_i but unaffected with respect to K_m for nucleotide substrate (Cozzarelli and Low, 1973; Clements *et al.*, 1975, and Table 8.2) clearly implies that the substrate and aryl binding sites are not strictly identical.

The capacity of the aryl binding site to accommodate the aromatic drug moiety supports the contention that it has a distinct hydrophobic character. We propose, on the basis of the affinity of this site for the aryl group and on the basis of several structure - activity relationships discussed below, that the major source of drug - enzyme binding energy in this region is derived from a *stacking* interaction of an aromatic ring of an amino acid residue of the enzyme with the aryl moiety. We have incorporated this hypothetical stacking mechanism into a specific, albeit speculative, model of drug binding at the aryl binding site; the model is depicted schematically in the upper left panel of Fig. 8.8. We specify in this model that the phenyl ring has a considerable degree of mobility, permitting it to assume a conformation commensurate with a proper 'stacking' interaction at the aromatic site, O. We have emphasised the necessity of aryl - hydrazino bond mobility on the basis of the observation that substituents which severely limit this mobility, i.e. $-NO_2$ and $-SO_2 CH_3$, either abolish or weaken profoundly the inhibitory activity of the arylhydrazinopyrimidine. The requirement for mobility about the phenyl - NH bond is clearly not an unrealistic concept, since in the hydrogen-bonded complex this latter bond is probably the only link in the pyrimidine - aryl bridge which is not firmly fixed relative to template.

We also postulate in our model of the aryl binding site the presence of two *secondary* sites of drug action, amino acid moieties R and Y; we distinguish the two by assigning R a hydrophobic character and Y a polar character; the presence of these groups at the active site would account for the apparent *dual* capacity of the aryl site to accommodate, with equal facility, hydrophobic (i.e. p-CH_3, C_2H_5) and hydrophilic (i.e. OH) aryl substituents. The presence of the two minor binding sites R and Y also can account for the anomalous behaviour of the alkyl- or halo-

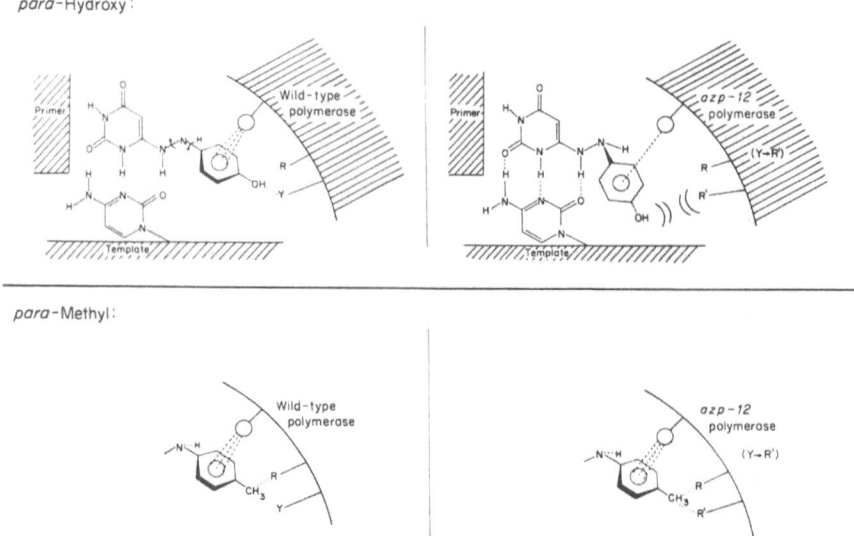

Figure 8.8 Model for the aryl binding site of *B. subtilis* DNA polymerase III and its mode of reaction with the aryl moiety. Mutant enzyme refers specifically to the $H_2 \cdot HPUra/H_2 \cdot HPIsocytosine$-resistant *azp-12* enzyme of Clements *et al.* (1975). Upper panels, binding of *p*-hydroxy derivatives; lower panels, binding of *p*-methyl derivatives

substituted, *p*-OH compounds described for the wild-type enzyme in Table 8.3. Inability of R and Y to bind simultaneously to the substituent(s) and the OH group, respectively, may yield a net *repulsive* interaction in which the efficiency of the primary phenyl binding is decreased.

The concepts of sites R and Y become less speculative when considered in the context of the effects of aryl substitution on the 'drug-resistant' polymerase derived from the *azp-12* mutant; indeed, these sites thoroughly explain the mechanism by which mutation *decreases* the potency of the *p*-OH inhibitors without affecting, negatively, the potency of compounds with H (phenylhydrazino-) or the hydrophobic alkyl substituents (CH_3 -, C_2H_5 - at the *p*- or *m*-position. This mechanism, which is depicted in Fig. 8.8, proposes that the *azp-12* mutation specifically results in the substitution of the hydrophilic Y group with a relatively hydrophobic group, R'. R' — in the case of the compounds containing the *p*-OH moiety — repels the latter, diminishing the facility and strength of the primary stacking reaction and, thus, inhibitor potency. Compounds containing the phenyl moiety alone, or alkyl- and halo-substituted aryl groups, are relatively hydrophobic, and the strength of their respective stacking reactions would presumably not be lessened by the presence of the R' group; indeed, the stacking may be *enhanced* by the presence of R'; in this context it is interesting to note the supersensitivity of the *azp-12* enzyme to the hydrophobic *p*-methyl analogue.

FUTURE STUDIES

The arylhydrazinopyrimidines are presently the only known DNA polymerase inhibitors which act via a specific capacity to recognise and react with a unique site on a replication-specific enzyme. Thus these drugs are unique reagents with which to dissect the structure and function of the replication-specific polymerases — at least those of Gram-positive bacteria — and, accordingly, we are exploiting them for this purpose. Specifically, we are synthesising new drug derivatives with particular emphasis on the development of irreversible types for covalently binding to the enzyme; we also are continuing the selection of drug-resistant site mutants of *B. subtilis* pol III in an effort to define in clearer detail the nature of the aryl binding site and its immediate environment.

The arylhydrazinopyrimidines are compounds which, via their resemblance to purine deoxyribonucleoside $5'$-triphosphates, possess structural characteristics that should accord them exceptionally facile access to the active sites of a spectrum of DNA polymerases. Therefore structural manipulation of the aryl and hydrazino moieties of the hydrazinopyrimidines may generate compounds which inhibit other distinct DNA polymerases — both prokaryotic and eukaryotic — with the same degree of selectivity observed for the Gram-positive bacterial polymerases. We are attempting to devise such compounds.

ACKNOWLEDGEMENTS

The authors are grateful to Dr Bernard Langley and Dr Alan Snow of Imperial Chemicals Industries, Ltd for gifts of inhibitors and for counsel regarding approaches to drug synthesis. Much of the authors' recent work described in this article was supported by U.S.P.H.S., N.I.H. Grants CA15915 (NCB) and GM21747 (GEW).

REFERENCES

Bazill, G. and Gross, J. (1972). *Nature New Biology*, 240, 82
Bazill, G. and Gross, J. (1973) *Nature New Biology*, 243, 241
Boyce, R. P. and Howard-Flanders, P. (1964). *Proc Nat. Acad. Sci. U.S.A.*, 51, 293
Brown, N. C. (1966). Ph. D. Thesis, Yale University, Graduate School
Brown, N. C. (1970). *Proc. Nat. Acad. Sci. U.S.A.*, 67, 1454
Brown, N. C. (1971). *J. Mol. Biol.*, 59, 1
Brown, N. C. (1972). *Biochim. Biophys. Acta*, 281, 202
Brown, N. C. and Handschumacher, R. E. (1966). *J. Biol. Chem.*, 241, 3033
Brown, N. C., Wisseman, C. and Matsushita, T. (1972). *Nature New Biology*, 237, 72
Clements, J., D'Ambrosio, J. and Brown, N. (1975). *J. Biol. Chem.*, 250, 522
Coulter, C. and Cozzarelli, N. (1975). *J. Mol. Biol.*, 91, 329
Cozzarelli, N. and Low, R. (1973). *Biochem. Biophys. Res. Commun.*, 57, 151
Gass, K. and Cozzarelli, N. (1973). *J. Biol. Chem.*, 248, 7688
Gass, K., Low, R. and Cozzarelli, N. R. (1973). *Proc. Nat. Acad. Sci. U.S.A.*, 70, 103
Gefter, M., Hirota, Y., Kornberg, T., Wechsler, J. and Barnoux, C. (1971). *Proc. Nat. Acad. Sci. U.S.A.*, 68, 3150

Low, R. Rashbaum, S. and Cozzarelli, N. (1974). *Proc. Nat. Acad. Sci. U.S.A.*, **71**, 2973
Low, R., Rashbaum, S. and Cozzarelli, N. (1976). *J. Biol. Chem.*, **251**, 1311
Mackenzie, J., Neville, M., Wright, G. E. and Brown, N. C. (1973). *Proc. Nat. Acad. Sci. U.S.A.*, **70**, 512
Matsushita, T., White, K. P. and Sueoka, N. (1971). *Nature New Biology*, **232**, 111
Moses, R. E. and Richardson, C. C. (1970). *Proc. Nat. Acad. Sci. U.S.A.*, **67**, 674
Neville, M. and Brown, N. (1972). *Nature New Biology*, **240**, 80
Wright, G. E. (1976). *J. Heterocyclic Chem.*, **3**, 539
Wright, G. E. and Brown, N. (1974). *J. Med. Chem.*, **17**, 1277
Wright, G. E. and Brown, N. (1976). *Biochim. Biophys. Acta*, **432**, 37

9
Structural and conformational studies on quinoxaline antibiotics in relation to the molecular basis of their interaction with DNA

M. J. Waring (Department of Pharmacology, University of Cambridge Medical School, Cambridge, UK)

INTRODUCTION

Research into drug action at the molecular level must first and foremost be concerned with the physical interaction between a drug and its receptor, and then attempt to explain the sequence of events which connect that interaction with the physiological response. It is commonly envisaged that the binding of the drug to its receptor provokes conformational changes in the latter which act as the immediate trigger leading to the biological effect. Obviously a *sine qua non* for understanding these events is a fairly detailed knowledge of the nature of the receptor and its conformation in the unperturbed state. Needless to say, the receptor is generally reckoned to be a macromolecule of some sort — quite likely (but not necessarily) a protein.

Thanks to the work which culminated in the model of Watson and Crick (1953) the nucleic acids (DNA in particular) have the distinction that they were the first really large macromolecular constituents of cells whose detailed structure and conformation could be accurately described. Thus, in so far as DNA can properly be regarded as a target for drug action, studies of its interaction with small molecules provide a uniquely propitious opportunity to probe the details of molecular interactions which should, if nothing else, serve as valuable models for drug—receptor interaction processes in general. In point of fact there is a wealth of evidence to suggest that binding to DNA, with consequent distortion of its structure and function, represents the fundamental site of action of a wide range of drugs employed in the chemotherapy of infectious and malignant disease (see, for example, Newton, 1970; Goldberg and Friedman, 1971; Waring, 1972; Corcoran and Hahn, 1975). So the topic of drug—nucleic acid interactions is of some considerable interest in its own right, quite apart from the light it may shed upon other pharmacologically important processes where the nature of the receptor is not so well defined.

But the very elegance of the Watson – Crick double-helical model of DNA presents problems as well as advantages in explaining the molecular basis of drug action. While it greatly facilitates the elucidation of conformational changes associated with drug binding, enabling correlation between distortion of structure and its functional consequences in favourable situations, there arises immediately the problem of discriminating between different types of DNA or DNA sequences. It is all very well to point to DNA as the target of action of selectively toxic antimicrobial or antitumour drugs, but whence their selectivity if all DNA molecules look much the same? This paper will be concerned with those two fundamental aspects of the drug – DNA interaction problem: on the one hand, the structural basis for binding of a particular class of antibiotics and the resulting perturbations of the DNA helix, and on the other hand, the question of selectivity in terms of preferential interaction with particular nucleotide sequences.

The Intercalation Model
A major landmark in the development of current ideas about drug – DNA interaction was the explicit formulation of the intercalation hypothesis by Lerman (1961). The germ of this idea can be discerned in earlier literature going back even beyond Watson and Crick, but it was Lerman's relatively precise model for the binding of aminoacridines to DNA which first established the concept of intercalation on firm ground. His model was patently aimed at providing an explanation at the molecular level for the production of frameshift mutations by proflavine and other acridines. In this regard it met with a good deal of success (reviewed in Waring, 1972). However, the potential applicability of the intercalation hypothesis to explain the binding to DNA of many other drugs was soon appreciated, and during the last fifteen years a considerable number of important chemotherapeutic drugs have been identified as intercalating agents. One of the first was ethidium bromide, a phenanthridine trypanocide now well known to molecular biologists as a classical intercalator and useful research tool (Fuller and Waring, 1964; Waring, 1975a). More recently the list has expanded greatly to include other antiprotozoal drugs, antimalarials, schistosomicides, antiviral agents and antitumour antibiotics, to name but a few (see reviews cited above).

By what criteria can the binding of a drug to DNA be identified as intercalative? Direct evidence in the form of a crystallographically determined structure for a true drug – DNA complex is still lacking even with the best-investigated examples, though the high-resolution structures determined for actinomycin – deoxyguanosine and ethidium – dinucleotide complexes by Sobell *et al.* (1971) and Tsai, Jain and Sobell (1975) provide powerful support for the assertion that those two drugs are efficient intercalators. In practically all other instances the evidence is necessarily somewhat indirect and rests largely on observations of analogous behaviour to the 'established' intercalating drugs, particularly ethidium. Two characteristic predictions of the intercalation model are of crucial significance as diagnostic aids, i.e. that the DNA helix should become locally unwound and physically extended as a result of the intercalation of the aromatic chromophore of the drug molecule between the DNA base-pairs (Lerman, 1961, 1964; Fuller and Waring, 1964; Waring, 1972). These (related) structural perturbations are amenable to experimental investigation by a number of techniques. The unwinding of the helix can be evidenced by the consequential removal and reversal of the supercoiling of closed circular duplex DNA, reflected in characteristic changes in the sedimentation coefficient and/or viscosity of such molecules (Crawford and Waring, 1967; Bauer and Vinograd, 1968). By this technique the relative helix-unwinding angles for binding of different drugs can be accurately determined (Waring, 1970, 1972, 1975b). The predicted extension of the DNA helix can be investigated by measuring changes in the viscosity of sonicated rod-like DNA fragments (Cohen and Eisenberg, 1969; Reinert, 1973). Neither of these techniques alone is sufficient to establish unequivocally an intercalative mode of binding, for non-intercalative unwinding of the DNA helix by steroidal diamines has been observed (Waring and Chisholm, 1972; Waring and Henley, 1975), and conversely viscosity enhancement indicative of helix extension by the antibiotic netropsin has been reported (Reinert, 1972), though no effect on the winding of the helix could be detected (Luck *et al.*, 1974; Wartell, Larson and Wells, 1974). However, where both types of experiment yield a positive result with good correspondence between theoretical predictions and experimental measurements, the conclusion of intercalation is generally considered justifiable (see, for example, Waring and Wakelin, 1974; Le Pecq *et al.*, 1975; and below).

Specificity of Intercalation
The realisation that intercalation into DNA may constitute the molecular mode of action of numerous drugs has provided a satisfactory basis for understanding their interference with nucleic acid synthesis via distortion of the structure and function of the DNA template, but it nevertheless highlights the question of their specificity — especially the origins of selective toxicity. How can the intercalation reaction endow a drug molecule with the capacity to discriminate between

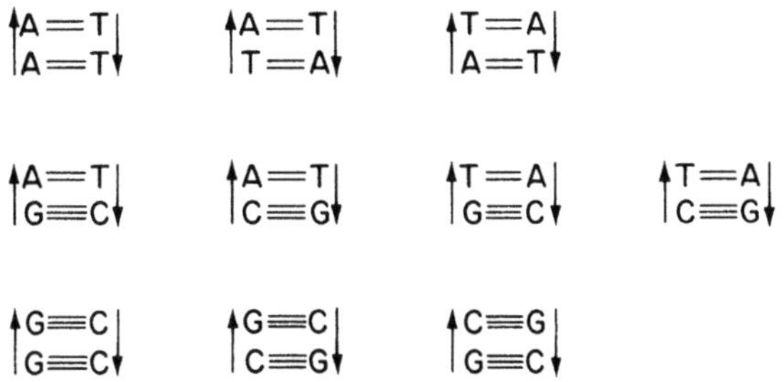

$$
\begin{array}{ccc}
\uparrow A=T \downarrow & \uparrow A=T \downarrow & \uparrow T=A \downarrow \\
\downarrow A=T \uparrow & \downarrow T=A \uparrow & \downarrow A=T \uparrow
\end{array}
$$

$$
\begin{array}{cccc}
\uparrow A=T \downarrow & \uparrow A=T \downarrow & \uparrow T=A \downarrow & \uparrow T=A \downarrow \\
\downarrow G\equiv C \uparrow & \downarrow C\equiv G \uparrow & \downarrow G\equiv C \uparrow & \downarrow C\equiv G \uparrow
\end{array}
$$

$$
\begin{array}{ccc}
\uparrow G\equiv C \downarrow & \uparrow G\equiv C \downarrow & \uparrow C\equiv G \downarrow \\
\downarrow G\equiv C \uparrow & \downarrow C\equiv G \uparrow & \downarrow G\equiv C \uparrow
\end{array}
$$

Figure 9.1 The ten distinguishable types of site for intercalation into DNA. Each illustration represents two adjacent hydrogen-bonded base-pairs in a DNA double helix, with the $5' \rightarrow 3'$ direction of the phosphodiester backbones shown by the arrows. From Waring (1972)

different DNAs or DNA sequences? For the simpler known intercalating drugs (and that is the vast majority) it is unreasonable to suppose that they might recognise more than the base-pairs on either side of the intercalation site, in which case there are only ten distinguishable types of potential site defined by ten unique dinucleotide sequences in each of the DNA strands (Fig. 9.1). In a polymer of random sequence any one of these sites would occur on average once per turn of the tenfold B-form DNA helix, i.e. at far too high a frequency to permit effective discrimination between regions of different genetic function within a single DNA molecule, still less between DNA molecules from different sources. Moreover, the evidence indicates that very few, if any, of the known intercalating agents are sufficiently specific to demand just one of the ten possible types of site. Actinomycin seems to display a strong preference for the GpC site (Wells and Larson, 1970; Sobell *et al.*, 1971) and ethidium may interact preferentially with pyrimidine(3'-5')purine sequences (Krugh and Reinhardt, 1975), but these preferences are far from absolute. Thus the intercalation reaction, at least in its ordinary form, is quite incapable of providing the level of discrimination needed for what may be termed biologically significant specificity, and it cannot account in molecular terms for the undoubted selective toxicity of the many useful chemotherapeutic agents which act in this way. Their selectivity (as opposed to their toxicity) must presumably be attributable to less sophisticated properties (Waring, 1975b).

The gist of these considerations is that the way to gain real specificity for interaction with defined, biologically significant DNA sequences is to combine multiple centres of specificity within one molecule. Müller and his collaborators have shown that where an intercalating chromophore manifests site-specificity at all it is typically (perhaps necessarily) for GC-rich sequences (Müller, Bünemann and Dattagupta, 1975; Müller and Crothers, 1975). By contrast, DNA-binding compounds which do not intercalate display, if anything, preferences for AT-rich

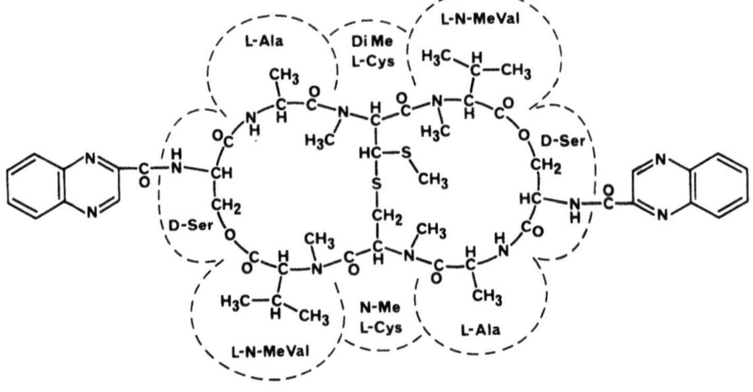

Figure 9.2 Structural formula of echinomycin (Dell *et al.*, 1975; Martin *et al.*, 1975)

sequences (Müller and Gautier, 1975). Thus by appropriate choice of intercalating chromophores judiciously linked to a 'spacer' bearing the right functional substituents it should be possible to design compounds which will bind preferentially, perhaps even with absolute specificity, to defined DNA nucleotide sequences considerably longer than those recognised by existing drugs.

That this approach is feasible, and has precedent in nature, is shown by our recent identification of the antibiotic echinomycin (Fig. 9.2) as a bifunctional intercalating agent — the first such substance ever described (Waring and Wakelin, 1974). The remainder of this article will deal briefly with the evidence for bifunctional intercalation of echinomycin and related antibiotics into DNA, then with attempts to discern essential and non-essential structural features which may affect the character and/or specificity of the interaction, and finally the development of a preliminary molecular model.

ECHINOMYCIN

Bifunctional Intercalation

The two tests outlined earlier were applied to establish that echinomycin binds to DNA in the fashion expected for an intercalating agent and that quantitative aspects of its effects on the macromolecular properties of DNA agree with those predicted for a hypothetical bifunctional intercalator. In Fig. 9.3 the effect of echinomycin on the sedimentation behaviour of circular DNA is shown, together with that of ethidium bromide for comparison. The classical removal and reversal of the supercoiling are clearly evident, and the equivalence binding ratio (Waring, 1970, 1972) for echinomycin occurs with 0.028 ± 0.004 antibiotic molecules bound per nucleotide — almost half the value found for ethidium under the same conditions (0.051 ± 0.007). Thus the helix-unwinding angle per DNA-bound echinomycin molecule is 1.82 ± 0.30 times that of ethidium. This value was checked by independent measurement of the crossover point of binding isotherms for closed and nicked circular PM2 DNA (Waring and Wakelin, 1974): here the unwinding angle of echinomycin was estimated to be 1.89 times that of ethidium.

Measurements of the viscosity of sonicated rod-like DNA fragments (left-hand panel of Fig. 9.4) revealed that binding of each echinomycin molecule extends the helix by about 6.3 Å, i.e. 1.87 ± 0.05 times the theoretical extension required to accommodate a single intercalated aromatic chromophore. As expected, the extension is approximately twice the values reported for proflavine and ethidium (Cohen and Eisenberg, 1969; Reinert, 1973).

The very good agreement between the results from these three tests leaves little room for doubt that both chromophores of echinomycin become intercalated when the antibiotic binds to DNA in a solvent of low ionic strength.

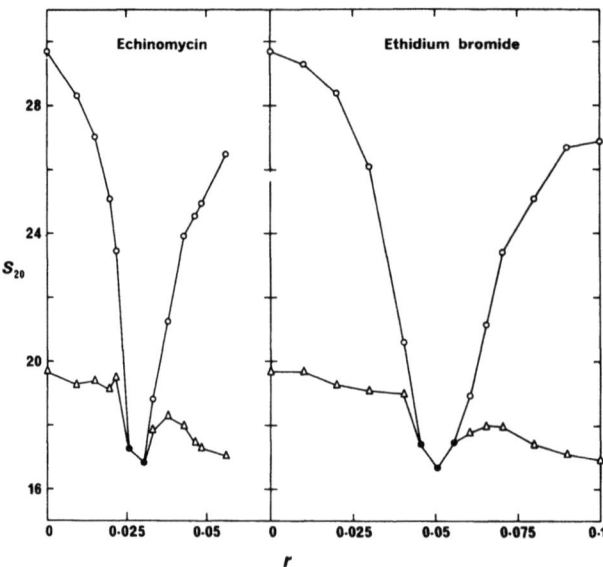

Figure 9.3 Effects of echinomycin and ethidium bromide on the sedimentation coefficient (S_{20}) of PM2 DNA at ionic strength 0.01, pH 7.0. The DNA preparations contained 80 – 90 per cent closed circular duplex molecules whose S_{20} is represented by O. The S_{20} of the nicked circles is shown by △, and when the two DNA components co-sedimented as a single unresolved boundary, the symbol ● is plotted. The abscissa represents the binding ratio r, drug molecules bound per DNA nucleotide. After Waring and Wakelin (1974)

However, when the experiments were repeated at moderate to high ionic strength, a peculiar change was observed; the helix extension fell progressively towards a value approaching that expected for ideal monofunctional intercalation (centre and right-hand panels of Fig. 9.4) and at the same time the equivalence binding ratio for PM2 DNA moved correspondingly closer to that observed with ethidium (Waring and Wakelin, 1974). It would appear that the bifunctional mode of reaction which occurs at low ionic strength is smoothly converted towards more nearly monofunctional interaction at ionic strength 0.5. At the intermediate ionic strength of 0.1 the characteristics of the binding process are almost exactly sesquifunctional ($1\frac{1}{2}$-fold).

Specificity in the Binding of Echinomycin to DNA

Further experiments were conducted in the buffer of low ionic strength (0.01) in order to investigate whether the novel bifunctional mode of binding of echinomycin might be associated with significant sequence-specificity, as anticipated in view of the considerations discussed above. Because of the low aqueous solubility of echinomycin (saturation occurs at about 5 μM) these and other experiments

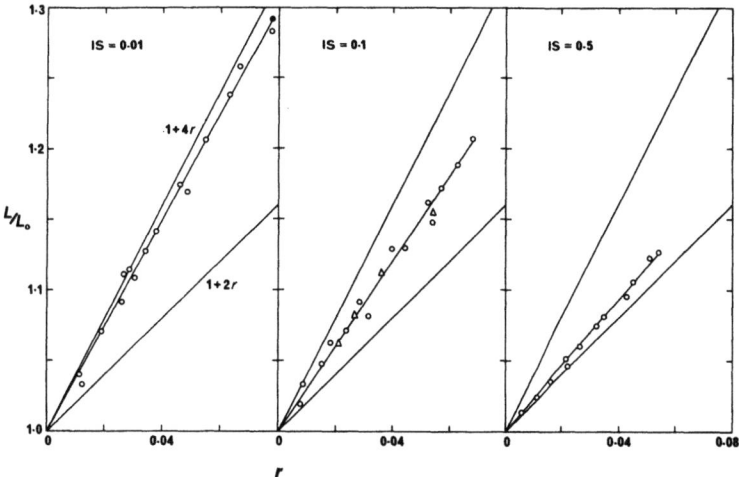

Figure 9.4 Relative increase in contour length L/L_0 of echinomycin – DNA complexes as a function of the binding ratio. L/L_0 was calculated from viscosity measurements on sonicated rod-like fragments of calf thymus DNA, M_r 5.4 × 10^5 (○) or 3.8 × 10^5 (△), as described by Cohen and Eisenberg (1969). The three panels show results from experiments at ionic strength (IS) 0.01 (left), 0.1 (centre) or 0.5 (right). Included in each panel are reference lines corresponding to the lengthening expected for ideal monofunctional intercalation ($1 + 2r$) and for ideal bifunctional intercalation ($1 + 4r$). The lines passing through the experimental points were fitted by the method of least squares and constrained to pass through the origin (0, 1). Their slopes correspond to $1 + (3.73 \pm 0.09)r$ (left); $1 + (2.99 \pm 0.09)r$ (centre); and $1 + (2.32 \pm 0.05)r$ (right). Reproduced by permission from Wakelin and Waring (1976)

demanding a knowledge of the binding ratio r had to be performed using a solvent-partition method specially developed for the purpose (Waring, Wakelin and Lee, 1975).

It was first established that echinomycin binds specifically to DNA, not RNA, and that it requires the presence of helical structure in the DNA (Waring and Wakelin, 1974). Scatchard plots for eight naturally occurring DNAs are shown in Fig. 9.5. They reveal that the binding does indeed differ depending upon the source of the DNA, but it does not correlate in any simple way with the gross base composition. Parameters of interaction derived from these plots are collected in Table 9.1. There seems to be a tendency for DNAs richer in G + C to bind the antibiotic more tightly — the highest binding constant was found for *Micrococcus lysodeikticus* DNA, the lowest for *Clostridium perfringens* DNA — but between these limits the association constant is not monotonically related to the mole fraction of G + C. In particular, a significant difference can be seen when the binding curves for *Escherichia coli* and *Salmonella typhimurium* DNAs are compared, yet these species share the same overall base composition. On the other hand, the parameters determined for calf thymus and nicked PM2 DNAs (both 42% G + C)

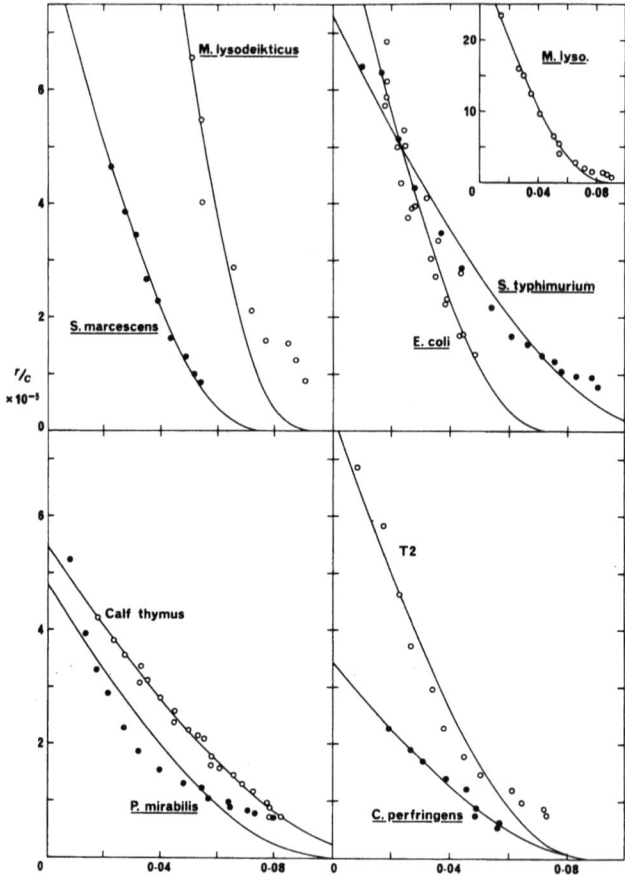

Figure 9.5 Effects of base composition on the binding of echinomycin to DNA. The data are presented in the form of the Scatchard (1949) plot, where r is the binding ratio (echinomycin molecules bound per DNA nucleotide) and c is the free antibiotic concentration. The ionic strength was 0.01, pH 7.0. For ease of comparison the same scale is used throughout, except for the inset (top right), where the data for *M. lysodeikticus* DNA are replotted with a contracted ordinate scale in order to include points at low values of r. The curves are theoretical, computed to fit Eq. (10) of McGhee and Von Hippel (1974) using the values of $K(0)$ and n listed in Table 9.1. Reproduced by permission from Wakelin and Waring (1976)

are practically the same, notwithstanding the extreme difference in their origins and genetic complexity. When the apparent frequencies of binding sites reflected in the site-size parameter n are compared, there is no relation at all to the base composition. For double-helical natural DNAs n lies within the range 9.5 ± 2.4 nucleotides per binding site.

Table 9.1 Parameters of interaction between echinomycin and nucleic acids

DNA	G + C (%)	$K(0)$ ($\times 10^{-5}$ M^{-1})	n
M. lysodeikticus	72	31.0	9.85
Serratia marcescens	58	8.71	11.61
E. coli	50	9.80	11.88
S. typhimurium	50	7.38	7.58
Calf thymus	42	5.48	7.17
Bacteriophage PM2 (nicked)	42	5.07	7.75
Proteus mirabilis	40	4.79	8.69
Bacteriophage T2	34	7.78	9.97
C. perfringens	30	3.44	9.46
Calf thymus (heat-denatured)	42	1.40	19.49
Bacteriophage fd	42	1.21	11.37
poly dG · poly dC	100	15.1	9.09
poly d(G–C)	100	5.53	5.48
poly d(A–T)	0	3.12	5.65

$K(0)$ and n are as defined by Eq. (10) of McGhee and Von Hippel (1974):

$$\frac{r}{c} = K(0)(1-nr)\left(\frac{1-nr}{1-(n-1)r}\right)^{n-1}$$

where r is the binding ratio (antibiotic molecules bound per DNA nucleotide) and c is the free antibiotic concentration. The site-size parameter n corresponds to the number of nucleotides occupied by a bound antibiotic molecule; as defined here, it is the *reciprocal* of the binding-site parameter which results from Scatchard (1949) analysis. $K(0)$ is the intrinsic association constant for binding to an isolated site, given by the intercept on the axis of r/c; in the treatment of Scatchard (1949) this intercept would be interpreted as K/n. The equation was solved by an iterative procedure which was made to recycle until $K(0)$ and n changed by less than 1 per cent. For details see Wakelin and Waring (1976).

In an effort to clarify the issue of specificity by studying simpler models the interaction between echinomycin and seven synthetic double-helical polymers was investigated. Four were found to interact barely at all, or only very weakly, with the antibiotic: poly dI · poly dC, poly d(I-C), poly dA · poly dT and poly rA · poly rU. The other three bound the antibiotic well (Fig. 9.6). The tightest binding was observed with poly dG · poly dC, whose binding constant was exceeded only by that of *M. lysodeikticus* DNA (Table 9.1). Poly d(G-C) yielded a binding constant of the same order as seen with several natural DNAs, while that of poly d(A-T) fell below the range found with native double-helical DNAs. Substantially higher levels of binding were attained with the two alternating polydeoxynucleotides than with other DNAs, reflected in the computed values of n (Table 9.1), suggesting that a potential binding site in these polymers might be formed by as little as 5-6 nucleotides ($2\frac{1}{2}$-3 base-pairs).

These results reveal that there is undoubtedly selectivity in the interaction between echinomycin and different DNA nucleotide sequences. Particularly striking is the failure of poly dA · poly dT to bind the antibiotic while its sequence isomer poly d(A - T) binds it well (Waring and Wakelin, 1974). Since the association constant for *M. lysodeikticus* DNA is twice as high as that for the best of the synthetic polynucleotides, poly dG · poly dC, it may be that the base sequence (or sequences) generating the optimum conditions for binding of echinomycin contains all four nucleotides. There are evidently considerable subtleties in the preference of echinomycin for available DNA binding sites and those preferences are clearly different from those of actinomycin, its nearest equivalent among previously studied DNA-binding drugs (Wells and Larson, 1970).

Whatever the exact nature of the selectivity inherent in echinomycin – DNA interaction, it must ultimately derive from a capacity to recognise distinct nucleotide sequences either by direct interaction between functional groupings on the antibiotic molecule and the base-pairs or indirectly via recognition of a local conformational peculiarity of the DNA associated with a particular type or types of sequence. The latter is a real possibility, at least in theory, based on

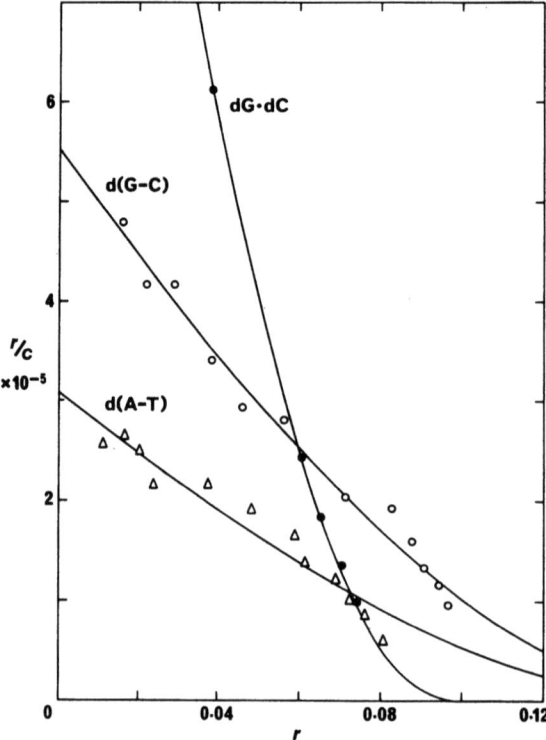

Figure 9.6 Interaction between echinomycin and synthetic polydeoxynucleotides. For details see the legend to Fig. 9.5. The theoretical curves correspond to the values of $K(0)$ and n listed in Table 9.1. Reproduced by permission from Wakelin and Waring (1976)

recent evidence for structural variations in the DNA helix originating from clustering of nucleotide-pairs of a given type (Bram, 1971a, b; Bram and Tougard, 1972). However, the large differences detected in the echinomycin-binding properties of the synthetic polynucleotides do not simply relate to what is known of their conformational characteristics in drawn fibres or in solution (Wakelin and Waring, 1976). Nevertheless, the possibility that polynucleotide polymorphism plays an important part in determining the suitability of DNA-binding sites for echinomycin must be borne in mind in any discussion of molecular models (see below).

Structural Determinants for Bifunctional Intercalation

In order to probe the role of the various parts of the echinomycin molecule as determinants of its DNA-binding properties a number of analogous compounds have been studied.

Role of the chromophores

Granted that in the complex the quinoxaline chromophores of the antibiotic are intercalated between the DNA base-pairs, the first question to ask is whether the chromophore moieties alone are effective intercalating agents. With the much simpler antimalarial drug chloroquine, for instance, the very similar (single) quinoline chromophore becomes intercalated (O'Brien, Allison and Hahn, 1966;

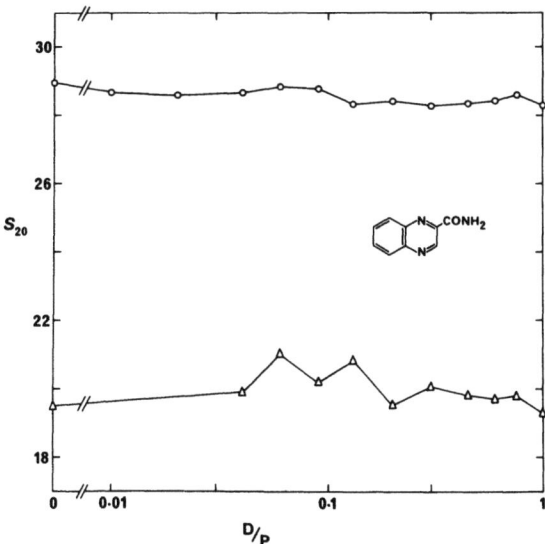

Figure 9.7 Sedimentation behaviour of PM2 DNA in the presence of quinoxaline-2-carboxamide. For details see the legend to Fig. 9.3. The abscissa represents the molar ratio of total ligand to DNA nucleotides (log scale). Unpublished experiment of L. P. G. Wakelin and M. J. Waring

Waring, 1970, 1975b). To answer this question the simplest possible analogue of the echinomycin chromophores, quinoxaline-2-carboxamide, was tested for possible effects on the supercoiling of circular DNA. No effect whatsoever could be detected (Fig. 9.7), even at ratios 40-fold higher than those required to cause complete relaxation of the supercoiling with echinomycin. In parallel experiments it was shown by equilibrium dialysis and examination of ultra-violet absorption spectra that no binding of quinoxaline-2-carboxamide to DNA could be detected.

A second substance considered as a potential analogue of echinomycin was the trypanocidal drug Bayer 7602, which contains two substituted quinoline chromophores linked by an ostensibly flexible five-atom 'spacer' chain. This drug is certainly capable of binding to DNA, but when tested as in Fig. 9.3 and 9.7 it was found only to remove but not reverse the supercoiling of PM2 DNA at relatively high D/P ratios (0.2 or greater), in no way mimicking the powerful effect of echinomycin (Wakelin and Waring, 1976). Evidently, therefore, the octapeptide ring of echinomycin plays more than a passive role in determining the strength and character of its interaction with DNA; it is not merely a convenient handle upon which two potentially intercalative chromophores are mounted.

Role of the peptide lactones

To investigate whether the integrity of the octapeptide ring is essential for DNA-binding, a derivative of echinomycin was prepared in which the lactone linkages

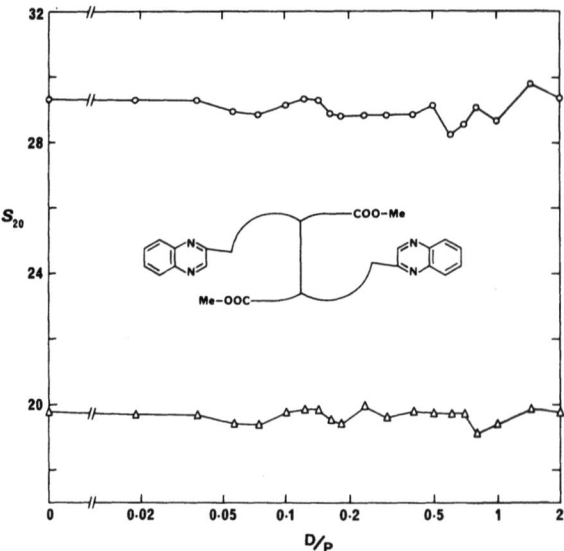

Figure 9.8 Sedimentation behaviour of PM2 DNA in the presence of echinomycinic acid dimethyl ester. For details see the legend to Fig. 9.3. The abscissa represents the molar ratio of total ligand (D) to DNA nucleotides (P) (log scale) Unpublished experiment of J. S. Lee

had been broken. These linkages are susceptible to cleavage by mild alkali (Keller-Schierlein, Mihailovic and Prelog, 1959), resulting in the formation of a dibasic carboxylic acid. This substance, echinomycinic acid, would not be expected to interact with DNA because of its anionic character at neutral pH, which would lead to highly unfavourable electrostatic forces in the vicinity of a polyanion such as DNA. Accordingly, the acid was converted to the stable dimethyl ester and the resulting uncharged product tested for interaction with circular DNA (Fig. 9.8). As with quinoxaline-2-carboxamide, no effect on the supercoiling could be detected at ratios far higher, in this case up to 100-fold, than those which substantially reduce the supercoiling with the intact antibiotic. Thus the integrity of the cyclic peptide appears to be essential for activity, perhaps by severely limiting its conformational flexibility. In this respect another parallel with actinomycin may be drawn, where again the pentapeptide lactones are known to be essential (Lackner, 1975).

Role of the cross-bridge

Another structural feature which might have significant influence on the conformation and activity of echinomycin is the dithioacetal cross-bridge across the two symmetrical halves of the octapeptide ring. It can be broken by treatment with methyl iodide, and preliminary tests with the product of cleavage indicate that the ability to bind to DNA is either severely reduced or lost altogether. However, a much more informative way in which to examine the role of the cross-bridge is provided by the availability of other naturally occurring antibiotics belonging to the quinoxaline series. That series can be divided into two groups: the quinomycins, of which echinomycin is a member, characterised by the possession of the dithioacetal cross-bridge (Dell *et al.*, 1975; Martin *et al.*, 1975), and the triostins, which are structurally homologous but possess a simple disulphide cross-bridge (Otsuka and Shoji, 1965; Katagiri, Yoshida and Sato, 1975). Thus triostin A (Fig. 9.9) provides a ready-made analogue of echino-

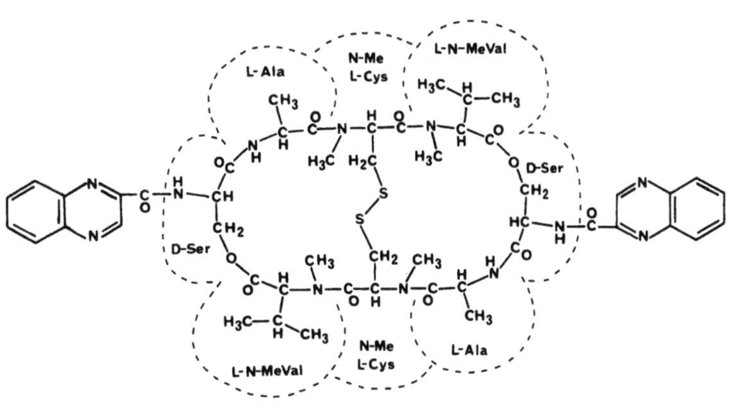

Figure 9.9 Structural formula of triostin A

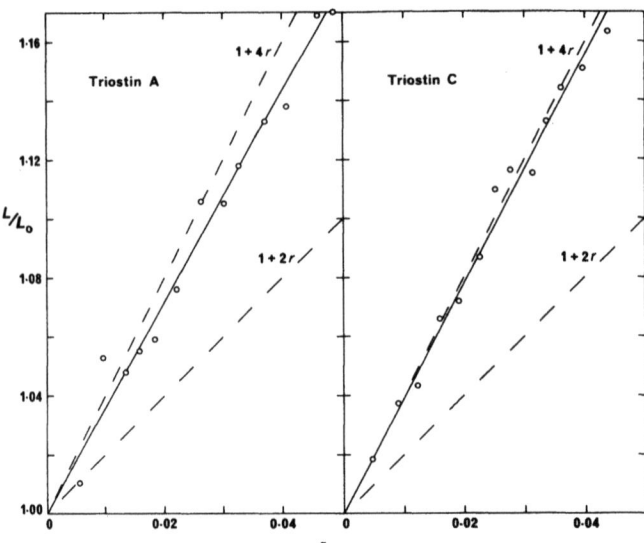

Figure 9.10 Effects of triostin antibiotics on the relative contour length of sonicated calf thymus DNA fragments. The ionic strength was 0.01, pH 7.0; other details are as described in the legend to Fig. 9.4. The slopes of the lines fitted to the experimental points correspond to the relations $1 + (3.57 \pm 0.17)r$ for triostin A (left) and $1 + (3.89 \pm 0.14)r$ for triostin C (right). Unpublished experiments of J. S. Lee

mycin in which the asymmetry imparted to the molecule by the —S—CH_3 grouping is lost and the cross-bridge is one bond longer. Other members of the quinoxaline series have amino acid replacements at the N-methyl valine sites; we have also performed a few experiments with triostin C, which has N, γ-dimethyl-*allo*-isoleucine at these positions (Otsuka and Shoji, 1965).

Both triostin A and triostin C behave as effective bifunctional intercalating agents. Judged by the DNA fragment-viscosity experiment they extend the helix by almost the theoretical value for a bifunctional process (Fig. 9.10; compare also the left-hand panel of Fig. 9.4). In the circular DNA-binding test the equivalence ratios for PM2 DNA were determined to be 0.028 ± 0.005 with both antibiotics, corresponding to a helix-unwinding angle 1.82 ± 0.4 times that of ethidium, in exact agreement with what was found for echinomycin (Fig. 9.3). Thus the precise length and constitution of the cross-bridge in echinomycin and triostin is not a crucial requirement as regards their capacity for bifunctional reaction (though its integrity probably is), and neither are the side-chains of the N-methyl valine residues — at least in respect of 'conservative' replacement.

The nature of the cross-bridge is not without significant influence on the binding to DNA, however. In Fig. 9.11 a set of Scatchard plots for triostin A – polynucleotide interaction is shown. These, together with the parameters of

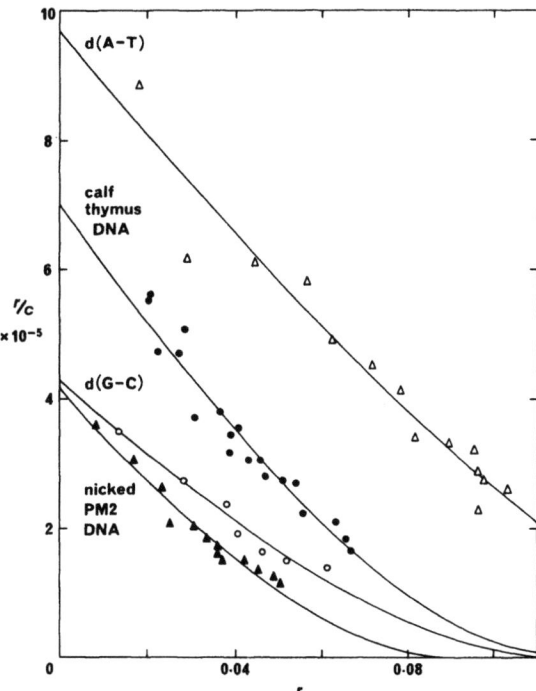

Figure 9.11 Scatchard plots for the binding of triostin A to nucleic acids. For details see the legend to Fig. 9.5. The theoretical curves correspond to the values of $K(0)$ and n listed in Table 9.2. Unpublished experiments of J. S. Lee

binding listed in Table 9.2, are for comparison with the corresponding data for echinomycin presented in Figs. 9.5 and 9.6 and Table 9.1. A number of important points emerge. Firstly, the parameters of interaction between triostin A and calf thymus DNA or nicked PM2 DNA are clearly different, whereas for echinomycin they were not. Secondly, triostin A binds better to heat-denatured calf thymus DNA than to the single-stranded DNA of phage

Table 9.2 Parameters of interaction between triostin A and nucleic acids

DNA	G + C (%)	$K(0)$ ($\times 10^{-5}$ M^{-1})	n
Calf thymus	42	7.00	7.29
Bacteriophage PM2 (nicked)	42	4.16	9.42
Calf thymus (heat-denatured)	42	1.53	22.82
Bacteriophage fd	42	0.60	21.07
poly d(G-C)	100	4.28	7.41
poly d(A-T)	0	9.70	4.76

fd, while the converse was found with echinomycin. Thirdly, the relative affinities of the two antibiotics for the alternating synthetic polynucleotides are completely interchanged; triostin A binds much better to poly d(A-T) than to poly d(G-C), whereas the reverse is true for echinomycin. This latter most important difference results mainly from a large change, over threefold, in the binding constant for poly d(A-T). It can only be concluded that the relatively slight difference in the nature of the cross-bridge, while not perceptibly affecting the geometrical characteristics of the antibiotic – DNA complex, nevertheless significantly alters whatever sequence-selectivity is associated with the interaction. This is clear proof of the active role played by the octapeptide ring in dictating the unique DNA-binding properties of these antibiotics. Whether the sulphur-containing cross-bridge is directly implicated in recognition processes involving the DNA base-pairs, or whether the extra bond in the triostin cross-bridge makes its presence felt by loosening the structure of an otherwise tightly constrained peptide ring, remains to be seen. Such questions can only be addressed in the light of evidence as to the three-dimensional structure of the antibiotics and their DNA complexes.

Conformational studies
The information needed for building a true picture of the stereochemical relation ship between the bound antibiotic molecule and its (distorted) DNA receptor is conformational data for both interacting species. With most problems in molecular pharmacology, evidence is available for the ligand but lacking for the receptor. Paradoxically, in the present situation there is sufficient information from the experiments described above to build quite an accurate model of the distorted receptor (DNA) and it is evidence on the conformation of the ligand (antibiotic) which is almost totally lacking. The ideal starting point for gaining an insight into the likely conformation of the DNA-bound antibiotic would be a crystal structure for the free species. Despite repeated attempts all efforts to produce crystals of echinomycin have thus far failed. Triostin A has been crystallised from solution in isoamyl acetate and X-ray diffraction data have been collected, but it appears that the molecule is too large (mol. wt., 1084) to yield to presently available direct methods of structure solution.

Accordingly, a theoretical study of conformational possibilities for the echino- mycin molecule has been undertaken, utilising such limited information as is available from nuclear magnetic resonance measurements (Dell *et al.*, 1975) and employing computational techniques applied previously to the structure of actinomycin D (De Santis, Rizzo and Ughetto, 1972a, b). The basis of the approach involves calculation of potential energy as a function of internal conformational parameters, i.e. angles of rotation about chemical bonds, the application of geometrical constraints imposed by the need to close the peptide ring and form the cross-bridge, and subsequent refinement to minimise the potential energy of the entire molecule using a method of steepest descent. It turned out that the cyclic nature of the octapeptide, and especially the need

Interaction of Quinoxaline Antibiotics with DNA 183

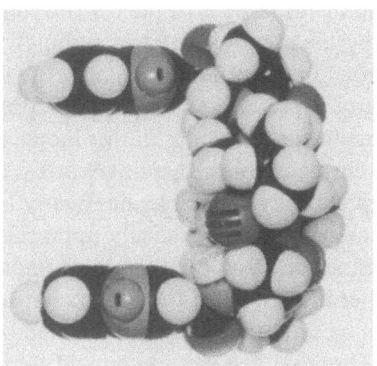

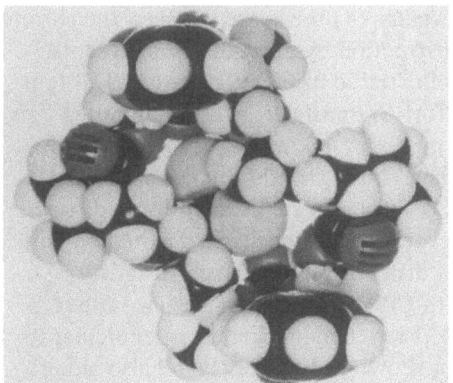 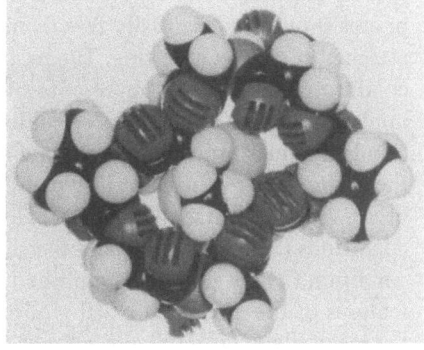

Figure 9.12 A space-filling (CPK) model of echinomycin. The top panel shows the molecule viewed from the 'side', i.e. roughly perpendicular to the average plane containing the peptide ring and the planes of the quinoxaline chromophores. In the two panels the model has been rotated approximately 90° about a vertical axis. On the lower left the chromophores project forward towards the viewer; on the right they project away from the direction of view and are completely obscured by the N-methylvalyl-O-seryl-alanyl sequences of the peptide ring. G. Ughetto and M. J. Waring (unpublished)

to establish the five-atom cross-link, imposed such stringent constraints on the allowed conformational possibilities that very few theoretical structures proved acceptable on purely energetic grounds.

This study is not yet complete, but sufficient data are available to build a model which can serve as a basis for discussion and refinement. Such a model, similar to (but not quite identical with) the most preferred theoretical structure, is illustrated in Fig. 9.12. All the peptide bonds are *trans*, as are also the lactone ester linkages. The two halves of the molecule have been considered to adopt a near-symmetrical disposition with respect to the central sulphur atom of the cross-bridge, as suggested by the pseudo-centre of symmetry implicit in the structural formula represented in Fig. 9.2. The asymmetric element in the formula, the —S—CH_3 group, presents something of a problem, since it can occupy any one of four possible orientations; in this model it has been positioned on the side away from the chromophores. It is noteworthy that the whole octapeptide ring, which is practically inflexible, lies nearly in a single plane.

The plausibility of this model depends crucially upon the extent to which it is compatible with the evidence on DNA binding. Most importantly, it stands or falls on the question whether it will permit the quinoxaline chromophores to be positioned so that they can be simultaneously intercalated between the DNA base-pairs. We can hypothesise that this would demand four properties of the structure: (1) the chromophores should lie on the same side of the peptide ring; (2) their planes should be approximately parallel; (3) the vertical distance between those planes should be an integral multiple (x) of 3.4 Å, i.e. the theoretical spacing required to accommodate x base-pairs; (4) the space between the chromophores should be essentially free from obstruction by any other substituents attached to the peptide ring. The model illustrated in Fig. 9.12 satisfies all four conditions. In essence it represents an effort to translate the best computed minimum-energy model into a 'real life' model by taking minor liberties with standard values for bond lengths and angles. In the strictly theoretical model the chromophores are not quite parallel; their planes are inclined towards each other with a dihedral angle of 35°. However, they are positioned in accord with conditions (1), (3) and (4), and the slight distortions introduced to satisfy condition (2) are easily accomplished with CPK or other models. Two other features of the model are worthy of note. Viewed along a line perpendicular to the mean plane of the chromophores (not shown in Fig. 9.12), and also along the quasi-dyad axis of the molecule (lower panels of Fig. 9.12), the structure displays the same chirality as DNA. Secondly, the side of the octapeptide ring bearing the chromophores presents a complete array of hydrophobic groups to face inwards towards the base-pairs in the groove of a DNA helix (left-hand panel of Fig. 9.12), leaving all of the peptide ring C=O groups directed outwards towards the solvent and the lactone oxygens close to where the polynucleotide backbones would lie (right-hand panel of Fig. 9.12). It must be admitted that this latter feature involves a 180° rotation of the peptide bond connecting one L-*N*-methylcysteine residue to L-alanine compared with the best theoretical model, but this rotation has the effect of preserving the quasi-rotational symmetry of the peptide ring.

Because the present model is only tentative, it would be premature at this stage to embark on discussion of likely contacts which might be involved as determinants of sequence selectivity. However, it may be noted that the NH components of the serine–chromophore amide bonds, as potential hydrogen bond donor groups, are obvious candidates for consideration in due course. The outstanding question for the present is the value of x defined in condition (3) above, i.e. the number of base-pairs sandwiched between the intercalated chromophores.

Neighbour Exclusion

It has long been suspected that when intercalating drug molecules interact with DNA, a neighbour-exclusion phenomenon operates to prohibit binding to sites adjacent to one already occupied (Crothers, 1968; Waring, 1972; McGhee and Von Hippel, 1974). In practical terms this means that intercalated chromophores would have to be separated by a minimum of *two* base-pairs, not one. This hypothesis, still subject to debate, takes on a new importance in the context of bifunctional intercalation. Is it, in fact, possible to fit two (or more) base-pairs between the chromophores of echinomycin? From the model illustrated in Fig. 9.12 the answer is clear: the space is just exactly right to accommodate two stacked base-pairs, since the computed distance between the C(2) atoms of the chromophores (i.e. the atoms linked to the peptide ring) is 10.2Å. Thus the structure of the antibiotic itself need not necessarily lead to conflict with the principle of neighbour exclusion. However, the issue does not end there. It was noted earlier that the levels of binding of echinomycin to poly d(A-T) and poly d(G-C) (and also of triostin A to poly d(A-T)) were surprisingly high. Calculations from the Scatchard plot data yielded values of n (Tables 9.1 and 9.2) suggesting that a sequence of only three nucleotide pairs (or even slightly fewer) might constitute a binding site. With a bifunctional mechanism of binding this would lead to serious conflict with the neighbour-exclusion principle, irrespective of the number of base-pairs sandwiched between the chromophores (Fig. 9.13). The reality of this dilemma is not proved, however, since it depends upon two assumptions: namely, that the mechanism of interaction with these synthetic polynucleotides is bifunctional as it is with natural DNAs under the same conditions, which has not been directly demonstrated; and also that the site-size parameter n is a valid measure of the occupancy of a polymeric lattice at saturation with ligand (McGhee and Von Hippel, 1974; Wakelin and Waring, 1976).

Prompted by these considerations, we have been led to investigate by other means the minimum distance between intercalating chromophores which will permit bifunctional interaction. A series of diacridine compounds have been synthesised in which two potentially intercalative 9-aminoacridine moieties are connected by a straight-chain aliphatic linkage of varying length (Fig. 9.14) (Canellakis *et al.*, 1976). Eight of these substances forming a homologous series were tested for their effects on the supercoiling of circular DNA and the viscosity of sonicated calf thymus DNA fragments. The results are summarised in Fig. 9.15. A clear transition from monofunctional to bifunctional interaction was observed when the length of the methylene bridge was increased from four to six —CH_2—

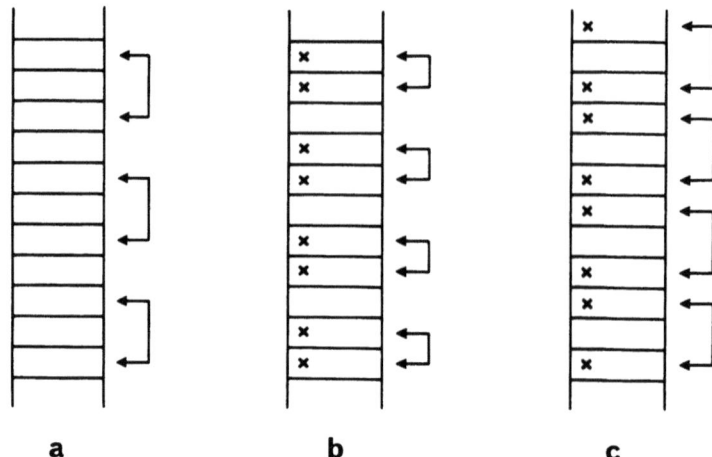

Figure 9.13 Schematic illustration of bifunctional interaction between echinomycin and helical polydeoxynucleotide assuming that the antibiotic occludes four (a) or three (b, c) nucleotide-pairs per bound molecule. The ladder represents the DNA helix and the antibiotic molecule is shown as a vertical line with its chromophores as horizontal arrowed lines. In (a) is represented the situation in which two base-pairs are sandwiched between the intercalated chromophores and four successive nucleotide-pairs constitute a binding site. In (b) and (c) the binding site contains only three nucleotide-pairs and the number of base-pairs sandwiched between the chromophores is either one (b) or two (c). Either of cases (b) and (c) necessitates violation of the neighbour-exclusion principle and the offending lattice positions are marked with a cross. Reproduced by permission from Wakelin and Waring (1976)

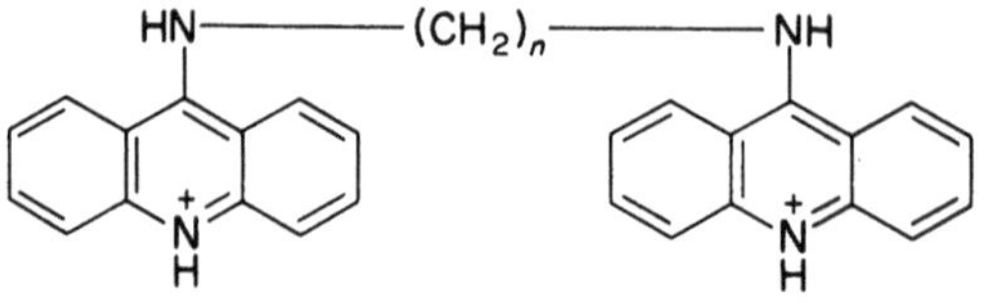

Figure 9.14 Generalised structural formula of dimeric 9-aminoacridine derivatives

groups. Compounds with four or fewer carbon atoms in the connecting chain yielded equivalence binding ratios for PM2 DNA of the same order as found for simple monomeric aminoacridines, and produced a helix extension closely approximating the $1 + 2r$ relation for ideal monofunctional intercalation. Compounds with six or more carbon atoms in the linkage yielded values, respectively, about half and double those found for the shorter derivatives. The compound with five carbon atoms in the chain yielded ambiguous results; its effect or circular DNA was intermediate between that of the two principal groups and it gave a curved plot of L/L_0 against D/P with slope changing from about 2 to 3.3 as the level of binding increased.

Interaction of Quinoxaline Antibiotics with DNA

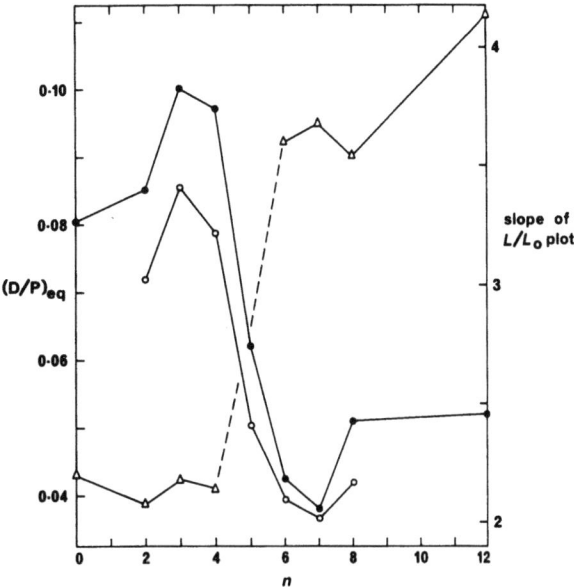

Figure 9.15 Variation of helix-unwinding angle and helix extension with length of the connecting chain $-(CH_2)_n-$ for simple dimeric 9-aminoacridine compounds. The left-hand ordinate shows the ligand/nucleotide ratio at equivalence (relaxation of the supercoiling) for PM2 DNA determined by ultracentrifugation (●), as in Fig. 9.3, or by a viscometric method (○), as described by Waring and Henley (1975). The left-hand ordinate records the slopes (△) of molecular extension plots like those in Fig. 9.4 and 9.10. The buffer was of ionic strength 0.01, pH 7.0. The points plotted for $n = 0$ are values determined for a comparable monomeric substance, 9-methylaminoacridine. Unpublished experiments of L. P. G. Wakelin, M. Romanos and M. J. Waring

Simple geometrical considerations and experiments with CPK space-filling models reveal that full extension of the C6 alkyl chain results in a maximum separation of 8.8 Å between the centres of the acridine chromophores, sufficient to accommodate one base-pair between them (the theoretical minimum would be 6.8 Å) but insufficient to accommodate two, which would require 10.2Å. Full extension of the C4 alkyl chain would provide a separation of only 6.3 Å, not enough to accommodate a single 3.4 Å thick base-pair, limiting this compound and the shorter homologues to monofunctional interaction. The important results are those for the C6 compound, which clearly are at variance with the prediction of the neighbour-exclusion hypothesis requiring a 'two-base-pair sandwich'. The position of the C5 compound can only be described as enigmatic; while geometrical considerations indicate that the separation between its chromophores could extend to 7.5 Å, it has not yet proved possible to build a satisfactory 'one-base-pair sandwich' model, though the experimental results (Fig. 9.15) suggest that its interaction with circular DNA may well have some bifunctional character. The difficulty of interpretation here may lie in adopting the simplistic view that straightforward geometrical ideas are adequate to explain the observations. In their study of a different series of diacridines having —NH— groups inserted into the spacer chain Le Pecq et al. (1975) concluded that bifunctional intercalation did not occur until the chain contained more than the six atoms which we find sufficient. It may require experimentation with a number of homologous series of compounds before the minimum separation between chromophores in a bifunctional intercalating agent can be stated with certainly. Or a precise molecular model for quinoxaline antibiotic.

ACKNOWLEDGEMENTS

It is a pleasure to record the contributions of my collaborators in this work, particularly Dr L. P. G. Wakelin, Dr G. Ughetto, Mr J. S. Lee, Mr M. Romanos, Mr D. Gauvreau and Mr D. Martin. These and other colleagues provided invaluable advice, assistance, criticism and samples of experimental materials. Original work reported here was supported by grants from the Medical Research Council, the Science Research Council and CIBA-Geigy Ltd. The synthesis of diacridines was financed by contract NOI-CM-12339, Division of Cancer Treatment, NCI, NIH, to Dr E. S. Canellakis of Yale University.

REFERENCES

Bauer, W. and Vinograd, J. (1968). *J. Mol. Biol.*, 33, 141
Bram, S. (1971a). *Nature, (London)* 232, 174
Bram, S. (1971b). *J. Mol. Biol.*, 58, 277
Bram, S. and Tougard, P. (1972). *Nature New Biol.*, 239, 128
Canellakis, E. S., Shaw, Y. H., Hanners, W. E. and Schwartz, R. A. (1976). *Biochim. Biophys. Acta*, 418, 277
Cohen, G. and Eisenberg, H. (1969). *Biopolymers*, 8, 45
Corcoran, J. W. and Hahn, F. E. (1975). *Antibiotics, III: Mechanism of Action of Antimicrobial and Antitumour Agents* (ed. J. W. Corcoran and F. E. Hahn), Springer-Verlag, Heidelberg.
Crawford, L. V. and Waring, M. J. (1967). *J. Mol. Biol.*, 25, 23
Crothers, D. M. (1968). *Biopolymers*, 6, 575
Dell, A., Williams, D. H., Morris, H. R., Smith, G. A., Feeney, J. and Roberts, G. C. K. (1975). *J. Amer. Chem. Soc.*, 97, 2497
De Santis, P., Rizzo, R. and Ughetto, G. (1972a). *Nature New Biol.*, 237, 94
De Santis, P., Rizzo, R. and Ughetto, G. (1972b). *Biopolymers*, 11, 279
Fuller, W. and Waring, M. J. (1964). *Ber. Bunsenges. Physik. Chem.*, 68, 805
Goldberg, I. H. and Friedman, P. A. (1971). *Ann. Rev. Biochem.*, 40, 775
Katagiri, K., Yoshida, T. and Sato, K. (1975). *Antibiotics, III: Mechanism of Action of Antimicrobial and Antitumour Agents* (ed. J. W. Corcoran and F. E. Hahn), Springer-Verlag, Heidelberg, p. 234
Keller-Schierlein, W., Mihailovic, M. L. and Prelog, V. (1959). *Helv. Chim. Acta*, 42, 305
Krugh, T. R. and Reinhardt, C. G. (1975). *J. Mol. Biol.*, 97, 133
Lackner, H. (1975). *Angew. Chem.* (English ed.), 14, 375

Le Pecq, J-B., Le Bret, M., Barbet, J. and Roques, B. (1975). *Proc. Nat. Acad. Sci. U.S.A.* 72, 2915
Lerman, L. S. (1961). *J. Mol. Biol.*, 3, 18
Lerman, L. S. (1964). *J. Cell. Comp. Physiol.*, 64 (Suppl. 1), 1
Luck, G., Triebel, H., Waring, M. and Zimmer, Ch. (1974). *Nucleic Acids Res.*, 1, 503
McGhee, J. D. and Von Hippel. P. H. (1974). *J. Mol. Biol.*, 86, 469
Martin, D. G., Mizsak, S. A., Biles, C., Stewart, J. C., Baczynskyj, L. and Meulman, P. A. (1975). *J. Antibiotics.*, 28, 332
Müller, W., Bünemann, H. and Dattagupta, N. (1975). *Eur. J. Biochem.*, 54, 279
Müller, W. and Crothers, D. M. (1975). *Eur. J. Biochem.*, 54, 267
Müller, W. and Gautier, F. (1975). *Eur. J. Biochem.*, 54, 385
Newton, B. A. (1970). *Adv. Pharmacol. Chemother.*, 8, 149
O'Brien, R. I., Allison, J. L. and Hahn, F. E. (1966). *Biochim. Biophys. Acta*, 129, 622
Otsuka, H. and Shoji, J. (1965). *Tetrahedron*, 21, 2931
Reinert, K. E. (1972). *J. Mol. Biol.*, 72, 593
Reinert, K. E. (1973). *Biochim. Biophys. Acta*, 319, 135
Scatchard, G. (1949). *Ann. N. Y. Acad. Sci.*, 51, 660
Sobell, H. M., Jain, S. C., Sakore, T. D. and Nordman, C. E. (1971). *Nature New Biol.*, 231, 200
Tsai, C., Jain, S. C. and Sobell, H. M. (1975). *Proc. Nat. Acad. Sci. U.S.A.*, 72, 628
Wakelin, L. P. G. and Waring, M. J. (1976). *Biochem. J.*, 157, 721
Waring, M. J. (1970). *J. Mol. Biol.*, 54, 247
Waring, M. J. (1972). *The Molecular Basis of Antibiotic Action* (by E. F. Gale, E. Cundliffe, P. E. Reynolds, M. H. Richmond and M. J. Waring), Wiley, London, p. 173
Waring, M. J. (1975a). *Antibiotics*, III: *Mechanism of Action of Antimicrobial and Antitumour Agents* (ed. J. W. Corcoran and F. E. Hahn), Springer-Verlag, Heidelberg, p. 141
Waring, M. J. (1975b). *Topics in Infectious Diseases*, Vol. 1: *Drug-Receptor Interactions in Antimicrobial Chemotherapy* (ed. J. Drews and F. E. Hahn), Springer-Verlag, Vienna, p. 77
Waring, M. J. and Chisholm, J. W. (1972). *Biochim. Biophys. Acta*, 262, 18
Waring, M. J. and Henley, S. M. (1975). *Nucleic Acids Res.*, 2, 567
Waring, M. J. and Wakelin, L. P. G. (1974). *Nature (London)*, 252, 653
Waring, M. J., Wakelin, L. P. G. and Lee, J. S. (1975). *Biochim. Biophys. Acta*, 407, 200
Wartell, R. M., Larson, J. E. and Wells, R. D. (1974). *J. Biol. Chem.*, 249, 6719
Watson, J. D. and Crick, F. H. C. (1953). *Nature (London)*, 171, 737
Wells, R. D. and Larson, J. E. (1970). *J. Mol. Biol.*, 49, 319

10
The receptor site for chloramphenicol *in vitro* and *in vivo*

Olaf Pongs (MRC Laboratory of Molecular Biology, Hills Road, Cambridge, UK)

INTRODUCTION

Chloramphenicol inhibits protein synthesis in Gram-negative and Gram-positive bacteria as well as in chloroplasts, blue-green algae and mitochondria (for a review, see Pestka, 1971). It was the first antibiotic to be synthesised by chemical methods (Controulis, Rebstock and Crooks, 1949). The molecule has a relatively simple structure, which consists of a propanediol moiety (III), carrying a p-nitrobenzene side-chain (I) and a dichloroacetyl side-chain (II) (Fig. 10.1).

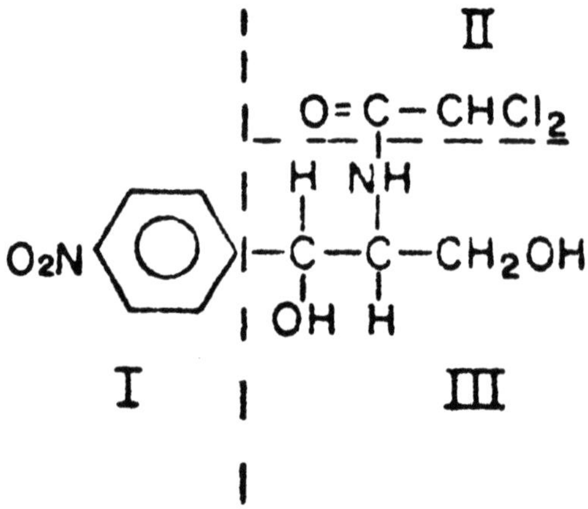

Figure 10.1 Structure of chloramphenicol, partitioned into three major sections

Structure – Activity Rules for Chloramphenicol Derivatives
The following general structure – activity rules can be deduced from the information available on numerous derivatives and analogues of this antibiotic (Hahn and Gund, 1975). (1) The aromatic nitro group can be replaced by electronegative substituents without loss of activity. The substitution, however, has to be in the

para position of the benzene ring (Rebstock, Tratton and Bambas, 1955; Hahn *et al.*, 1956; Kolosov *et al.*, 1961). (2) The propanediol moiety has two asymmetric carbon atoms, which allow four possible stereoisomers; only the naturally occurring D-(−)-*threo* stereoisomer, i.e. chloramphenicol, has strong bacteriostatic properties (Maxwell and Nickel, 1954). (3) Though the acyl side-chain is essential for activity, it is the site where variations have been introduced into the molecule most frequently (Kolosov *et al.*, 1961). This is probably due to the relative ease with which the dichloroacetyl side-chain can be replaced by other substituents. The rule of thumb for these substitutions is that increases in the size of the substituent decrease potency of the drug (Hansch *et al.*, 1973). Recently we took advantage of the relatively simple chemistry of acyl side-chain substitutions and replaced the dichloroacetyl by an iodoacetyl side-chain, which yielded the chloramphenicol analogue monoiodoamphenicol (Bald, Erdmann and Pongs, 1972). This chloramphenicol analogue has very similar properties to those of chloramphenicol *in vitro* and *in vivo*, but with one important difference. Whereas chloramphenicol binds reversibly to its receptor site, monoiodoamphenicol has the potential, not only to bind, but also to react at the same receptor site. Looking at the structure of monoiodoamphenicol from a different point of view, it can be regarded as a derivative of iodoacetamide. It then becomes immediately apparent that monoiodoamphenicol carries a chemically reactive iodoacetyl side-chain, which can undergo nucleophilic displacement reactions with a properly oriented amino acid functional group in the binding region of monoiodoamphenicol. Since monoiodoamphenicol and chloramphenicol compete for the receptor site on the ribosome, monoiodoamphenicol could be employed as an affinity probe to investigate the molecular nature of this site (Pongs, Bald and Erdmann, 1973).

The Mode of Action of Chloramphenicol

It has been shown that chloramphenicol inhibits peptidyl-puromycin formation in intact bacteria (Nathans, 1964). Furthermore, protein synthesis is resistant to chloramphenicol in a mixed system of yeast ribosomes and *Escherichia coli* supernatant, but not in one of *E. coli* ribosomes and yeast supernatant (So and Davie, 1963). These data imply that the site of action of chloramphenicol is on the ribosome, where the drug inhibits peptide bond formation. Studies on the effect of chloramphenicol on ribosomes *in vitro* showed the following: (1) there is one preferential binding site for chloramphenicol (and for monoiodoamphenicol as well) on the large subunit of the ribosome (Vazquez, 1964; Fernandez-Munoz *et al.*, 1971); (2) binding of 3'-terminal fragments of aminoacyl-tRNA, such as C-A-C-C-A (Leu), to ribosomes is inhibited by chloramphenicol, whereas binding of 3'-terminal fragments of peptidyl-tRNA is not (Pestka, 1969; Celma, Monro and Vazquez, 1971; Fernandez-Munoz *et al.*, 1971); (3) puromycin and chloramphenicol prevent each other from binding to the ribosome. The binding sites, however, are not identical, since the type of inhibition is non-competitive

(Fernandez-Munoz et al., 1971; Vazquez, 1974). Apparently, these data clearly indicate that chloramphenicol binds in the A-site of the ribosomal peptidyl-transferase centre and, thereby, inhibits peptide bond formation.

This notion is illustrated in Fig. 10.2, which summarises the general mode of action of chloramphenicol in protein synthesis. It should be pointed out that Fig. 10.2 does not imply a direct interference of chloramphenicol with transpeptidation, as is the case for puromycin. There are two alternatives which should be kept in mind for a further discussion of the mode of action of chloramphenicol: (1) inhibition or disturbance of functional attachment of the aminoacyl end of aminoacyl-tRNA could account for inhibition of peptide bond formation; (2) chloramphenicol does not directly block transpeptidation but inhibits the conversion of peptidyl-tRNA into the puromycin-susceptible donor state (Weber and DeMoss, 1969).

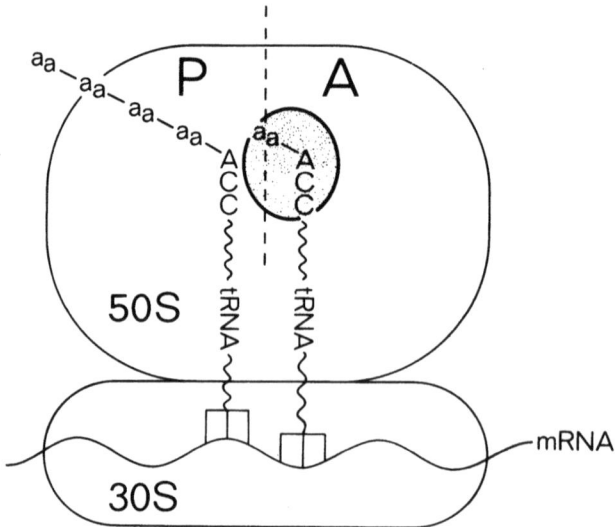

Figure 10.2 Illustration of the general mode of action of chloramphenicol on the ribosome. 'A' represents the puromycin-resistant tRNA binding site of the ribosome and 'P' the puromycin-sensitive tRNA binding site. The encircled shaded area indicates the site where chloramphenicol probably interferes with accommodation of aminoacyl-tRNA and with transpeptidation. For a further discussion see text

Experiments whose results are summarised in Table 10.1 show that the effect of chloramphenicol on polynucleotide-directed protein synthesis is a function of template used. Polypeptide synthesis directed by poly(U) is substantially more resistant to the action of chloramphenicol than is peptide synthesis directed by poly(A) or by phage mRNA. About a 150-fold higher concentration of chloramphenicol is needed to significantly inhibit poly(U)-dependent polyphenylalanine synthesis as compared with phage mRNA synthesis. It is interesting to

Table 10.1 Chloramphenicol inhibition of *in vitro* polypeptide synthesis as a function of template

Template	Concentration (μM) of chloramphenicol causing an inhibition of 50%
poly (A)	15
poly(C)	3
poly(U)	1000
f2 mRNA	6

Values represent averages from various published data (Vazquez, 1964; Pestka, 1971; Hahn and Gund, 1975; Pongs *et al.*, 1975)

compare these inhibition data with the binding constant of chloramphenicol to *E. coli* 70 S ribosomes. This binding constant is 2×10^{-6} M at 0°C (Fernandez-Munoz *et al.*, 1971), which corresponds to a binding constant of about 10^{-5} M at 37°C. This value is not compatible with the *in vitro* inhibition data reported in Table 10.1. A concentration of 3×10^{-6} M is sufficient to reduce poly(C)-directed polyproline synthesis by 50 per cent. This concentration is about one order of magnitude below the apparent binding constant of chloramphenicol to 70 S ribosomes in the absence of mRNA and tRNA. On the other hand, a 10^{-3} M concentration of chloramphenicol is needed to reduce poly(U)-directed polyphenylalanine synthesis by 50 per cent. This is a concentration which is about two orders of magnitude higher than the apparent binding constant of chloramphenicol. Therefore one has to conclude that *in vitro* studies on the receptor site of chloramphenicol should be interpreted with some caution, if they were carried out with 70 S ribosomes in the absence of mRNA, tRNA and factors. Furthermore, the data suggest either that the action of chloramphenicol at its receptor site strongly depends on the nature of the aminoacyl-tRNA present in the ribosomal A-site or that certain aminoacyl-tRNAs compete much more efficiently than others with chloramphenicol for its receptor site on the ribosome. The former point of view is favoured by the author for the following reasons.
(1) The receptor site of chloramphenicol is apparently different in the presence and absence of mRNA/tRNA (*vide supra*). (2) Chloramphenicol prevents polysome breakdown (Das, Goldstein and Kanner, 1966). (3) Monoiodoamphenicol-labelled 70 S ribosomes are completely inactive for f2 mRNA-directed synthesis, but are still active with respect to poly(U)-directed polyphenylalanine synthesis (Pongs *et al.*, 1975). Thus monoiodoamphenicol-labelled 70 S ribosomes also exhibit the peculiar template-dependent activities that ribosomes do in the presence of chloramphenicol. (4) Affinity labelling studies on the chloramphenicol receptor site of 70 S ribosomes yield different results *in vitro* and *in vivo* (Pongs and Messer, 1976).

In summary, it is proposed that the chloramphenicol receptor site is near the ribosomal site which binds aminoacyl-tRNA in the peptidyltransferase centre of the ribosome. The receptor site, however, is not *identical* with this particular active site of the ribosome. On the other hand, occupation of the receptor by the drug leads to an inhibition of functional attachment of aminoacyl-tRNA in the ribosomal A-site and, thereby, to an inhibition of transpeptidation. The degree of this inhibition apparently depends on the specific situation on each ribosome during protein synthesis. This would mean that inhibition of protein synthesis by chloramphenicol is not a straightforward all-or-none process, since bound Phe-tRNA^{Phe}, for instance, makes ribosomes more resistant to chloramphenicol than other aminoacyl-tRNAs. In the extreme case, this could lead to a situation where some ribosomes are susceptible to the action of chloramphenicol and others are not. Such a case will be actually discussed below for the action of monoiodoamphenicol *in vivo*.

MOLECULAR NATURE OF THE CHLORAMPHENICOL RECEPTOR SITE *IN VITRO*

So far, attempts have not been successful to isolate chloramphenicol-resistant strains of *E. coli* in which resistance resides in an altered ribosome structure. Therefore studies on the molecular nature of the chloramphenicol receptor site were confined to biochemical means. Two main experimental techniques have been applied, so far, to study the chloramphenicol receptor site of the *E. coli* ribosome. Ribosomal proteins can be split off from ribosomes by incubation with LiCl (Homann and Nierhaus, 1971). Incubation of 70 S ribosomes with 0.8 M LiCl yields proteindeficient ribosomal core particles and a corresponding split protein fraction (Nierhaus and Nierhaus, 1973). These ribosomal core particles have lost their ability to bind chloramphenicol, but have retained their ability to bind the 3'-terminal fragment of peptidyl-tRNA C-A-C-C-A (*N*-acetyl-Leu). This is a clear indication that chloramphenicol does not bind in the ribosomal P-site as has been recently proposed (Hahn and Gund, 1975). Rebinding of proteins L6, L11 and L16 to these ribosomal core particles restores the chloramphenicol receptor site (Nierhaus and Nierhaus, 1973). If protein L16 alone is rebound to the core particles, chloramphenicol binding is already significantly stimulated. Similar experiments with protein L6 or with protein L11 did not give comparable results. These observations suggest that protein L16 is intimately involved in the chloramphenicol receptor site and that proteins L6 and L11 are less so. However, reconstitution experiments are hampered by the fact that it is difficult in these experiments to distinguish between direct and indirect effects. Thus it is not clear whether protein L16 is an integral part of the chloramphenicol receptor site or whether it merely generates a conformation of the ribosome which in turn restores the chloramphenicol receptor site.

One way out of this ambiguity is to undertake affinity labelling studies of the chloramphenicol receptor site. As already pointed out, the dichloroacetyl moiety of chloramphenicol can be readily replaced by a variety of substituents. One such replacement is that by iodoacetyl, which yields monoiodoamphenicol (Bald et al., 1972). Another similar one is that by bromoacetyl, which yields monobromamphenicol (Sonenberg, Wilchek and Zamir, 1973). (The latter compound, somewhat erroneously, is often referred to in the literature as bromamphenicol.) Both chloramphenicol analogues have in common the fact that they possess chemically reactive α-haloacetyl side-chains. Accordingly, they were used as affinity probes of the ribosomal receptor site (Sonenberg et al., 1973; Pongs et al., 1973).

Since it had to be established that monoiodoamphenicol was a true analogue of chloramphenicol, its general mechanism of action was compared with that of chloramphenicol (Pongs et al., 1975; Pongs and Messer, 1976). Similar concentrations of monoiodoamphenicol and of chloramphenicol inhibit cell growth of E. coli. Addition of monoiodoamphenicol to cell cultures of E. coli results in an immediate cessation of protein synthesis, whereas DNA synthesis remains unaffected. In vitro, monoiodoamphenicol binds to 70 S ribosomes. Its binding constant is about one order of magnitude lower than that of chloramphenicol (Pongs et al., 1973). Equilibrium dialysis experiments showed that chloramphenicol as well as lincomycin compete with monoiodoamphenicol for the same binding site. Furthermore, monoiodoamphenicol inhibits f2mRNA- and poly(U)-dependent polypeptide synthesis like chloramphenicol (Pongs et al., 1975). All these data together clearly indicate that monoiodoamphenicol can be regarded as a sensible affinity probe of the chloramphenicol receptor site.

Fewer studies have been carried out with monobromamphenicol. Its binding and reaction with ribosomes was mainly studied with 50 S subunits, where a strong competition between chloramphenicol and monobromamphenicol was not apparent (Sonenberg et al., 1973). In this context, it should be noted that the affinity of monoiodoamphenicol as well as of chloramphenicol is one order of magnitude higher to 70 S ribosomes than to 50 S subunits. This indicates either that upon dissociation of ribosomes into subunits the conformation of the chloramphenicol receptor site becomes altered or that the 30 S subunit contributes a share to the receptor site.

The above experiments established that monoiodoamphenicol both bound to and reacted specifically at the chloramphenicol receptor site of the ribosome. Analysis of the monoiodoamphenicol-labelled ribosomal proteins should, therefore, reveal which protein is near or at the receptor site. The results showed that the primary target of the monoiodoamphenicol-labelling reaction was protein L16 (Pongs et al., 1973). Some radioactivity of label was also detected in proteins S3, L6, L14 L24 and L26/27. Thus the labelling data indicated that monoiodoamphenicol had preferentially reacted with protein L16 of the large ribosomal subunit. This result is in very good agreement with the reconstitution experiments discussed above. It could be concluded, therefore, that protein L16 is located at the ribosomal chloramphenicol receptor site.

In recent years, considerable knowledge has been accumulated on the structure and function of the ribosome (for a recent review, see, for instance, Wittmann, 1976). This makes it possible to locate protein L16, and thus a part of the chloramphenicol receptor site, on the ribosome and to relate protein L16 to the functions of the ribosomal peptidyltransferase centre (Pongs et al., 1974). Studies with N-bromoacetyl-phenylanalyl-tRNA showed that under appropriate ionic conditions this tRNA binds to the ribosomal A-site and, thereby, reacts with protein L16 (Pellegrini, 1973). This result implies that protein L16 is part of the A-site of the ribosomal peptidyltransferase centre. Since monoiodoamphenicol also reacted with protein L16, it is concluded that the chloramphenicol receptor site is indeed at the ribosomal A-site.

Binding of bromoacetyl-phenylalanyl-tRNA or of p-nitrophenyl-carbamyl-phenylalanyl-tRNA in the P-site leads to labelling of protein L27 plus the additional proteins L2, L16 and L14 as major products (Oen et al., 1973; Czernilofsky et al., 1974). These data indicate that protein L16 is located in the peptidyltransferase centre such that it can not only be labelled by reactive tRNA analogues which are bound in the A-site but also by tRNA analogues which are bound in the P-site. It is interesting that proteins L14 and L27, which are among the major P-site labelled proteins, are labelled by monoiodoamphenicol to some extent (vide supra). The reaction of monobromamphenicol with 50 S subunits resulted in the preferential attachment of this label to proteins L2 and L27 (Sonenberg et al., 1973). This apparent contradiction of the monoiodoamphenicol-labelling results might be explained on the basis of the preceding data in the following way. The nature of the chloramphenicol receptor site depends considerably on the incubation conditions. Different mRNA templates and aminoacyl-tRNAs as well as 70 S ribosomes or 50 S subunits all exhibit different aspects of apparently one and the same receptor site. Therefore it is proposed that the receptor site is of composite nature, and does not simply consist of one protein.

If one considers the available information on the composition of the peptidyltransferase centre as summarised in Fig. 10.3, the complex nature of the chloramphenicol receptor site becomes more apparent. Protein L16 should be very close to proteins L2 and L27 as well as to proteins L6 and L11. Alterations in the relationship of one protein to another as well as conformational changes in this domain of the ribosome would be expected to have a major impact on the outcome of affinity labelling experiments. Therefore it is not inconceivable that monoiodoamphenicol and monobromamphenicol bind at exactly the same site; but the major target of one label could be a minor one of the other and vice versa. Monoiodoamphenicol labels predominantly protein L16 and to a small extent protein L27, which is one of the major proteins labelled by monobromamphenicol. All these data are only compatible with the view that the chloramphenicol receptor site is actually a domain, which covers the area of the peptidyltransferase centre, which is indicated in Fig. 10.2 and which consists of proteins L2, L11, L16 and L27 as depicted in Fig. 10.3.

Recently, outstanding topographical data on the 50 S subunit were obtained by electron microscopic studies of complexes between ribosomal subunits and specific antibody fragments against single ribosomal proteins. These data allow a more vivid illustration of the chloramphenicol receptor site as is shown in Fig. 10.4.

Determinants of protein L16 against specific antibody fragments are very close to those of proteins L7/12 and L11. As indicated in Fig. 10.4, proteins L7/12 represent the common binding site for all the translation factors, which are involved in tRNA movement on the ribosome. Protein L11, together with proteins L2, L6 and L27, belongs to the peptidyltransferase centre of the ribosome (Pongs et al., 1974).

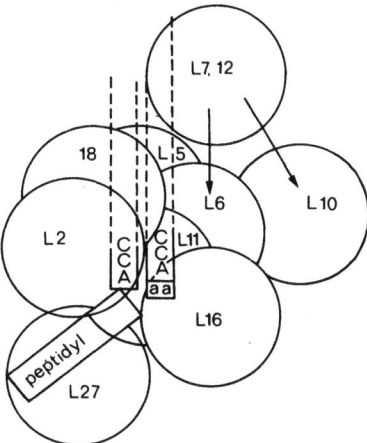

Figure 10.3 Arrangement of ribosomal proteins, 5 S RNA and tRNA in the peptidyltransferase centre of the ribosome as described by Pongs et al. (1974). Protein L16 is close to the 3'-terminal end of aminoacyl-tRNA (CCA aa) and proteins L2 and L27 are close to the 3'-terminal end of peptidyl-tRNA, For further details see text

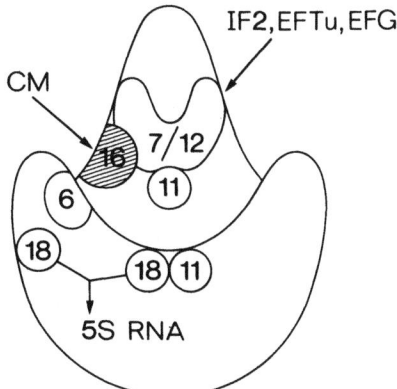

Figure 10.4 Three-dimensional model of the chloramphenicol receptor site on the 50 S ribosomal subunit, showing the location of proteins L6, L7/12, L11, L16 and L18, according to Stöffler and Tischendorf (1975). Protein L16 has been shaded as chloramphenicol binding protein in order to emphasise its proximity to proteins L7/12, the binding site of translation factors IF2, EFTu and EFG

THE CHLORAMPHENICOL RECEPTOR SITE *IN VIVO*

One might expect from the preceding discussion of *in vitro* affinity labelling experiments that addition of monoiodoamphenicol to a growing culture of *E. coli* would result in an immediate cessation of protein synthesis, whereas other macromolecular syntheses should not be directly affected. This was indeed observed (Pongs and Messer, 1976). Furthermore, it could be demonstrated that, similarly to chloramphenicol, one molecule of monoiodoamphenicol is sufficient to inhibit one ribosome.

Monoiodoamphenicol was reactive enough *in vivo* to become covalently attached to the ribosome. Moreover, it did not react with cell components other than the ribosome. Though the amount of label incorporated into ribosomal protein was proportional to the degree of inhibition of protein synthesis, more than one protein reacted with monoiodoamphenicol. Electrophoretic analyses of the proteins labelled *in vivo* led to the conclusion that predominantly an acidic protein, tentatively protein S6, and to a lesser extent two basic proteins, L16 and L24, had been labelled. Thus the *in vitro* and *in vivo* results are only compatible with respect to protein L16. Although a 1:1 stoicheiometry between label and ribosome could be deduced from the dosage-response curve, three different ribosomal proteins became labelled. This finding again suggests that the chloramphenicol receptor site is composed of more than one ribosomal protein of the peptidyltransferase centre.

Protein S6 is a fractional protein (Weber, 1972). It is readily washed off during purification of ribosomes. This might explain why *in vitro* studies with monoiodoamphenicol demonstrated proteins L16 and L24 as part of the receptor site, but not protein S6 (Pongs and Messer, 1976).

The *in vivo* affinity labelling experiments showed another interesting feature. Monoiodoamphenicol was only partially bacteriocidal. In other words, the *irreversible* inhibition (in contrast to the overall inhibition) of ribosomal protein synthesis by monoiodoamphenicol was not complete. The rate of protein synthesis after monoiodoamphenicol treatment always resumed at a rate which was 40 per cent of that of the control, even if the time of incubation of *E. coli* cells with the drug was increased up to 6 h or the concentration of the drug was raised up to 1000 μg/ml. Therefore only 60 per cent of the ribosomes in one cell were susceptible to the irreversible inhibition by monoiodoamphenicol. The kinetics of recovery of the rate of protein synthesis after monoiodoamphenicol treatment revealed another unexpected result. The rate remained constant over a period of 35 min. Thereafter it switched without any observable delay and apparently spontaneously to an exponential rate of protein synthesis which was like that of control cultures. This must mean either that new ribosomes are not synthesised prior to the observed switch or that newly synthesised ribosomes do not take part in protein synthesis before this switch occurs. Monoiodoamphenicol treatment and subsequent removal of the drug leaves 40 per cent of the total ribosomes in the cell functional. But they are now committed to synthesise protein at a constant rate. Exponential growth as well as DNA synthesis can only resume after sufficient amounts of protein have been synthesised.

In summary, the *in vivo* affinity labelling data demonstrate that the chloramphenicol receptor site consists of more than ⌄ne protein and that not all ribosomes alike are susceptible to an affinity reaction, although inhibition of protein synthesis by the drug is complete. This observation means in molecular terms that the receptor site of all ribosomes in *E. coli* is not the same. As discussed in the preceding paragraph, the actual receptor site on a ribosome is highly dependent on the momentary functional status of the ribosome in protein synthesis.

ACKNOWLEDGEMENTS

I am greatly indebted to Drs R. Bald, V. A. Erdmann, G. Stöffler and G. Wischnath, who so invaluably contributed to the research summarised in this paper. This work was supported by the Deutsche Forschungsgemeinschaft.

REFERENCES

Bald, R., Erdmann, V. A. and Pongs, O. (1972). *FEBS Lett.*, 28, 149
Celma, M. L., Monro, R. and Vazquez, D. (1971). *FEBS Lett.*, 13, 247
Controulis, M., Rebstock, M. C. and Crooks, H. M. (1949). *J. Amer. Chem. Soc.*, 71, 2458
Czernilofsky, A. P., Collatz, E. E., Stöffler, G. and Küchler, E. (1974). *Proc. Nat. Acad. Sci. U.S.A.*, 71, 230
Das, H. K., Goldstein, A. and Kanner, L. C. (1966). *Mol. Pharmacol.*, 2, 158
Fernandez-Munoz, R., Monro, R. E., Torres-Pinedo, R. and Vazquez, D. (1971). *Eur. J. Biochem.*, 23, 185
Hahn, F. E. and Gund, P. (1975). *Topics in Infectious Diseases* (ed. J. Drews and F. E. Hahn), Springer, Vienna, p. 245
Hahn, F. E., Hayes, J. E., Wisseman, C. L., Hopps, H. E. and Smadel, J. E. (1956). *Antibiot. Chemother.*, 6, 531
Hansch, C., Nakamoto, K., Gorin, M., Denisevich, P., Garrett, E. R. and Won, C. H. (1973). *J. Med. Chem.*, 16, 917
Homann, H. E. and Nierhaus, K. H. (1971). *Eur. J. Biochem.*, 20, 249
Kolosov, M. N., Shemiakin, M. M., Khokhlov, A. S. and Gurevich, A. I. (1961). *Khimia Antibiotikov* I, Iedatoto Akademii Nauk USSR
Maxwell, R. E. and Nickel, V. S. (1954). *Antibiot. Chemother.*, 4, 289
Nathans, D. (1964). *Proc. Nat. Acad. Sci. U.S.A.*, 51, 585
Nierhaus, D. and Nierhaus, K. H. (1973). *Proc. Nat. Acad. Sci. USA*, 70, 2224
Oen, H., Pellegrini, M., Eilat, D. and Cantor, C. (1973). *Proc. Nat. Acad. Sci. USA*, 70, 2799
Pellegrini, M. (1973). Ph.D. dissertation, Columbia University, New York
Pestka, S. (1969). *Proc. Nat. Acad. Sci. USA*, 64, 709
Pestka, S. (1971). *Ann. Rev. Microbiol.*, 25, 487
Pongs, O., Bald, R. and Erdmann, V. A. (1973). *Proc. Nat. Acad. Sci. USA*, 70, 2229
Pongs, O., Bald, R., Erdmann, V. A. and Reinwald, E. (1975). *Topics in Infectious Diseases* (ed. J. Drews and F. E. Hahn), Springer, Vienna, p. 179
Pongs, O., Nierhaus, K. H., Erdmann, V. A. and Wittmann, H. G. (1974). *FEBS Lett.*, 40, S 28
Pongs, O. and Messer, W. (1976). *J. Mol. Biol.*, 101, 171

Rebstock, M. C., Tratton, C. D. and Bambas, L. L. (1955). *J. Amer. Chem. Soc.*, 77, 24
So, A. G. and Davie, E. W. (1963). *Biochemistry*, 2, 132
Sonenberg, N., Wilchek, M. and Zamir, A. (1973). *Proc. Nat. Acad. Sci. USA*, 70, 1423
Stöffler, G. and Tischendorf, G. W. (1975). *Topics in Infectious Diseases* (ed. J. Drews and F. E. Hahn), Springer, Vienna, p. 117
Tischendorf, G. W., Zeichhardt, H. and Stöffler, G. (1975). *Proc. Nat. Acad. Sci. USA*, 72, 4201
Vazquez, D. (1964). *Biochim. Biophys. Acta*, 114, 277
Vazquez, D. (1974). *FEBS Lett.*, Suppl. 40, 63
Weber, H. J. (1972). *Molec. Gen. Genet.*, 119, 233
Weber, M. J. and DeMoss, J. A. (1969). *J. Bacteriol.*, 97, 1099
Wittmann, H. G. (1976). *Eur. J. Biochem.*, 61, 1

11
The mechanism of cytochrome P450-catalysed drug oxidations

V. Ullrich (Department of Physiological Chemistry, University of the Saarland, Homburg-Saar, German Federal Republic)

INTRODUCTION

Most compounds involved in the metabolism of cells, organs and organisms are hydrophilic in nature, possessing polar groups capable of undergoing a variety of metabolic reactions. Lipophilic molecules, like steroids or the fat-soluble vitamins, are in the minority. These latter compounds consist, in substantial part, of aromatic or alicyclic rings and/or aliphatic side-chains. These hydrocarbon groups are metabolically rather inert and in fact only one group of enzymes, the mono-oxygenases, can attack aromatic or aliphatic C — H bonds. Mono-oxygenases use molecular oxygen and two electrons from an external donor to introduce an oxygen atom into organic substrates according to the equation (Mason, 1957):

$$RH + O_2 + DH_2 \rightarrow ROH + D + H_2O$$

where RH represents substrate and DH_2 represents reduced electron donor. Such enzymes play an important role in the formation and transformation of steroids, bile acids, amino acids or vitamins (Ullrich, 1972). Micro-organisms using lipophilic compounds as the sole carbon source rely on the presence of mono-oxygenases for the initial oxidation of the substrate to alcohols, which can be further oxidised with concomitant production of chemical energy.

In the examples discussed so far, the products of mono-oxygenation are further metabolised. In contrast, there are a number of mono-oxygenases which have as their only function the conversion of lipophilic compounds to more hydrophilic and, hence, excretable forms. This is known to occur with steroids and a large number of lipophilic compounds which are foreign to the organism and enter the body with food, by respiration or absorption through the skin. Examples of such compounds include food additives, natural plant constituents such as alkaloids or terpenes, industrial organic chemicals and an increasing number of drugs. The mono-oxygenase system responsible for the oxidation of these compounds may be regarded as a detoxifying system, since without it an accumulation of these compounds in hydrophobic parts of the body would lead to disturbances of physiological functions. The designation 'detoxifying system' should, however, be avoided, since today we know that the same system can also potentiate the toxicity of compounds, depending on their chemical structure.

Since other features of this drug mono-oxygenase system are also rather unusual, its nature and mechanism of action have elicited considerable interest. It is the purpose of this contribution to summarise the current results and ideas on the mechanism and to relate them to pharmacological, toxicological and even medical problems involved in drug metabolism.

THE OCCURRENCE AND THE STRUCTURE OF THE DRUG MONO-OXYGENASE SYSTEM

According to an earlier hypothesis by Brodie, Gillette and LaDu (1958), only terrestrial animals were thought to require the enzymic outfit for the oxidation of lipophilic compounds, since they are preferentially exposed to these chemicals. Since then corresponding activities have also been detected in fish (Pedersen, Hershberger and Juchau, 1974), and in view of the contamination of surface water it is not surprising that even marine species contain activities. Table 11.1 lists a number of species from the North Sea in which mono-oxygenase activities could be detected. As a test the O-dealkylation of the fluorogenic substrate 7-ethoxycoumarin was used (Ullrich and Weber, 1972). From the organs tested only the hepatopancreas and the small intestine showed O-dealkylation activity. In higher animals and in man the liver contains the highest drug mono-oxygenase activity. Small intestine (Wattenberg, Leong and Strand, 1962; Lehrmann, Ullrich and Rummel, 1973) contains considerably less, but when calculated on the basis

Table 11.1 O-Dealkylation activity for 7-ethoxycoumarin in organ homogenates of various marine species

Species	Organ	Specific activity (nmol/mg protein)
Myoxocephalus scorpius	liver	0.21
	intestine	0.60
Zoarces viviparus	liver	0.08
Carcinus maenas	hepatopancreas	0.04
	intestine	0.02
Eupagurus bernhardus	hepatopancreas	0.06
Buccinium undatum	hepatopancreas	0.11
Ciona intestinalis	hepatopancreas	0.014

After preparation the organs were immediately homogenised and the mixture was passed through a gauze cloth. The values represent averages of 3–4 preparations.

of the single cell, the activity of the intestinal mucosal cell is comparable to that of the hepatocyte. Lung (Wattenberg and Leong, 1965) and skin (Alvares et al., 1973) are also active, but heart and brain are not. This is demonstrated in Table 11.2 for the different organs of mice by measuring the O-dealkylation activity in total homogenates. It is evident that only those organs which are considered by the pharmacologist as the 'ports of entry' of foreign compounds into the organism contain activity.

Table 11.2 Organ distribution of 7-ethoxycoumarin O-dealkylation activity in the mouse

Organ	Activity per organ (nmol min^{-1})	% of total activity
Liver	147	86.5
Small intestine	15	8.5
Skin	7	4
Lung	0.7	1
Kidney	0.1	0.1
Brain	0	0
Heart	0	0

The activity was determined fluorometrically in organ homogenates as described by Ullrich and Weber (1972), except for small intestine and skin, which were incubated in substrate solution for 10 min. By surface reflectance fluorimetry it was established that the reaction was linear with time. The umbelliferone formed was eluted from the tissue by ether extraction.

The intracellular localisation has invariably been in the endoplasmic reticulum membranes. These membranes contain a cytochrome which, from its unusual carbon monoxide complex, has been termed cytochrome P450 (Omura and Sato, 1964). The same cytochrome had been identified as the oxygen and substrate binding component from steroid hydroxylases (Estabrook, Cooper and Rosenthal, 1963) and it is now established that it also has the same function in the drug mono-oxygenase system. The transfer of the electrons is mediated by an FAD- and FMN-containing NADPH-dependent reductase (Iyanagi and Mason, 1973), and by recombination of these two components the drug mono-oxygenase activity could be reconstituted (Lu, Junk and Coon, 1969; Strobel et al., 1970).

One of the most interesting aspects of cytochrome P450 is its broad substrate specificity. In view of the almost endless number of lipophilic chemicals, the question arose whether all compounds are metabolised by a simple cytochrome P450 or whether a variety of specific enzymes exist. There was already evidence from various research groups that pretreatment of animals with drugs which could act as inducers of the mono-oxygenase system leads to changes in the liver microsomal fractions with respect to activities towards, several substrates as well as in the product patterns (Conney et al., 1969; Frommer et al., 1972; Kuntzman, 1969).

Table 11.3 Effect of inhibitors on the O-dealkylation activity for 7-ethoxycoumarin in rat liver microsomes after various pretreatments

Pretreatment	Specific activity	% Inhibition by		
		Metyrapone (2×10^{-5} M)	Naphthoflavone (2×10^{-5} M)	Tetrahydrofuran (10^{-2} M)
None (controls) ♂	0.7 ± 0.2	52 ± 10	10 ± 5	15 ± 6
None (controls) ♀	0.4 ± 0.2	5 ± 3	12 ± 5	48 ± 20
Phenobarbital (3 d)	2.2 ± 0.6	72 ± 12	7 ± 5	4 ± 2
3,4-Benzpyrene (2 d)	5.4 ± 2.0	2 ± 5	90 ± 6	2 ± 5
Ethanol (20 d)	0.9 ± 0.2	7 ± 3	10 ± 5	79 ± 10

Data are taken from Ullrich et al. (1975). The specific activity is expressed as nmol (mg protein)$^{-1}$ min^{-1}.

For the substrate 7-ethoxycoumarin, we could show that after various pretreatments the activity could be inhibited differently by the three compounds metyrapone, naphthoflavone and tetrahydrofuran (Ullrich, Weber and Wollenberg, 1975) (Table 11.3). The observed differences in the pattern of inhibition do not accord with the presence of only one species of cytochrome P450 fractions in liver microsomes and revealed that even up to seven species may be present (Welton and Aust, 1974; Haugen, van der Hoeven and Coon, 1975). According to our results, 7-ethoxycoumarin is a substrate for at least three forms of cytochrome P450. Thus we would suggest that the different forms have an overlapping substrate specificity but show a preference for certain groups of compounds. Thus the 3,4-benzpyrene-induced cytochrome P450 (or P448) shows greater activity towards aromatic compounds, phenobarbital-induced cytochrome P450 towards aliphatic compounds (Ullrich, 1968; Frommer, Ullrich and Staudinger, 1970) and ethanol-induced cytochrome P450 possibly for more hydrophilic compounds such as ethers or alcohols.

The use of inhibitors provides a convenient test for the presence of the multiple forms. If one applies these inhibitors to the study of the drug mono-oxygenase activity in human liver biopsies the results given in Table 11.4 are obtained. Although it is not established and even unlikely that the cytochrome P450 species in humans are identical with those in rats, the different patterns of inhibition in the various patients indicate that many cytochrome P450 species must also exist in humans. There is not yet a clear-cut answer with regard to the biological signi-

Table 11.4 O-Dealkylation activities for 7-ethoxycoumarin in human liver needle biopsies

Patient (sex)	Age	Specific activity	Metyrapone	% Inhibition by Tetrahydrofuran	Naphthoflavone
S., T. (m)	32	0.10	27	52	16
L., E. (f)	47	0.12	37	38	10
A., E. (m)		0.12	33	42	32
Z., A. (f)	55	0.00	–	–	–
B., E. (f)	63	0.10	22	25	33
R., R. (f)	25	0.02	0	100	0
M., M. (m)	21	0.15	27	51	31
R., G. (m)	30	0.35	16	41	0
B., H. (m)	38	0.04	28	70	46
S., K. (f)	70	0.14	33	34	84
C., P. (m)	47	0.30	30	28	22
C., K. (m)	57		48	52	27
Z., J. (m)	20	0.13	20	35	95
F., K. (m)	29	0.04	10	67	17
S., K. (m)	41	0.05	22	44	19
F., H. (m)	40	0.04	15	80	33
K., A. (m)	63	0.02	0	10	72
B., J. (m)		0.03	39	50	0
W., A. (m)	66	0.02	5	25	70

The activity is expressed as nmol umbelliferone formed per mg of protein per minute in a 500 g supernatant. The fluorometric assay was performed in a microcuvette of 0.1 ml volume (Ullrich and Weber, unpublished).

ficance of the multiple forms, but as a general rule one can assume that higher affinities for a substrate can only be achieved by increasing the substrate specificity of an enzyme. Since the efficacy of cytochrome P450 in metabolising foreign compounds is directly related to its affinity, it is apparent that a multiplicity of this cytochrome represents an evolutionary advantage. The existence of various forms of cytochrome P450 explains the different patterns of metabolites in microsomes from different origins or the multiphasic kinetic behaviour, but it does not appear to affect the mechanism of the system, which seems to be identical for all cytochromes P450.

THE MECHANISM OF CYTOCHROME P450 CATALYSIS

The Substrate Binding Reaction

In general, enzyme catalysis starts with the formation of an enzyme–substrate complex. This was also established for cytochrome P450 by spectroscopic studies on the interaction of substrates with the oxidised cytochrome. Additions of lipophilic compounds result in spectral changes which are characterised by a shift of the

Soret absorption band around 420 nm to a new absorption at about 390 nm (Remmer et al., 1966) The dissociation constant characterising this spectral change corresponded to the K_m of the mono-oxygenation reaction (Schenkman, Remmer and Estabrook, 1967), in accordance with the classical concept of enzyme – substrate complex formation. Using the soluble cytochrome P450 from camphor-oxidising bacteria as a model, it was found that the oxidised cytochrome with the 420 nm Soret band is a low-spin complex, whereas the 390 nm absorbing species is also ferric cytochrome P450 but in a high-spin state (Peisach and Blumber, 1970). This was also confirmed in microsomes but only about 30 per cent of the cytochrome P450 reacted with the substrate cyclohexane (Waterman, Ullrich and Estabrook, 1973), as a consequence of the heterogeneity of cytochrome P450. Recent work on model complexes has further characterised the enzyme – substrate complex as a five-coordinated complex, whereas the 420 nm species is a hexa-coordinated complex (Koch et al., 1975). The ligand in the fifth position is probably a sulphide group from a cysteinyl residue in the apoprotein, whereas the sixth ligand in the substrate-free cytochrome may be a water molecule (Griffin and Peterson, 1975). The mercaptide ligand would be unique for a haemoprotein and could explain many of the unusual spectral properties of cytochrome P450.

In view of this coordination chemistry, the substrate binding reaction can be formulated as shown in Fig. 11.1

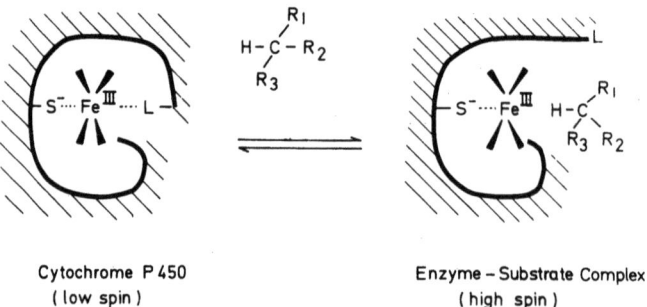

Cytochrome P 450   Enzyme – Substrate Complex
(low spin)   (high spin)

Figure 11.1 Scheme for substrate binding to cytochrome P450

The Reduction of the Enzyme – Substrate Complex

Oxygen can bind only to the ferrous cytochrome P450, and, hence, the reduction of the ferric cytochrome P450 – substrate complex is a very important stage in the reaction sequence. The enzymatic reduction of cytochrome P450 can be monitored by the formation of its carbon monoxide complex at 450 nm (Gigon, Gram and Gillette, 1969). These reduction kinetics are biphasic and consist of a fast phase, which corresponds to the reduction of the enzyme – substrate complex, and a slow phase representing the reduction of free cytochrome (Diehl, Schädelin and Ullrich 1970). In the absence of carbon monoxide (which shifts the equilibrium towards the reduced form) there seems to be hardly any electron transfer to the free cytochrome, in agreement with the very low redox potential – in the

The Mechanism of Cytochrome P450-Catalysed Drug Oxidations 207

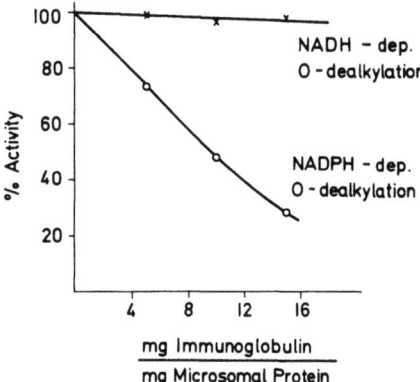

Figure 11.2 Effect of anti-(NADPH-cytochrome P450 reductase) antibody on the NADH- and NADPH-dependent O-dealkylation of 7-ethoxycoumarin in rat liver microsomes. Microsomes from phenobarbital pretreated rats were used. The antibody preparation was kindly donated by Dr Omura and prepared according to Morimoto *et al.* (1976)

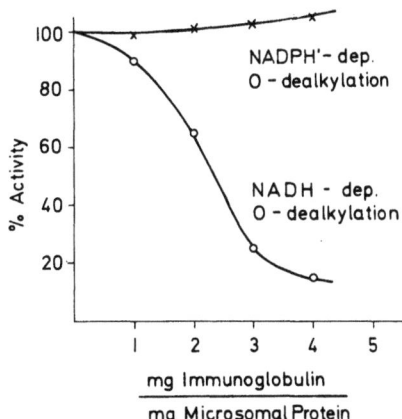

Figure 11.3 Effect of anti-(NADH-cytochrome b_5 reductase) antibody on the NADH- and NADPH-dependent O-dealkylation of 7-ethoxycoumarin in rat liver microsomes. The antibody preparation was kindly donated by Dr Omura

region of 380 mV — for low-spin cytochrome P450 (Waterman and Mason, 1970). The high-spin enzyme–substrate complex has a considerably higher potential (Wilson, Tsibris and Gunsalus, 1973), which could explain why NADPH-oxidation is greatly enhanced in the presence of substrates. The first-order rate constant for the reduction of the enzyme–cyclohexane complex has been calculated as $1.1\ \text{s}^{-1}$ by computer simulation of the reduction kinetics (Diehl *et al.*, 1970). This

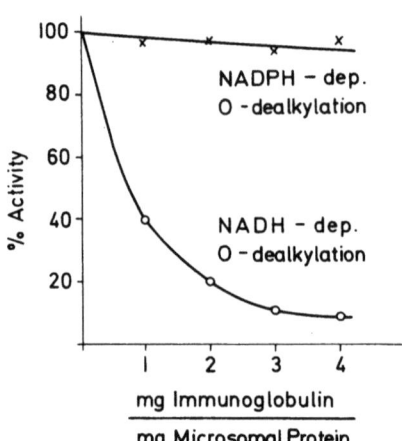

Figure 11.4 Effect of anti-(cytochrome b_5) antibody on the NADH- and NADPH-dependent O-dealkylation of 7-ethoxycoumarin in rat liver microsomes. The antibody preparation was kindly donated by Dr Omura and was prepared according to Mannering, Kuwahara and Omura (1974)

is supported by the finding that increasing the electron flow to the cytochrome by providing a second pathway involving NADH increases the hydroxylation rate (Staudt, Lichtenberger and Ullrich, 1974). The electron transport chain from NADH does not involve the NADPH-cytochrome P450 reductase but rather NADH-cytochrome b_5 reductase and cytochrome b_5. This could be established by the use of antibodies, as shown in Figs. 11.2 - 11.4. The coordination chemistry of the reduced cytochrome is less well known, since electron paramagnetic resonance (EPR) is not applicable to ferrous complexes. Since the mercaptide anion is expected to complex less well to ferrous iron than to ferric iron, the reduced enzyme-substrate complex may possibly contain a sulphydryl group at the fifth coordination position. (Fig. 11.5).

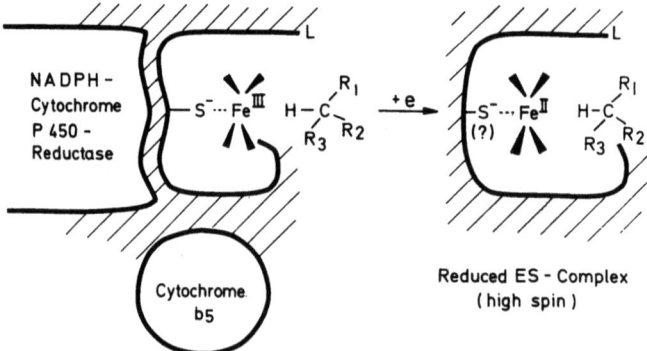

Figure 11.5 Scheme for the reduction of the cytochrome P450-substrate complex

The Oxygen Activation Process

A coordinatively unsaturated ferrous cytochrome can be expected to add oxygen in a very rapid reaction to yield an oxy complex. This has been found with cytochrome P450 from camphor-grown bacteria (Gunsalus, 1970; Ishimura, Ullrich and Peterson, 1971) but not yet with microsomal cytochrome P450, although a 440 nm band in a difference spectrum has been attributed to an oxy complex by Estabrook and associates (Estabrook et al., 1971). The spectral and magnetic properties of the oxy complex are almost identical with those of oxy-haemoglobin and oxy-myoglobin. Certainly, the bound oxygen molecule in these species cannot be regarded as sufficiently activated to hydroxylate C — H bonds. The actual activation process occurs by transfer of a second electron to the oxy complex. Details of this reaction are not yet known and only indirect evidence has been accumulated for the structure of the active oxygen. From its chemical reactivity an oxenoid structure is very likely (Ullrich and Staudinger, 1968). This term characterises a complex which can transfer an oxygen atom with strongly electrophilic properties to an acceptor molecule. Since peracids are known to exhibit very similar properties to those of the enzymic active oxygen of monooxygenases, a peroxide structure was discussed (Ullrich and Staudinger, 1968). On the other hand the O — O bond may be liable enough to undergo proton-catalysed splitting with formation of water and a ferric oxygen atom complex, in which higher oxidation states of iron may participate in the stabilisation of the oxygen atom (Fig. 11.6).

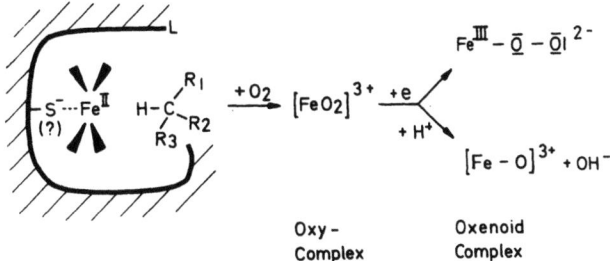

Oxy-   Oxenoid
Complex   Complex

Figure 11.6 Scheme for the oxygen activation reaction of cytochrome P450

Recent approaches towards the elucidation of the structure of active oxygen have been based on the use of oxidising agents as substitutes for molecular oxygen and NADPH. Thus it was found that cytochrome P450 can catalyse hydroxylations by using cumene hydroperoxide as a source of active oxygen (Rahimtula and O'Brien, 1974). Unfortunately, this experiment does not allow discrimination between the two postulated structures. Certain steroid hydroxylations in liver microsomes can be mediated in the presence of periodate (Hrycay et al., 1975), which indeed favours the $[FeO]^{3+}$ structure, but it is not clear whether periodate oxidises the iron to the pentavalent state or whether periodate serves as an oxygen atom donor for the ferric cytochrome P450. Drug hydroxylations are not catalysed by this compound (V. Ullrich, unpublished). The latter mechanism has been proposed for a mono-oxygenation that we observed with iodosobenzene (Lichtenberger, Nastainczyk and Ullrich, 1976). In the presence of this compound cytochrome P450 could catalyse the hydroxylation of cyclohexane and the O-dealkylation of 7-ethoxycoumarin. These reactions showed similar affinity differences for the various cytochrome P450 species to those of the oxygen- and NADPH-dependent reaction, so the active site of the cytochrome must be involved. The simplest explanation for the action of iodosobenzene would be that it is able to transfer its oxygen atom to the substrate via cytochrome P450.

The Oxygen Atom Transfer Reaction

In contrast to the high substrate and product specificities of some cytochrome P P450-dependent steroid hydroxylases, the mono-oxygenation of drugs usually leads to several products. Generally it can be concluded that the product pattern formed is the result of the attack by an electrophilic oxygen species on the substrate. Hydroxylating model systems such as trifluoroperacetic acid lead to a product pattern very similar to that of the enzymatic reactions (Ullrich et al., 1967; Frommer and Ullrich, 1971), indicating that with small substrate molecules steric factors do not greatly influence the product distribution. This situation changes if larger molecules are used as substrates. In this case the pattern of products is even altered when microsomes induced by different pretreatments are used (Conney et al., 1969). The last step in the reaction sequence which completes the cycle can be formulated as shown in Fig.11.7.

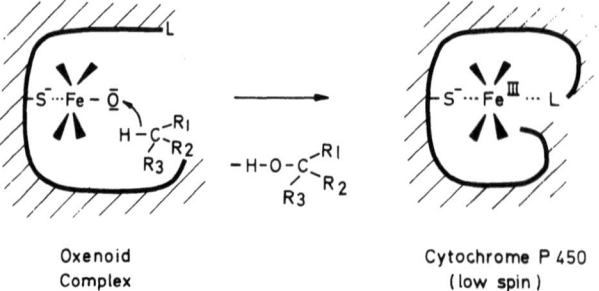

Oxenoid Complex   Cytochrome P 450 (low spin)

Figure 11.7 Scheme for the oxygen atom transfer from the oxenoid complex of cytochrome P450 to the substrate

THE FORMATION OF TOXIC METABOLITES

Alcohols and phenols are the most common products of the mono-oxygenation reaction. Very often, however, the oxygen atom transfer leads to unstable intermediates which can undergo subsequent reactions. Examples are the dealkylation of alkyl groups at heteroatoms, which are believed to proceed via hydroxylations at the α-carbon atom. Phenols may often, if not always, be products of rearrangements of arene oxide intermediates (Jerina et al., 1968) and arene oxides may be isolated only if the rearomatisation energy is low enough. Since arene oxides are rather reactive electrophiles, further reactions with water by formation of dihydrodiols or with glutathione to form conjugates may occur. Under certain conditions even reactions with thiol groups of proteins or amino groups of nucleic acids resulting in covalent binding of the metabolites may take place (Waterfall and Sims, 1973). Such a chemical alteration of nucleic acids may lead to mutagenesis or carcinogenesis. The effects of covalent binding to proteins are more difficult to evaluate and pathological reactions are difficult to predict.

CONCLUSIONS

The mechanism of cytochrome P450 seems to be gradually unravelling, but still a number of questions remain open. Part of these remaining problems may be interesting only to chemists, who wonder about the unique coordination chemistry of this cytochrome and the electronic structure of the oxenoid complex. The biochemists are still struggling with the isolation of the membrane-bound components and are trying to reconstitute the system. This has become considerably more complicated by the known existence of multiple forms of cytochrome P450. Also the mode of regulation of the biosynthesis of cytochrome P450 and the reductase is far from being understood. Most relevant, however, seems to be the toxification reactions which arise from the unspecificity of the system. The number of chemicals we are exposed to is increasing every day. Some of them may be reactive *per se* and can be easily identified. Many of the others seem harmless at first sight, but may be metabolised to reactive intermediates in the body, perhaps with resultant irreversible damage. Since the majority of malignant tumour growth may be traced back to environmental factors, it seems worthwhile to elucidate the mechanism of action of this cytochrome completely as a step towards understanding the relationship between the structure of a compound and its potential toxicity.

REFERENCES

Alvares, A. P., Leigh, S., Kappas, A., Levin, W. and Conney, A. H. (1973). *Drug Metab. Disposition*, 1, 386

Brodie, B. B., Gillette, J. R. and LaDu, B. N. (1958). *Ann. Rev. Biochem.*, 27, 427

Conney, A. H., Levin, W., Jacobson, M., Kuntzman, R., Cooper, D. Y. and Rosenthal, O. (1969). *Microsomes and Drug Oxidations* (ed. Gillette, Conney, Cosmides, Estabrook, Fouts and Mannering), Academic Press, New York, p. 279

Diehl, H., Schädelin, J. and Ullrich, V. (1970). *Hoppe-Seyler's Z. Physiol. Chem.*, 351, 1359

Estabrook, R. W., Cooper, D. Y. and Rosenthal, O. (1963). *Biochem. Z.*, 338, 741

Estabrook, R. W., Hildebrandt, A. G., Baron, J., Netter, K. J. and Leibman, K. (1971). *Biochem. Biophys. Res. Commun.*, 42, 132

Frommer, U. and Ullrich, V. (1971). *Z. Naturforschg.*, 26b, 322

Frommer, U., Ullrich, V. and Staudinger, Hj. (1970). *Hoppe-Seyler's Z. Physiol. Chem.*, 351, 903

Frommer, U., Ullrich, V., Staudinger, Hj. and Orrenius, S. (1972). *Biochim. Biophys. Acta,* 280, 487
Gigon, P. L., Gram, T. E. and Gillette, J. R. (1969). *Molec. Pharmacol.,* 5, 109
Griffin, B. W. and Peterson, J. A. (1975). *J. Biol. Chem.,* 250, 6445
Gunsalus, I. C. (1970). Conference on cytochrome P450, Philadelphia
Haugen, D. A., van der Hoeven, T. A. and Coon, M. J. (1975). *J. Biol. Chem.,* 250, 3567
Hrycay, E., Gustafsson, J. A., Ingelmann-Sundberg, M. and Ernster, L. (1975). *Biochem. Biophys. Res. Commun.,* 66, 357
Ishimura, Y., Ullrich, V. and Peterson, J. A. (1971). *Biochem. Biophys. Res. Commun.,* 42, 140
Iyanagi, T. and Mason, H. S. (1973). *Biochemistry,* 12, 2297
Jerina, D., Daly, J. W., Landis, W., Witkop, B. and Udenfriend, S. (1968). *J. Amer. Chem. Soc.,* 90, 6523
Koch, St., Tang, S. C., Holm, R. H., Frankel, R. B. and Ibers, J. A. (1975). *J. Amer. Chem. Soc.,* 97, 916
Kuntzman, R. (1969). *Ann. Rev. Pharmacol.,* 9, 21
Lehrmann, Ch., Ullrich, V. and Rummel, W. (1973). *Naunyn-Schmiedeberg's Arch. Pharmacol.,* 276, 89
Lichtenberger, F., Nastainczyk, W. and Ullrich, V. *Biochem. Biophys. Res. Commun.,* 70, 939
Lu, A. Y. H., Junk, K. W. and Coon, M. J. (1969). *J. Biol. Chem.,* 244, 3714
Mannering, G. J., Kuwahara, S. and Omura, T. (1974). *Biochem. Biophys. Res. Commun.,* 57, 476
Mason, H. S. (1957). *Adv. Enzymol.,* 19, 79
Morimoto, T., Matsuura, S., Sasaki, S., Tashiro, Y. and Omura, T. (1976). *J. Cell. Biol.,* 68, 189
Omura, T. and Sato, R. (1964). *J. Biol. Chem.* 239, 2370
Pedersen, M. G., Hershberger, W. K. and Juchau, M. R. (1974). *Bull. Environment. Contam. Toxicol.,* 12, 481
Peisach, J. and Blumberg, W. E. (1970). *Proc. Nat. Acad. Sci. USA,* 67, 172
Rahimtula, A. D. and O'Brien, P. J. (1974). *Biochem. Biophys. Res. Commun.,* 60, 440
Remmer, H., Schenkman, J. B., Estabrook, R. W., Sasame, H. A., Gillette, J. R., Cooper, D. Y., Narasimhulu, S. and Rosenthal, O. (1966). *Molec. Pharmacol.,* 2, 187
Schenkman, J. B., Remmer, H. and Estabrook, R. W. (1967). *Molec. Pharmacol.,* 3, 113
Staudt, H., Lichtenberger, F. and Ullrich, V. (1974). *Eur. J. Biochem.* 46, 99
Strobel, H. W., Lu, A. Y. H., Heidema, J. and Coon, M. J. (1970). *J. Biol. Chem.,* 245, 4851
Ullrich, V. (1968). *Hoppe-Seyler's Z. Physiol. Chem.,* 350, 357
Ullrich, V. (1972). *Angew. Chem. (Int. Ed.).* 11, 701
Ullrich, V. and Staudinger, Hj. (1968). *Biochemie des Sauerstoffs* (ed. Hj. Staudinger and B. Hess), Springer, Berlin
Ullrich, V. and Weber P. (1972). *Hoppe-Seyler's Z. Physiol. Chem.,* 353, 1171
Ullrich, V., Weber, P. and Wollenberg, P. (1975). *Biochem. Biophys. Res. Commun.,* 64, 808
Ullrich, V., Wolf, J., Amadori, E. and Staudinger, Hj. (1967). *Hoppe-Seyler's Z. Physiol. Chem.,* 349, 85
Waterfall, J. F. and Sims, P. (1973). *Biochem. Pharmacol.,* 22, 2469
Waterman, M. R. and Mason, M. S. (1970). *Biochem. Biophys. Res. Commun.,* 39, 450
Waterman, M. R., Ullrich, V. and Estabrook, R. W. (1973). *Arch. Biochem. Biophys.,* 155, 355
Wattenberg, L. W. and Leong, J. L. (1965). *Fed. Proc.,* 24, 494
Wattenberg, L. W., Leong, J. L. and Strand, P. J. (1962). *Cancer Res.,* 22, 1120
Welton, A. F. and Aust, S. D. (1974). *Biochem. Biophys. Res. Commun.,* 56, 898
Wilson, G. S., Tsibris, J. C. M. and Gunsalus, I. C. (1973). *J. Biol. Chem.,* 248, 6059

12
Interaction of ouabain and cassaine with $Na^+ + K^+$ — ATPase and its relationship to their inotropic actions

Thomas Tobin (Equine Drug Research Program, Department of Veterinary Science, University of Kentucky, Lexington, Ky.) and Tai Akera (Department of Pharmacology, Michigan State University, East Lansing, Mich.)

INTRODUCTION

Sodium – potassium – activated ATPase (ATP phosphohydrolase E.C. 3.6.1.3) is a membrane-bound enzyme which is thought to be closely related to, if not identical with, the sodium pump activity of cell membranes. *In vivo*, this enzyme pumps sodium out of and potassium into the cell and it has therefore, during its transport cycle, access to both sides of the cell membrane (Post *et al.*, 1969). The transport function of $Na^+ + K^+$-ATPase is required for volume control in the cell, but it also subserves many other cellular functions (Post, 1968).

The normal reaction cycle of the sodium pump of red cell membranes is shown in Fig. 12.1. Three sodium ions are pumped out of the cell and two potassium ions are pumped into the cell with the concomitant hydrolysis inside the cell of one ATP molecule to ADP and inorganic phosphate (P_i). This reaction requires Mg^{2+} inside the cell and is specifically inhibited, from outside the cell only, by low concentrations of cardiac glycosides such as ouabain (Post, 1968).

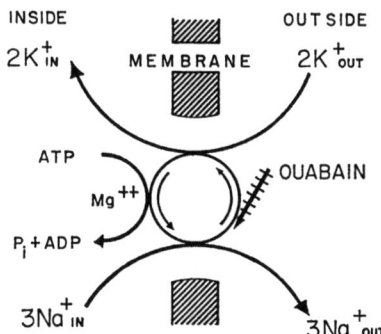

Figure 12.1 Stoicheiometry and localisation of the sodium and potassium pump in human erythrocytes. Reprinted by permission from Post (1968)

213

If cells are broken and their plasma membrane fragments isolated, this pump activity appears as a magnesium-dependent, sodium- and potassium-stimulated ATPase whose activity is specifically inhibited by cardiac glycosides such as ouabain. If these membrane fragments are incubated with Mg^{2+}, $[\gamma\text{-}^{32}P]$ ATP and 100 mM potassium ion, a slowly accumulating and stable phosphorylation of the membranes is observed (Fig. 12.2). If sodium ion is substituted for potassium ion, there is an immediate increase of about tenfold in the level of labelling of these membranes, followed by a slow increase, as before (Post, Sen and Rosenthal, 1965).

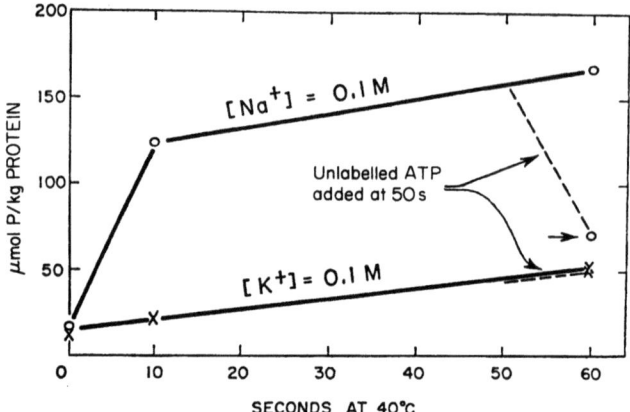

Figure 12.2 Onset and turnover of Na^+-dependent labelling of kidney membranes. The initial volume for each experiment was 1.1 ml. The reaction was started with 0.5 μmol of Mg-$[\gamma\text{-}^{33}P]$ ATP in 0.1 ml. It was stopped with acid, and radioactivity was measured in the washed precipitate. The values at zero time were determined by adding acid before $[\gamma\text{-}^{32}P]$ ATP. For two points, unlabelled MgATP, 5 μmol in 0.1 ml, was added at 50 s. This reduced the specific activity of the $[\gamma\text{-}^{32}P]$ ATP to one-eleventh of the initial value. The labelling shown by the *unmarked arrow* was calculated by adding one-eleventh of the increment in labelling at 60 s due to sodium ion to the labelling at 60 s in the presence of potassium ion. Reprinted by permission from Post *et al.* (1965)

At 0°C the Na^+-stimulated ^{32}P labelling of these membranes turns over relatively slowly, as may be demonstrated by adding unlabelled ATP to the system (Fig. 12.2). It is thus possible to directly observe the action of K^+ on it, as shown in Fig. 12.3. In this experiment, the phospho-enzyme was first formed in the presence of Na^+ and Mg^{2+} and $[\gamma\text{-}^{32}P]$ ATP, then isolated by the addition of excess cold EDTA, which blocks the Mg^{2+}-requiring phosphorylation reaction. Under these conditions the sodium-stimulated ^{32}P labelling of the membrane decays slowly with a half-life of about 8 s. If, however, a small amount of K^+ is added to the system, the rate at which the phospho-enzyme breaks down is greatly accelerated (Fig. 12.3), suggesting a potassium-accelerated dephosphorylation

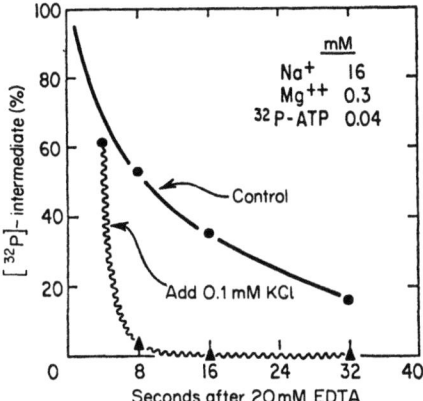

Figure 12.3 Dephosphorylation of the phosphorylated intermediate by K^+. The temperature was $0°C$. Reprinted by permission from Post (1968)

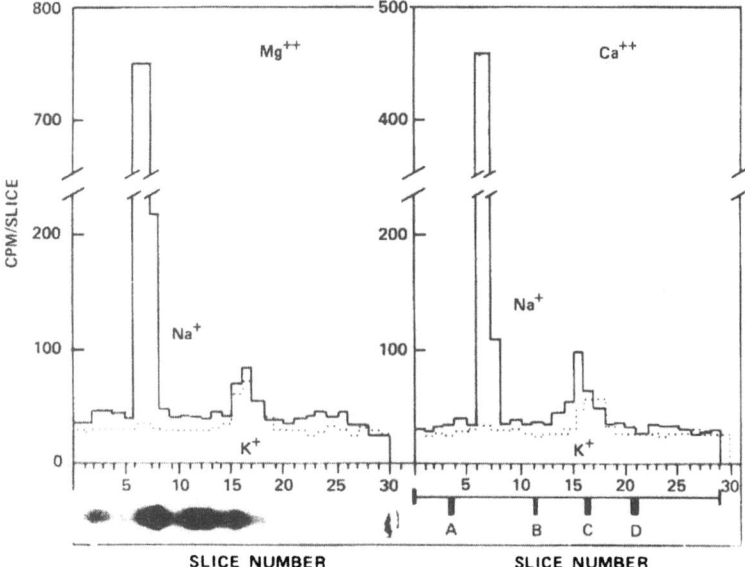

Figure 12.4 Gel electrophoresis of rat brain ATPase phosphorylated in the presence of Mg^{2+} or Ca^{2+}. Rat brain ATPase was phosphorylated by $[\gamma\text{-}^{32}P]$ ATP in the presence of 100 mM Na^+ or 100 mM K^+ and either 1 mM Mg^{2+} or 1 mM Ca^{2+}. Phosphorylation was for 5 s at $0°C$, and denaturation, washing and electrophoresis were performed as described in Tobin et al. (1975). Mg^{2+}-stimulated labelling was 500.6 pmol ^{32}P/mg protein, while Ca^{2+}-stimulated labelling was 247 pmol ^{32}P/mg protein. The solid lines show radioactivity observed in each slice when labelling was performed in the presence of Na^+, the dotted lines labelling in the presence of K^+. The lower panels show the staining patterns of the ATPase preparations (right-hand panel) or migration distances of thyroglobulin (A), ovalbumin (B), catalase (C) or lysozyme (D) standards. Reprinted by permission from Tobin et al. (1975)

(Post, 1968). Thus the experiments of Figs. 12.2 and 12.3 present evidence that the reaction cycle of Na$^+$ + K$^+$-ATPase involves a Na$^+$-stimulated phosphorylation of these membranes and a K$^+$-accelerated hydrolysis of the phospho-enzyme complex.

If membrane preparations phosphorylated in the presence of Na$^+$, Mg^{2+} and [γ-^{32}P] ATP are solubilised in sodium dodecyl sulphate (SDS) and run on acrylamide gels at pH 2.4, the material whose phosphorylation is stimulated by Na$^+$ runs as a single band with an apparent molecular weight of about 95 000 (Tobin, Akera and Brodie 1975) (Fig. 12.4). This phosphorylated material has been identified as a β-aspartyl phosphate group (Post and Orcutt, 1973). Thus the Na$^+$-stimulated phosphorylation of the plasma membrane observed in the earlier experiments appears to be associated with the phosphorylation of aspartic acid residues in membrane polypeptides of about 95 000 molecular weight. This reaction cycle is summarised in Fig. 12.5.

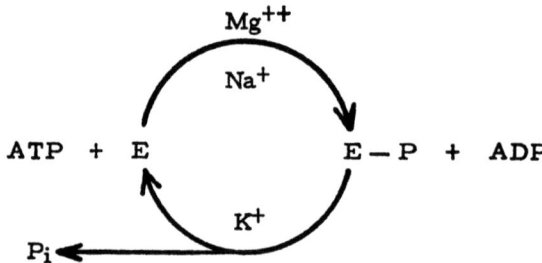

Figure 12.5 A partial reaction sequence for formation and breakdown of a phosphorylated intermediate in (Na$^+$ + K$^+$)-ATPase. Reprinted by permission from Post (1968)

THE EFFECTS OF OUABAIN

As pointed out earlier, both the sodium pump and the sodium – potassium-ATPase activity of broken membranes are very specifically inhibited by cardiac glycosides such as ouabain. The availability in the mid-1960s of [^{3}H]-ouabain made it possible to study the interaction of ouabain with this enzyme in detail. The right-hand panel of Fig. 12.6 shows an experiment in which guinea-pig kidney Na$^+$ + K$^+$-ATPase was incubated with micromolar concentrations of [^{3}H]-ouabain in the presence of Na$^+$, Mg^{2+} and various nucleotide triphosphates. In the presence of Na$^+$, Mg^{2+} and [^{3}H]-ouabain no significant binding of [^{3}H]-ouabain to these membrane preparations was observed. At indicated zero time, however, the nucleotides were added and binding commenced. In the presence of low concentrations of ATP and CTP binding increased rapidly, peaked at about two minutes, and then declined slowly. Nucleotides other than ATP and CTP were less effective in supporting [^{3}H]-ouabain binding, though ADP also supported a significant level of [^{3}H]-ouabain binding. The left-hand panel of Fig. 12.6 shows

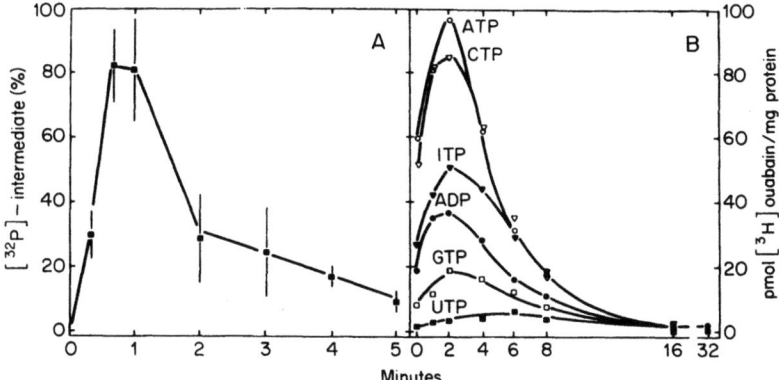

Figure 12.6 Time course of [γ-^{32}P] ATP-dependent labelling and nucleotide-supported [^{3}H]-ouabain binding to Na$^+$ + K$^+$-ATPase. (A) Guinea-pig kidney enzymes were incubated with 100 mM Na$^+$ and 5 mM Mg^{2+} at 37°C. At indicated zero time 25 μM [γ-^{32}P] ATP was added to start the labelling reaction. The reaction was stopped with trichloroacetic acid. (■-■) shows the amount of ^{32}P-labelling of the enzyme at the indicated time points. Labelling is expressed as a percentage of peak labelling for each of four different experiments which averaged 122 pmol ^{32}P/mg protein. (B) At indicated zero time the binding reaction was started by the addition of 50 μM of each of the indicated nucleotides and stopped by centrifugation at the indicated time points. The symbols show the binding of [^{3}H]-ouabain supported by each of the nucleotides with no deductions made for background labelling. Reprinted by permission from Tobin et al. (1974)

that under these conditions the phosphorylation of these membranes by [γ-^{32}P] ATP is also transient, consistent with the concept that the [^{3}H]-ouabain binding observed in Fig. 12.6 requires prior phosphorylation of the enzyme (Tobin et al., 1974).

Though the experiment of Fig. 12.6 is suggestive, there are a number of problems with the conclusion that [^{3}H]-ouabain binding in the presence of Na$^+$, Mg^{2+} and ATP requires phosphorylation of the enzyme by ATP. In the first place, with the exception of ATP, all of the nucleotides used in the experiment of Fig. 12.6 are very poor substrates for the overall Na$^+$ + K$^+$-ATPase activity. Secondly, it seems rather unlikely that the ADP-stimulated binding observed in Fig. 12.6 can be explained on the basis of a direct phosphorylation from ADP. Therefore, in an effort to resolve these discrepancies we studied the action of a non-phosphorylating analogue of ATP, β-γ-methylene ATP, on the binding of [^{3}H]-ouabain to guinea-pig kidney Na$^+$ + K$^+$-ATPase.

β,γ-Methylene ATP is an analogue of ATP in which the terminal bridge oxygen of the nucleotide molecule has been replaced by a methylene group. This analogue is structurally similar to ATP and binds to the enzyme but is not hydrolysed by it, presumably because the terminal phosphonate group cannot be transferred to the enzyme. Use of this analogue should therefore allow one to distinguish between effects due to the binding of ATP (which would be mimicked by β-γ-methylene ATP) and those due to both binding and phosphorylation as shown by authentic ATP.

The experiment of Fig. 12.7 was designed to reveal any tendency of β-γ-methylene ATP to inhibit [^{3}H]-ouabain binding to Na$^+$ + K$^+$-ATPase. Na$^+$ and Mg^{2+} were required in the system to stimulate phosphorylation by ATP. To stimulate [^{3}H]-ouabain binding to the enzyme in the presence of Na$^+$ and Mg^{2+}, 1 mM inorganic phosphate was included in the system (Tobin and Sen, 1970). Under these conditions [^{3}H]-ouabain binding equilibrated at about 40 per cent of the level observed in the presence of Na$^+$, Mg^{2+} and ATP. At 15 min this binding was challenged by the addition of either ATP or β-γ-methylene ATP. As shown in Fig. 12.7, ATP produced a prompt increase in the equilibrium level of [^{3}H]-ouabain binding, while β,γ-methylene ATP produced an equally prompt decline to zero in the equilibrium level of [^{3}H]-ouabain binding. The experiment shows that the β,γ-methylene analogue of ATP is strongly inhibitory to P_i-suppor-

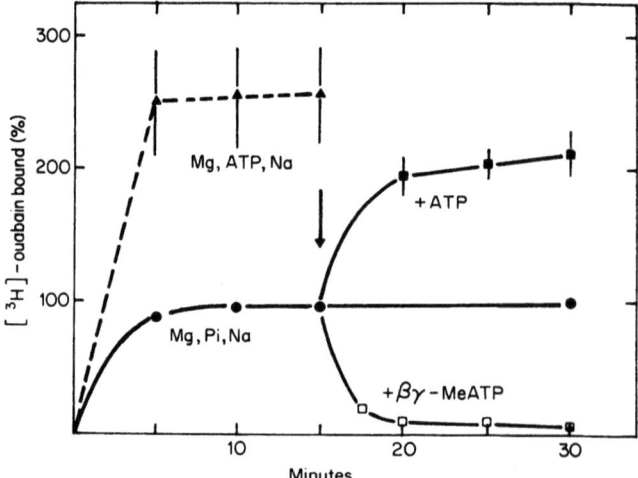

Figure 12.7 Inhibition of the equilibrium level of [^{3}H]-ouabain binding by β,γ-methylene-ATP. Guinea-pig kidney enzymes were incubated with 5×10^{-7} M [^{3}H]-ouabain at 37°C. The binding reaction was started by the addition of 4 mM Mg^{2+} at zero time and stopped at the indicated times. (●-●) shows binding in the presence of 4 mM Mg^{2+}, 1 mM P., and 60 mM Na$^+$. After 15 min, binding in the presence of Na$^+$, Mg^{2+} and P_i was challenged by the addition of 3 mM ATP (■-■) or 3 mM β,γ-methylene-ATP (□-□). (▲-▲) shows [^{3}H]-ouabain binding in the presence of 60 mM Na$^+$, 3 mM Mg^{2+} and 5 mM ATP and (♦) shows binding in the presence of 4 mM Mg^{2+}, 1 mM P_i and 2.5×10^{-4} M unlabelled ouabain. Binding in the presence of Na$^+$, Mg^{2+} and P_i at 30 min was arbitrarily taken as 100 per cent. Maximal binding (4 mM Mg^{2+}, 1 mM P_i without Na$^+$) averaged 94.2 pmol [^{3}H]-ouabain/mg protein. Reprinted by permission from Tobin et al. (1973)

ted [^{3}H]-ouabain binding. Broadly similar observations have been made with
α, β-methylene ADP and β, γ-imido ATP. These experiments are thus consistent
with the idea that in the presence of Na$^+$ and ATP phosphorylation of this
enzyme is required to support [^{3}H]-ouabain binding to these membranes
(Tobin et al., 1974).

Most of the experiments and experimental designs for the [^{3}H]-ouabain
binding experiments presented up to this point were based on the premise that
the interaction of [^{3}H]-ouabain with the cardiotonic steroid binding site of
Na$^+$ + K$^+$-ATPase was readily reversible. However, reports from other laboratories
suggested that [^{3}H]-ouabain binding, in the hands of other workers, was essentially
irreversible. This led us to examine the factors which determined the rate at
which [^{3}H]-ouabain dissociated from its binding sites on this enzyme. The first
variable that we investigated was temperature, as shown in Fig. 12.8. It turned out
that [^{3}H]-ouabain binding to guinea-pig kidney enzyme is highly temperature-
dependent, binding being relatively labile ($t_{\frac{1}{2}}$ = 3 min) at 37°C, but very stable
($t_{\frac{1}{2}}$ = 9 h) at 0°C (Tobin and Sen, 1970). This finding has turned out to be of
considerable practical importance, since it allows one to stabilise or labilise the
enzyme-ouabain complex simply by varying the temperature; this has become
an important manoeuvre in studies on the Na$^+$ + K$^+$-ATPase - ouabain interaction.

Another important variable which affects the rate of dissociation of the ouabain-
enzyme complex is the species and tissue from which the enzyme is prepared.

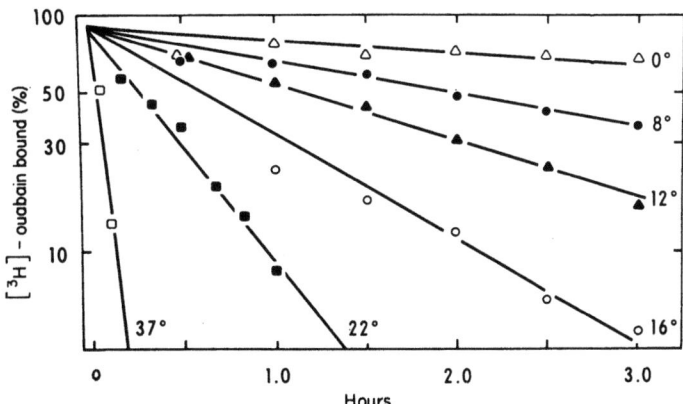

Figure 12.8 Stability of enzyme–ouabain complex at different temperatures.
Enzyme, 4 mM MgCl$_2$, 1 mM H$_3$PO$_4$ and 2.5 x 10^{-7} M [^{3}H]-ouabain were
incubated for 20 min at 37°C. The tubes were then cooled to the indicated
temperature and 10 mM EDTA and 5 x 10^{-4} M unlabelled ouabain added.
The reaction was stopped by centrifugation at the indicated time points. At
22 and 37°C only unlabelled ouabain was added. At 37°C the reaction was
stopped by rapidly freezing (20 s) the tubes in an acetone–dry ice mixture.
After thawing at 0°C, the tubes were centrifuged as before. The pH of the
system did not change (7.4 ± 0.1 pH units) with temperature. Reprinted by
permission from Tobin and Sen (1970)

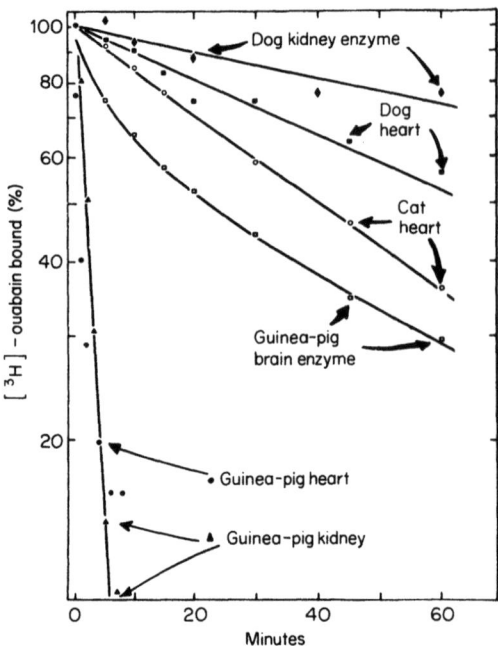

Figure 12.9 Dissociation of enzyme–ouabain complex in different tissues and species: [^{3}H]-ouabain–enzyme was formed and its dissociation followed as described by Tobin et al. (1972b). The symbols indicate the percentage of the binding at zero time in a given tissue remaining at the times indicated. The enzymes prepared from different tissues were as follows: ▲, guinea-pig kidney; ●, guinea-pig heart; ○, guinea-pig brain; ■, dog heart; ♦, dog kidney; ○, cat heart. Reprinted by permission from Tobin et al. (1972b)

Figure 12.9 shows an experiment in which we compared the rates of dissociation of [^{3}H]-ouabain from $Na^+ + K^+$-ATPase preparations from a number of tissues at 37°C. The experiment shows that [^{3}H]-ouabain dissociates rapidly and at approximately similar rates from guinea-pig heart and kidney enzymes, but more slowly from dog heart and kidney $Na^+ + K^+$-ATPases (Tobin, Henderson and Sen, 1972b; Tobin and Brody, 1972).

The observation that the rate of dissociation of [^{3}H]-ouabain from cardiac $Na^+ + K^+$-ATPase obtained from different species is variable and slow raised an interesting possibility concerning the rate of loss of ouabain-induced inotropy in certain species. The most straightforward model which one can assume for $Na^+ + K^+$-ATPase as the cardiotonic receptor for cardiac glycosides would be a simple occupancy model. If this were the case, the rates of dissociation of the ouabain–enzyme complex observed in Fig. 12.9 should be rate-limiting for the offset of ouabain-dependent inotropy in perfused hearts. From a survey of the literature it was readily apparent that ouabain-induced inotropy in guinea-pig hearts decayed at just about the same rate as [^{3}H]-ouabain binding to guinea-pig heart ATPase in the experiment of Fig. 12.9. Therefore the test of the simplest possible receptor model for the cardiotonic action of ouabain involving $Na^+ + K^+$-ATPase in perfused hearts was to determine whether the rates of dissociation observed in Fig. 12.9 are comparable with the rates of offset of inotropic responses due to ouabain.

Because Langendorff perfusion experiments are done under specific temperature and ionic conditions, we repeated the experiments of Fig. 12.9 under conditions applicable to the perfusion experiments. The data of Fig. 12.10 show that when conditions appropriate to perfusion experiments were used (temperature 27°C; binding supported by Na^+, Mg^{2+} and ATP; 5 mM K^+ present in the system; Akera et al., 1973), the rate at which [^{3}H]-ouabain dissociated from these ATPase preparations was somewhat slower than previously. However, clear

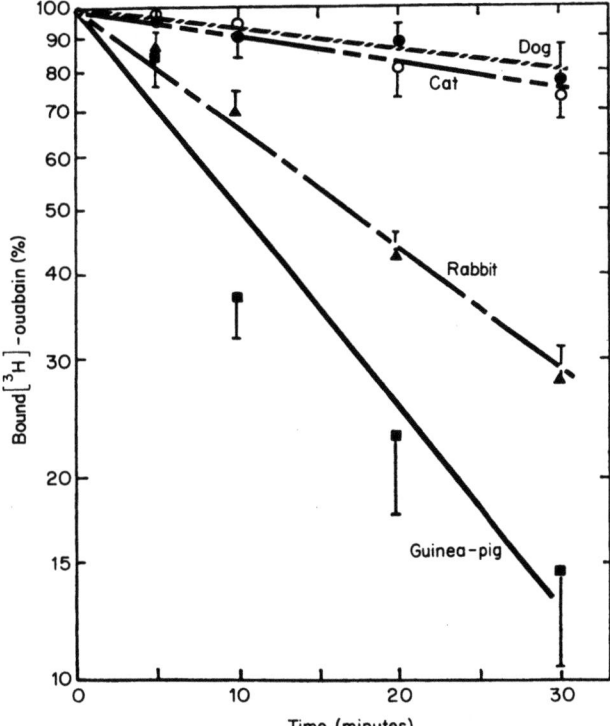

Figure 12.10 Dissociation of [^{3}H]-ouabain from cardiac $Na^+ + K^+$-ATPase in vitro at 27°C. Bound [^{3}H]-ouabain was expressed as the percentage of that immediately after the addition of unlabelled ouabain in each enzyme preparation. ●, dog; ○, cat; ▲, rabbit; and ■ guinea-pig. Each point represents the mean of five experiments. Vertical lines indicate SEM. Reprinted by permission from Akera et al. (1973)

separations in rates of dissociation from the ATPases chosen were observable, allowing comparison with inotropy decay rates (Akera et al., 1973).

Figure 12.11 shows the rates at which inotropy due to ouabain was lost in perfused guinea-pig, rabbit, kitten and puppy hearts. Inotropy was lost rapidly in the guinea-pig and rabbit hearts, consistent with the rapid dissociation of ouabain from $Na^+ + K^+$-ATPase in these tissues. Inotropy was lost relatively slowly, however, in the perfused puppy and kitten hearts, consistent with the relatively slow dissociation of $[^3H]$-ouabain from its binding sites on $Na^+ + K^+$-ATPase in these tissues. This relationship is underscored in Fig. 12.12, where the half-times for dissociation and loss of inotropy are compared. The experiment shows a good correlation between the rates of loss of inotropy and the rates of dissociation of $[^3H]$-ouabain from $Na^+ + K^+$-ATPase over the range accessible with currently

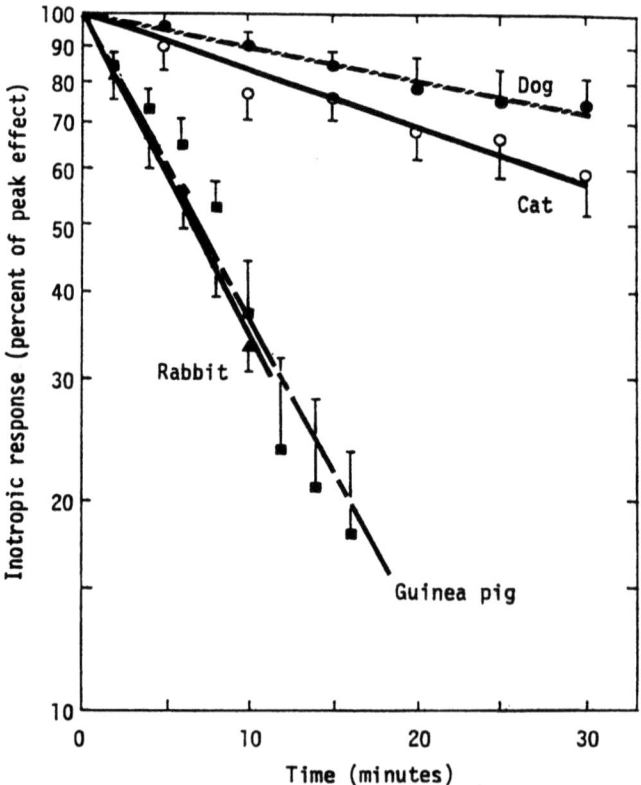

Figure 12.11 Washout of positive inotropic effect of ouabain in Langendorff preparations at 27°C. The maximal positive inotropic effect was arbitrarily set at 100 per cent. ● Dogs; ○ cats; ▲ rabbits; and ■ guinea-pigs. Each point represents the mean of four experiments. Vertical lines indicate SEM. Reprinted by permission from Akera et al. (1973)

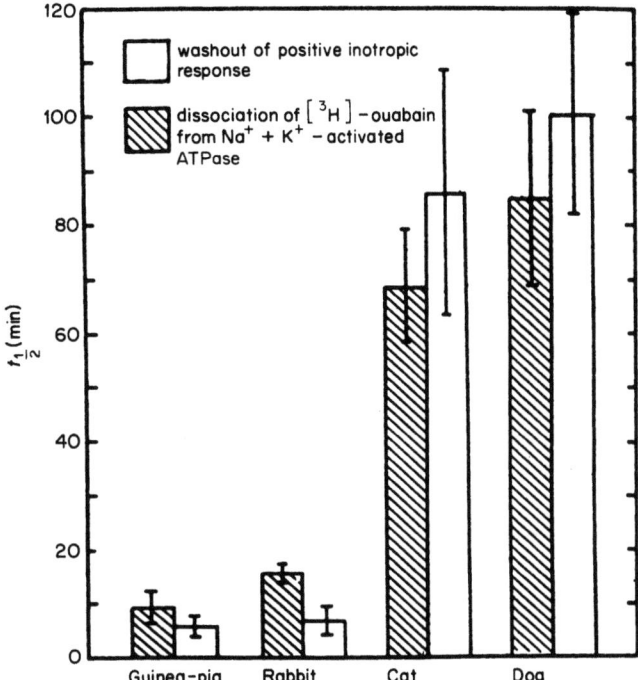

Figure 12.12 Half-times of the inotropic effect of ouabain and the dissociation of [^{3}H]-ouabain from cardiac (Na$^+$ + K$^+$)-activated ATPase at 27°C. Half-time was calculated from Fig. 12.10 and 12.11 by fitting a linear regression line to the data obtained in each experiment. Mean of four (inotropic data) and five (dissociation data) experiments in each species, respectively. Vertical lines indicate SEM. Reprinted by permission from Akera et al. (1973)

available techniques. The experiment is consistent with the concept that Na$^+$ + K$^+$-ATPase is the cardiotonic receptor for cardiac glycosides, that occupancy of the receptor is closely linked to the inotropic effect and that the rate at which glycosides dissociate from this receptor is rate-limiting for offset of the inotropic effect of these drugs (Akera et al., 1973).

Other studies in this area have shown that the time course of both onset and offset of ouabain-induced inotropy in guinea-pig heart tissue is associated with the binding and dissociation of ouabain from cardiac Na$^+$ + K$^+$-ATPase. Concomitant with these increases and decreases in ouabain binding, the ability of cardiac slices to take up ^{86}Rb is also lost and then recovered. These experiments and others (Ku et al., 1974a; Ku et al., 1975, 1976; and Post et al., 1969) comprise a substantial body of evidence which suggests that inhibition of Na$^+$ + K$^+$-ATPase by cardiac glycosides is closely linked to development of their positive inotropic effects (Akera and Brody, 1975).

THE EFFECTS OF CASSAINE

Comparative studies on the cardiac glycosides suggest the existence of several structural requirements for their cardiotonic actions. These requirements are generally considered to be a cyclopentanoperhydrophenanthrene nucleus with A/B *cis*, B/C *trans* and C/D *cis* fusion of the four-ring structure, a C_{14}-OH group and an unsaturated lactone ring in the β configuration on C17 (Kahn, VanAtta and Johnson, 1963). The erythrophleum alkaloids, however, share many of the pharmacological actions of the cardiac glycosides while satisfying none of these structural requirements (Fig. 12.13). In particular, the erythrophleum group of alkaloids are cardiotonic and cardiotoxic like the cardiac glycosides and are also specific inhibitors of monovalent cation transport and of $Na^+ + K^+$-ATPase (Bonting *et al.*, 1964; Peters, Rabin and Wasserman, 1974).

To further investigate the hypothesis that inhibition of $Na^+ + K^+$-ATPase can account for the positive inotropic effects of various groups of drugs we examined the interactions of cassaine with $Na^+ + K^+$-ATPase in some detail.

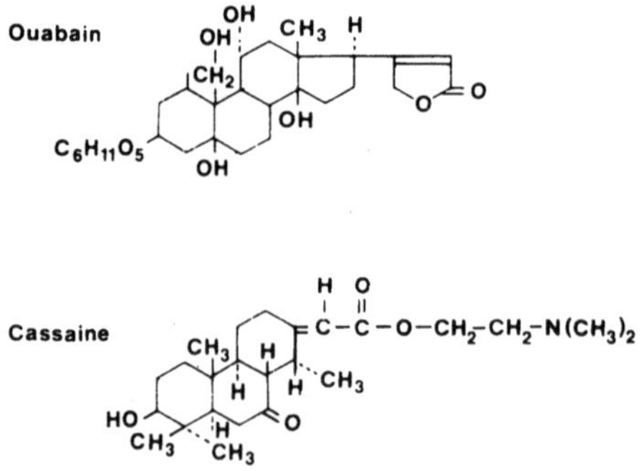

Figure 12.13 Structural formulae of ouabain and cassaine

These studies commenced with the working hypothesis that, because of the structural differences outlined, the interaction of cassaine with $Na^+ + K^+$-ATPase would be distinguishable from that of the cardiac glycosides. It was further hoped that such differences in interaction at the enzymatic level would be reflected in differences in the cardiotonic effects of cassaine. Thus, it might be possible to correlate events at the enzymatic level with those occurring at the level of the perfused heart, and these studies might provide further evidence in support of the possibility that $Na^+ + K^+$-ATPase is the positive inotropic receptor for the cardiac glycoside and erythrophleum alkaloid group of drugs.

Figure 12.14 shows inhibition of rat brain $Na^+ + K^+$-ATPase by cassaine and ouabain. In this experiment cassaine had about one-fourth of the apparent affinity of ouabain for this enzyme preparation. Further, the dotted line in Fig. 12.14 shows that preincubation of the enzyme with cassaine in the absence of K^+ does not increase the apparent affinity of cassaine for this enzyme. This

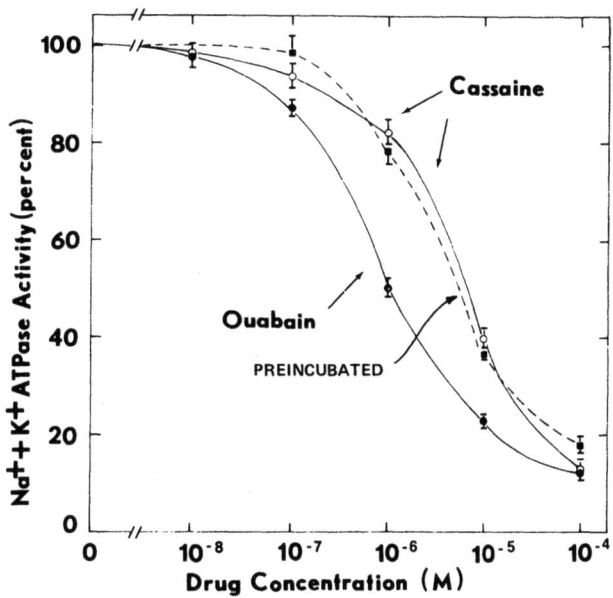

Figure 12.14 Inhibition of rat brain $Na^+ + K^+$-ATPase by ouabain and cassaine. About 30 µg of enzyme was incubated with the indicated concentrations of cassaine or ouabain in the presence of 100 mM Na^+, 15 mM K^+, 5 mM Mg^{2+} and 50 mM Tris HCl buffer, pH 7.6 at 37°C. The ATPase reaction was started by the addition of 5 mM ATP and stopped 10 min later. The solid circles (●-●) show inhibition in the presence of the indicated concentrations of ouabain, the open circles (○-○) inhibition in the presence of indicated concentrations of cassaine. The solid squares (■-■) show inhibition when the enzyme was preincubated with the indicated concentrations of cassaine, $Na^+ + K^{2+}$ and ATP for 10 min and the ATPase reaction started by adding K^+. $Na^+ + K^+$-ATPase activity is expressed as a percentage of that observed in the absence of ouabain which averaged 185.5 ± 9.0 µmol P_i/mg protein/h. Reprinted by permission from Tobin et al. (1975)

is in marked contrast to what is observed with ouabain, where preincubation can increase the apparent I_{50} for ouabain on this enzyme up to tenfold. In the case of ouabain this effect depends on the stability of the enzyme – ouabain complex (Akera, 1971), so one interpretation of this effect is that the cassaine – enzyme complex is considerably less stable than the ouabain – enzyme complex.

Figure 12.15 shows a direct test of the ability of cassaine to displace [^{3}H] -ouabain from its binding sites on $Na^+ + K^+$-ATPase. In this experiment rat brain $Na^+ + K^+$- ATPase was incubated with low concentrations of [^{3}H] -ouabain of high specific activity in the presence of Na^+, Mg^{2+} and ATP. At the time points indicated by the arrows cassaine was added either before, with or after the [^{3}H] -ouabain. The experiment shows that these low concentrations of cassaine do decrease the binding of [^{3}H] -ouabain to this enzyme and that the amount of

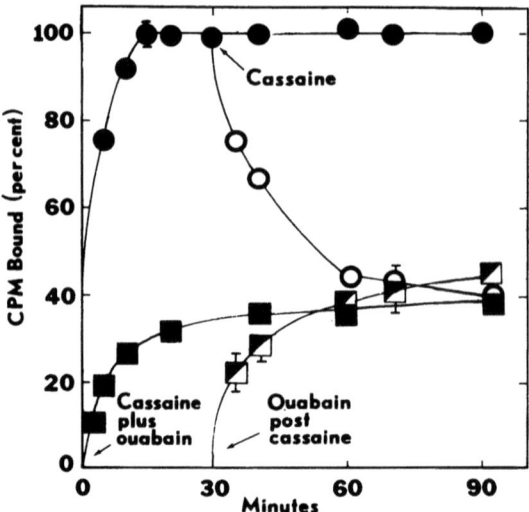

Figure 12.15 Effect of cassaine on [^{3}H]-ouabain binding to Na$^+$ + K$^+$-ATPase. Rat brain enzyme was incubated at 37°C in the presence of 100 mM Na$^+$, 0.2 mM Mg^{2+} and 5 mM ATP. The solid circles show the radioactivity bound when tracer amounts (0.3 × 10^{-9} M) of [^{3}H]-ouabain were added to the binding system. The solid squares show radioactivity bound when the same concentrations of cassaine and [^{3}H]-ouabain were added together. The half squares (◨◨) show radioctivity bound when the [^{3}H]-ouabain was added 30 min after the cassaine. The points are the mean ± SEM of four separate experiments with radioactivity bound expressed as a percentage of that bound at 90 min in the presence of Na$^+$, Mg^{2+} and ATP, which averaged 11.8 ± 1.0 pmol [^{3}H]-ouabain/mg protein. Reprinted by permission from Tobin et al. (1975)

this decrease was essentially independent of the sequence of addition of the ligands. The experiment suggests that the interactions of low concentrations of cassaine with this enzyme are fully reversible and is consistent with the idea that cassaine and ouabain may compete for the same binding sites on this enzyme.

While the data of Fig. 12.15 may suggest a direct displacement of [^{3}H]-ouabain from its binding sites on this enzyme by cassaine, other ligands of this enzyme such as Na$^+$ and ATP (and the ATP analogues) can readily displace [^{3}H]-ouabain from its binding sites on this enzyme by what appear to be indirect or allosteric interactions (Tobin and Sen, 1970; Tobin, Banerjee and Sen, 1970, Tobin et al., 1974). We therefore next investigated the actions of cassaine on the intermediate steps of the Na$^+$ + K$^+$-ATPase reaction to choose between these possibilities. The rationale behind this approach was that if cassaine produced its effects by binding at the ouabain-binding site of Na$^+$ + K$^+$-ATPase, one might expect its actions on the intermediate steps of the reaction cycle of this enzyme to be similar to those of ouabain. Because radiolabelled cassaine was not available

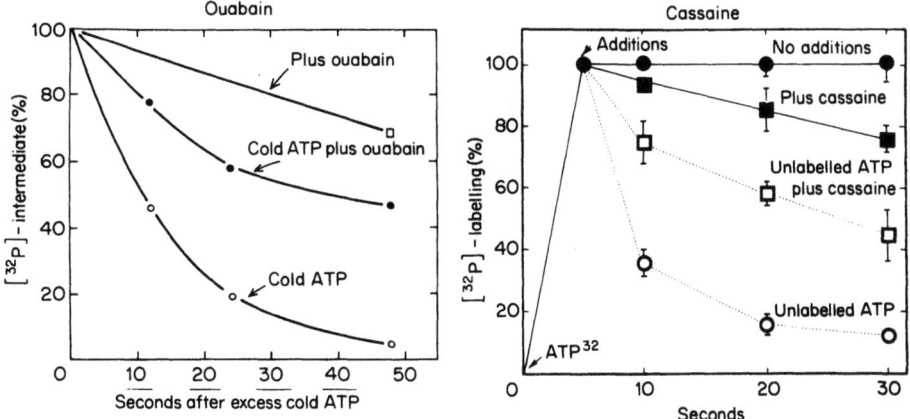

Figure 12.16 In the experiment shown in the left-hand panel guinea-pig kidney Na$^+$ + K$^+$-ATPase was phosphorylated from [γ-^{32}P] ATP with Mg^{2+} and Na$^+$. Once formed, E-P was isolated at indicated zero time by the addition of unlabelled ATP (open circles), or unlabelled ATP plus 2.5 × 10^{-4} M ouabain (solid circles). The open square shows the level of E-P when ouabain alone was added to the system at zero time. Reprinted by permission from Sen et al. (1969).

The right-hand panel shows the actions of cassaine on E-P formed similarly in rat brain ATPase. The solid circles show the steady state levels of E-P, the solid squares levels of E-P in the presence of 1 × 10^{-4} M cassaine. The open circles show spontaneous turnover of the phosphorylated intermediate when it was isolated by the addition of unlabelled ATP, while the open squares show its turnover in the presence of unlabelled ATP and 1 × 10^{-4} M cassaine. Reprinted by permission from Tobin et al. (1975)

to us, we used an indirect method following ^{32}P labelling of this enzyme from [γ-^{32}P] ATP as described by Sen, Tobin and Post (1969).

Figure 12.16 compares the reactivity of ouabain and cassaine with the phosphorylated intermediate of Na$^+$K$^+$-ATPase. The left-hand panel shows the reaction of guinea-pig kidney phosphoenzyme with ouabain at 0°C. In this experiment the phosphorylated intermediate was first formed in the presence of Na$^+$, Mg^{2+} and [γ-^{32}P] ATP. Then, at indicated zero time, the ^{32}P phosphoenzyme was isolated by the addition of excess unlabelled ATP and the spontaneous turnover of E-P exposed. When ouabain was added to the system with the unlabelled ATP, the turnover of the phosphoenzyme was slowed. However, if ouabain alone was added to the system, the amount of E-P present also declined, in apparent contradiction to the ability of ouabain to stabilise E-P. Other experiments have shown that this action is due to the generation of a dephosphoenzyme resistant to rephosphorylation (Sen et al., 1969). Thus this experiment shows that ouabain interacts readily with the phosphoenzyme, slows its turnover and then gives rise to a form of the enzyme which is not readily rephosphorylated. Since ouabain binding is virtually irreversible at 0°C, this resistance to rephosphorylation results in essentially complete inhibition of turnover (Sen et al., 1969).

The right-hand panel of Fig. 12.16 shows that essentially the same results were observed with cassaine. Cassaine alone reduces the steady state level of E-P in much the same manner as ouabain. The spontaneous turnover of the phosphoenzyme was also slowed by cassaine. The experiment shows that the qualitative actions of cassaine and ouabain on the spontaneous turnover and steady state levels of the phosphoenzyme are similar.

Figure 12.17 shows a further parallelism in the actions of ouabain and cassaine on the phosphorylated intermediate of $Na^+ + K^+$-ATPase. In the left-hand panel of Fig. 12.17 $Na^+ + K^+$-ATPase was phosphorylated in the presence of Na^+, Mg^{2+}, [γ-^{22}P] ATP and ouabain. Phosphorylation was essentially complete at 3 s and then the level of the phosphoenzyme slowly declined owing to the ouabain present. When the ouabain-treated phosphoenzyme was challenged with K^+, the dephosphorylation obtained was only partial, showing that in the presence of ouabain a K^+-resistant phosphoenzyme accumulates. This action of ouabain on E-P is typical of the cardiac glycosides (Sen et al., 1969; Post et al., 1969). The

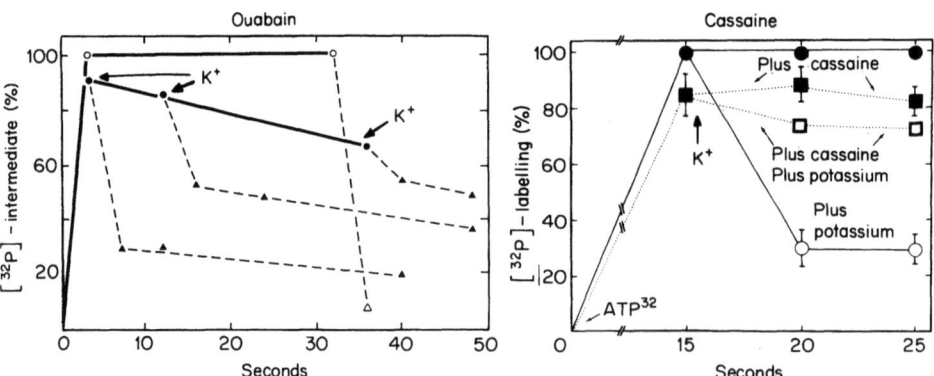

Figure 12.17 Resistance of ouabain or cassaine-treated phospho-enzymes to dephosphorylation by K^+.

The left-hand panel shows the effect of ouabain on the K^+-sensitivity of E-P. The solid circles show levels of E-P when this enzyme was phosphorylated from [γ-^{32}P] ATP, Mg^{2+} and Na^+ in the presence of 2.5×10^{-4} M ouabain. At the time points indicated by the arrows 15 mM K^+ was added to the system, and the solid triangles show the subsequent levels of E-P observed. The open circles and open triangle show steady state levels of E-P and the action of K^+ in the absence of added ouabain. Reprinted by permission from Sen et al. (1969).

The right-hand panel shows a similar experiment with cassaine. The solid circles show the steady state level of E-P when in the presence of Na^+, Mg^{2+} and ATP, the open circles the levels of E-P after addition of K^+ at 15 s. The solid squares show steady state levels of E-P when cassaine (1×10^{-4} M) was added to the system 5 s after the addition of [γ-^{32}P] ATP. The open squares show the effect of K^+ (added at 15 s) on the cassaine-treated phospho-enzyme. Reprinted by permission from Tobin et al. (1975)

right-hand panel of Fig. 12.17 shows that qualitatively similar results are obtained with cassaine. When the enzyme was phosphorylated in the presence of cassaine, the steady state level of the phosphoenzyme was reduced, much as was observed with ouabain. If this cassaine-reacted phosphoenzyme was then challenged with K^+, it was found to be largely resistant to K^+, in contrast to the native phosphoenzyme. The experiments show that with respect to potassium ion the actions of both ouabain and cassaine on the phosphorylated intermediate of $Na^+ + K^+$-ATPase are similar.

From the similarity of the cassaine- and ouabain-induced patterns of reactivity of the phosphoenzyme, it is probably reasonable to conclude that cassaine produced its effects by interacting with and stabilising a configuration of this enzyme similar to that stabilised by ouabain. However, if cassaine stabilised a configuration of this enzyme similar to that stabilised by ouabain, it can then antagonise $[^3H]$-ouabain binding (Fig. 12.15) only by interacting directly at the cardiotonic

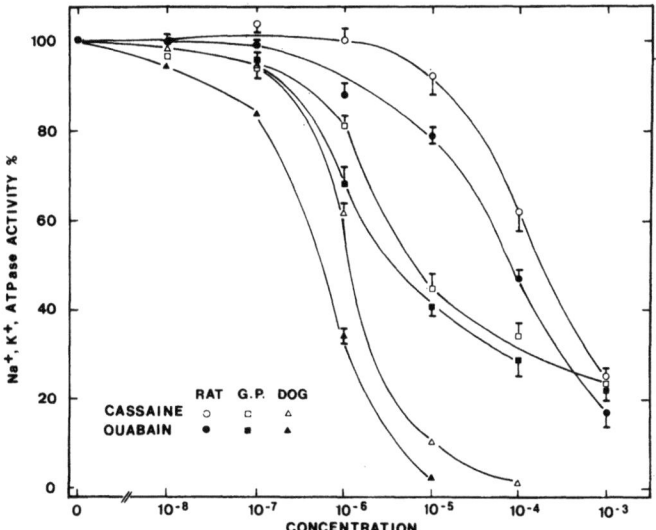

Figure 12.18 Inhibition of dog, guinea-pig (G.P.) and rat heart ATPases by cassaine or ouabain. Rat and guinea-pig heart $Na^+ + K^+$-ATPases were prepared as described by Akera et al. (1969), while the dog heart ATPase was prepared as described by Pitts, Lane and Schwartz (1973). Their $Na^+ + K^+$-ATPase activity was then assayed under standard conditions (100 mM Na^+, 15 mM K^+) in the presence of the indicated concentration of cassaine and ouabain. The solid triangles, squares and circles show inhibition of the dog, guinea-pig and rat enzyme preparations of ouabain. The open triangles, squares and circles show inhibition of these enzymes by the indicated concentrations of cassaine. All points are the mean ± SEM of determinations on four different enzymes except for the dog heart preparation, where only the points at 1×10^{-6} M are from four individual determinations. Reprinted by permission from Tobin et al. (1975)

steroid binding sites of $Na^+ + K^+$-ATPase. If cassaine does interact directly with the cardiotonic steroid binding sites of $Na^+ + K^+$-ATPase, one might then expect species-dependent differences in the sensitivity of different $Na^+ + K^+$-ATPase to cassaine, since the glycoside binding sites on $Na^+ + K^+$-ATPase are the only binding sites on this enzyme which show substantial species-dependent differences in ligand affinity (Tobin et al., 1972b; Tobin and Brody, 1972; Akera et al., 1969). Testing this hypothesis, Fig. 12.18 shows that similar species-dependent differences in sensitivity to cassaine are observed in dog, guinea-pig and rat heart ATPases. These experiments are therefore consistent with the idea that cassaine produces its inhibition of $Na^+ + K^+$-ATPase by interacting at the cardiotonic steroid binding site of $Na^+ + K^+$-ATPase.

At this point the data suggest that cassaine interacts with $Na^+ + K^+$-ATPase at the cardiotonic steroid binding site of this enzyme and the interaction appears to be qualitatively quite similar to that of ouabain. The only major quantitative

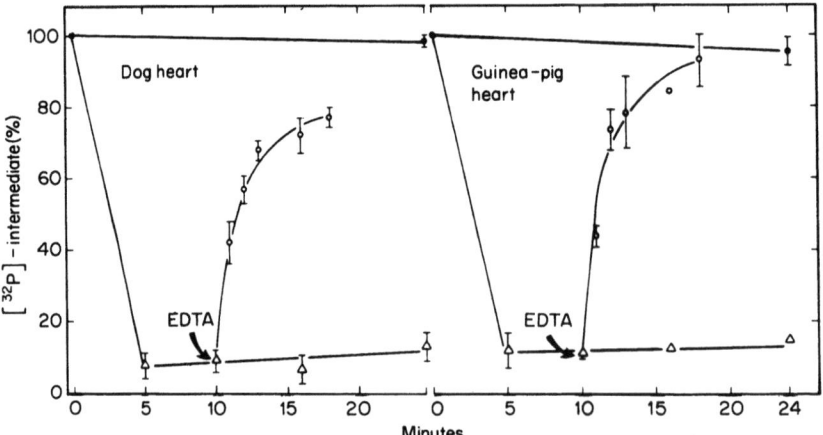

Figure 12.19 Rates of recovery of phosphorylation in cassaine-inhibited guinea-pig and dog heart enzymes. The left-hand panel shows the results of experiments with dog heart enzymes, the right-hand panel experiments with guinea-pig heart enzymes. About 150 μg of each enzyme was incubated with 100 mM Na^+ and 0.2 mM Mg^{2+} at 37°C. The experiment was started at indicated zero time by the addition of 1.0 mM UTP, with or without 1×10^{-4} M cassaine in the system. The solid circles show the labelling (after 4 s) from [γ-^{32}P] ATP added with 10 mM EDTA and 12 mM Mg^{2+} at the indicated times after UTP alone. The open triangles show the labelling observed in the presence of cassaine plus UTP at the indicated times. The open circles show the labelling observed in the presence of cassaine plus UTP when the 10 mM EDTA was added at 10 min; labelling with Mg^{2+} and [γ-^{32}P]-ATP was for 4 s, and labelling in the presence of 100 mM K^+ was subtracted as background labelling. The experiments with the dog heart enzyme are shown as the mean ± SEM of four individual experiments, those with the guinea-pig heart as the means ± SEM of three experiments. Maximal K^+-sensitive ^{32}P incorporation was 159 ± 26 pmol ^{32}p/mg protein in the guinea-pig heart enzymes. Reprinted by permission from Tobin et al. (1975)

difference suggested by these experiments is the implication of Fig. 12.16 that the enzyme – cassaine complex is less stable than the enzyme – ouabain complex. We therefore decided to investigate the rates of dissociation of the cassaine – enzyme complex in an attempt to identify a quantitative difference between the interactions of cassaine and ouabain with cardiac $Na^+ + K^+$-ATPase.

We estimated the rate of dissociation of cassaine from $Na^+ + K^+$-ATPase indirectly (Fig. 12.19) by the method used to demonstrate dissociation of strophanthidin bromacetate from this enzyme (Tobin et al., 1973). In this method cassaine was bound to the enzyme in the presence of Na^+, Mg^{2+} and UTP. UTP was used instead of ATP because it phosphorylates $Na^+ + K^+$-ATPase, but does not interfere significantly with the subsequent phosphorylation of this enzyme from ATP under appropriate conditions (Tobin et al., 1973; Tobin et al., 1972a). In this way cassaine was allowed to bind to this enzyme in the presence of Na^+ and UTP and the cassaine – enzyme complex was then isolated by the addition of EDTA. Under these conditions the ability of the enzyme to accept a phosphate group from $[\gamma-^{32}P]$ ATP after exposure to cassaine was recovered relatively rapidly and completely in the guinea-pig enzyme; more slowly and less completely in the dog heart enzyme (Fig. 12.19). The data suggest that cassaine dissociates rapidly from the guinea-pig enzyme in the presence of Na^+, UTP and excess EDTA and somewhat more slowly from dog heart ATPase.

The half-lives of the enzyme–cassaine estimated from the data of Fig. 12.19 are much shorter than the 10 and 95 min half-lives reported for the ouabain – enzyme complexes at 27°C in these species (Fig. 12.10). If the basis of the cardiotonic actions of cassaine is indeed its reversible interaction with the cardiotonic steroid binding site of $Na^+ + K^+$-ATPase, then one would expect the rates of offset of the positive inotropic responses due to cassaine to be (a) much faster than the rates of offset of the positive inotropic actions of ouabain, and (b) faster in the guinea-pig heart than in the dog heart. Figure 12.20 shows that the rates of guinea-pig heart than in the dog heart. Figure 12.20 shows that the rates of offset of the ouabain-induced positive inotropic effects in dog and guinea-pig hearts are about 10 and 55 min, respectively, in good agreement with data previously reported by Akera et al. (1973). However, if cassaine was substituted for ouabain as the inotropic agent, the half-lives of the inotropic effects were much shorter, about 2.5 min in the guinea-pig and 9.5 min in the dog heart preparation. These much faster offsets of cassaine-dependent inotropy are consistent with the lower apparent affinity of cassaine for cardiac $Na^+ + K^+$-ATPase preparations in Fig. 12.14 and the rapid recovery of guinea-pig and dog heart enzymes from inhibition by cassaine shown in Fig. 12.19.

In conclusion, it appears that the only quantitative difference between the interaction of cassaine and ouabain with $Na^+ + K^+$-ATPase is the faster dissociation rate of cassaine from the cardiotonic steroid binding site. This difference at the enzymatic level is reflected at the tissue level in the offset of cassaine-induced inotropy being four to five times faster than the offset of ouabain-induced inotropy. These observations make it very likely that the offset rates

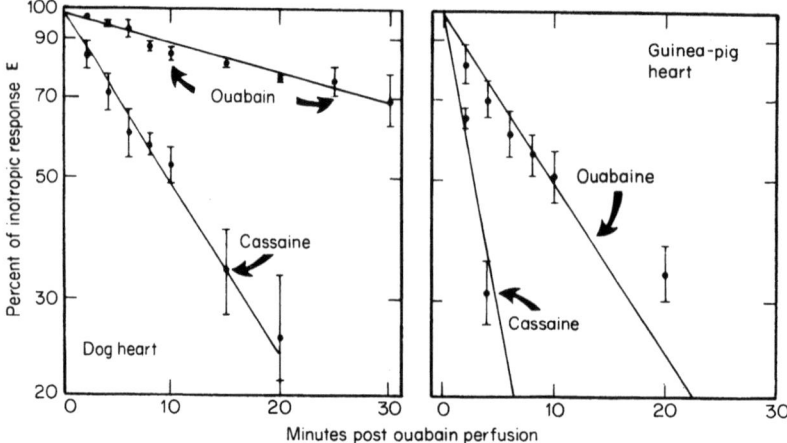

Figure 12.20 Rates of offset of ouabain- and cassaine-induced inotropic effects in dog and guinea-pig hearts. The left-hand panel shows experiments on puppy hearts, the right-hand panel experiments on guinea-pig hearts. Langendorff preparations of these hearts were perfused with Krebs–Henseleit solution containing 6×10^{-7} M drug (puppy hearts) or 1.2×10^{-6} M drug (guinea-pig hearts). After 20 min of drug perfusion the hearts were switched to drug-free solution and the rates of loss of the inotropic response measured. The guinea-pig heart data are the means ± SEM of five separate experiments, with ouabain producing a 35 ± 6.0 percent increase in cardiac contractile force and cassaine a 51 ± 3.0 per cent increase. The puppy heart experiments are shown as the means of four experiments, with ouabain producing a 34 ± 4.6 per cent inotropic response and cassaine a 23.0 ± 5.0 per cent inotropic response. Reprinted by permission from Tobin et al. (1975)

observed with ouabain are in fact determined by the rates of dissociation of ouabain from the $Na^+ + K^+$-ATPase and not due to diffusion barriers. If the rates of offset observed with ouabain were due to diffusion barriers, one would expect essentially similar rates with cassaine rather than the much faster dissociation rates observed. Thus the rapid offset rates of cassaine-induced inotropy correlate well with what is known about the interaction of cassaine with the $Na^+ + K^+$-ATPase (Peters et al., 1974) and are in good agreement with the concept that the rate of dissociation of these drugs from the cardiotonic steroid binding site of $Na^+ + K^+$-ATPase is rate-limiting for the offset of their pharmacological effects in perfused hearts (Akera et al., 1973).

ACKNOWLEDGEMENTS

Published as paper No. 76-4 with the permission of the Dean and Director and from the Equine Drug Research Program, Department of Veterinary Science, University of Kentucky, Lexington, Ky. 40506. This work was supported by grants from the Michigan Heart Association, Grant HL 16055 and HL 16052-01 from the National Institutes of Health, and General Research Support Grant NIH-RR-05623-04 to the College of Veterinary Medicine, Michigan State University, from the National Institutes of Health, and Grant BMS 74-18512 from the National Science Foundation. The technical help of Mrs Annie Han is gratefully acknowledged.

REFERENCES

Akera, T. (1971). *Biochim. Biophys. Acta,* **249**, 53
Akera, T., Baskin, S. I., Tobin, T. and Brody, T. M. (1973). *Naunyn-Schmiedebergs Arch. Pharmacol.,* **277**, 151
Akera, T. and Brody, T. M. (1975). *Life Sci.,* **18**, 135
Akera, T., Larsen, F. S. and Brody, T. M. (1969). *J. Pharmacol. Exp. Therap.,* **170**, 17
Bonting, S. L., Hawkins, N. M. and Canady, M. R. (1964). *Biochem. Pharmacol.,* **13**, 13
Kahn, J. B., VanAtta, R. A. and Johnson, G. L. (1963). *J. Pharmacol. Exp. Therap.,* **147**, 215
Ku, D., Akera, T., Pew, C. L. and Brody, T. M. (1974a). *Naunyn-Schmiedebergs Arch. Pharmacol.,* **295**, 185
Ku, D., Akera, T., Tobin T. and Brody, T. (1974b). *Res. Commun. Chem. Pathol. Pharmacol.,* **9**, 431
Ku, D., Akera, T., Tobin, T. and Brody, T. M. (1975). *Naunyn-Schmiedebergs Arch. Pharmacol.,* **240**, 113
Ku, D., Akera, T., Tobin, T. and Brody, T. M. (1976). *J. Pharmacol. Exp. Therap.* (in press)
Peters, T., Rabin, R. H. and Wasserman, O. (1974). *Eur. J. Pharmacol.,* **26**, 166
Pitts, B. J. R., Lane, L. K. and Schwartz, A. (1973). *Biochem. Biophys. Res. Commun.,* **53**, 1060
Post, R. L. (1968). *Regulatory Functions of Biological Membranes* (ed. J. Jarnefelt), Elsevier, Amsterdam, p. 163
Post, R. L., Kume, S., Tobin, T., Orcutt, B. and Sen, A. K. (1969). *J. Gen. Physiol.,* **545**, 306
Post, R. L. and Orcutt, B. (1973). *Organization of Energy Transducing Mambranes* (ed. M. Nakao and L. Packer), Tokyo University Press, Tokyo, p. 35
Post, R. L., Sen, A. K. and Rosenthal, A. S. (1965). *J. Biol. Chem.,* **240**, 1437
Sen, A. K., Tobin, T. and Post, R. L. (1969). *J. Biol. Chem.,* **244**, 6596
Tobin, T., Akera, T. and Brody, T. M. (1975). *Biochim. Biophys. Acta,* **389**, 117
Tobin, T., Akera, T. and Brody, T. M. (1976). *Biochim. Biophys. Acta* (in press)
Tobin, T., Akera, T., Ku, D. and Lu, M. C. (1973). *Molec. Pharmacol.,* **9**, 676
Tobin, T., Akera, T., Lee, C. Y. and Brody, T. M. (1974). *Biochim. Biophys. Acta,* **345**, 102
Tobin, T., Banerjee, S. P. and Sen, A. K. (1970). *Nature,* **225**, 745
Tobin, T., Baskin, S. I., Akera, T. and Brody, T. M. (1972a). *Molec. Pharmacol.,* **8**, 256
Tobin, T. and Brody, T. M. (1972). *Biochem. Pharmacol.,* **21**, 1533
Tobin, T., Henderson, R. and Sen, A. K. (1972b). *Biochim. Biophys. Acta,* **274**, 551
Tobin, T. and Sen. A. K. (1970). *Biochim. Biophys. Acta,* **198**, 120

13
Adenylate cyclase: actions and interactions of regulatory ligands

C. Londos and M. Rodbell (Membrane Regulation Section, Laboratory of Nutrition and Endocrinology, National Institute of Arthritis, Metabolism and Digestive Diseases, National Institutes of Health, Bethesda, Maryland, USA)

INTRODUCTION

The discovery of adenylate cyclase systems has provided a means for study of hormone action *in vitro* under controlled conditions. By 1960 it had been established by Sutherland and his associates (Sutherland and Rall, 1960) that the only ingredients necessary to elicit a hormonal effect on the enzyme were magnesium ion, ATP, hormone and membranes bearing the enzyme. This seemingly simple system, in which hormone was shown to increase the V_{max} of adenylate cyclase, soon became considerably more complex when it was shown that several of the basic assay components exerted multiple effects on the enzyme. While such effects have contributed to a confusing body of literature on adenylate cyclase, they have led also to the elucidation of certain regulatory features of the enzyme system. In this report we shall present a brief review of the current ideas and controversies regarding the interaction of several regulatory ligands with adenylate cyclase, followed by some more recent data which may help to resolve at least one of these controversies.

Working with different hormone-sensitive adenylate cyclase systems, several groups observed that increasing divalent cation (Me^{2+}) concentrations (Mg^{2+} or Mn^{2+}) in excess of that required to form the productive substrate complex, MeATP, resulted in stimulation of enzyme activity (Birnbaumer, Pohl and Rodbell, 1969; Rosen and Rosen, 1969; Burke, 1970; Drummond and Duncan, 1970; Drummond, Severson and Duncan, 1971). It was postulated that the enzyme systems contained separate metal-binding sites, and that hormones regulated enzyme activity by increasing the affinity of the putative metal ion site for the metal ion (Birnbaumer *et al.*, 1969). Calcium inhibited activity, presumably by binding to the metal-binding site (Birnbaumer *et al.*, 1969; Drummond and Duncan, 1970). That such effects might be due to factors other than a direct action of Me^{2+} on the enzyme system was proposed by de Haen (1974), who explained the data of Birnbaumer *et al.* (1969) and of Drummond *et al.* (1971) with a model in which increasing the metal ion concentration increased activity by chelating free substrate, ATP^{4-}, which was considered to be a potent inhibitor.

The model of de Haen has been modified recently by Rendell et al. (1975), who fitted steady state kinetic data on the hepatic system to a model in which free protonated substrate served as inhibitor. In these models hormones act by inducing an enzyme state which is less susceptible to inhibition by uncomplexed substrate. However, in a more recent report, also based on computer fitting of kinetic data, the notion that free substrate is a potent inhibitor has been disputed. Garbers and Johnson (1975) have fitted data obtained with brain adenylate cyclase to a model in which metal ions act at a separate metal ion-binding site on the enzyme system. Since different models can provide apparently acceptable fits to kinetic data, the question of how increasing metal ion concentrations activate adenylate cyclase systems seems unresolved. Later in this report we hope to shed new light on this controversy.

Studies of the binding of glucagon to its receptor in liver membranes led to the discovery of a nucleotide regulatory site on adenylate cyclase (Rodbell et al., 1971 a, b). Briefly, it was found that ATP or, at much lower concentrations, GTP increased the rate of dissociation of glucagon from its receptor and increased stimulation of the enzyme by the hormone. Subsequent studies revealed that, in several tissues sensitive to a variety of hormones (including prostaglandins), activation of adenylate cyclase by hormones is dependent upon the presence of low concentrations of guanine nucleotides, and that synergism can be demonstrated between the actions of hormones and guanine nucleotides (for a review, see Rodbell et al., 1975). This role of nucleotides was unsuspected and was only revealed by the seemingly odd observation that they affected the binding of a hormone to its receptor.

In the absence of hormone, GTP is a weak activator of adenylate cyclase systems. Recently Gpp(NH)p, a nucleotidase-resistant analogue of GTP, has been found to stimulate to high activity all eukaryotic membrane-bound adenylate cyclase systems tested (Harwood, Low and Rodbell, 1973; Glossmann and Gips, 1974; Lefkowitz, 1974; Londos et al., 1974; Spiegel and Aurbach, 1974; Londos and Rodbell, 1975; Pfeuffer and Helmreich, 1975; Salomon et al., 1975; Schramm and Rodbell, 1975). Prior to the discovery of the stimulatory effects of Gpp(NH)p, fluoride ion was the only agent other than hormones which caused marked stimulation of adenylate cyclase activity, and the only agent which could stimulate detergent-dispersed preparations. As a result of the activating effects of Gpp(NH)p, its actions at a site intimately linked to the expression of hormone action, and its ability to activate detergent-dispersed enzyme, the nucleotide analogue has supplanted fluoride in in vitro studies. Another important feature of the actions of Gpp(NH)p is that, like fluoride, its effects are either slowly reversible or irreversible. Interestingly, the effects of both fluoride and guanine nucleotides are found only in adenylate cyclase systems from a membrane source. Neither agent activates the enzyme in *Escherichia coli* (Tao and Lipmann, 1969; Londos et al., 1974), in *Bacillus pertussis* (E. Hewlitt, personal communication), or the cytosol adenylate cyclase found in rat seminiferous tubules (Braun and Dods, 1975; C. Londos, unpublished observations).

Guanine nucleotide binding sites have been characterised in plasma membranes from several tissues, primarily with the use of labelled Gpp(NH)p (Spiegel and Aurbach, 1974; Glossmann, 1975a; Pfeuffer and Helmreich, 1975; Salomon and Rodbell, 1975) and, in one case, with labelled GTP (Lefkowitz, 1975). As observed with adenylate cyclase activation, the binding sites are relatively specific for guanine nucleotides and display kinetic constants for binding which are strikingly similar to those seen for enzyme activation.

The actions of Gpp(NH)p and GTP differ in that when adenylate cyclase systems are washed free of the analogue, the enzyme remains in an activated state. This persistence of the activated state has permitted a comparison of the relationship between bound nucleotide and adenylate cyclase activity, a relationship found to be linear with the hepatic enzyme system (Salomon et al., 1975) and nearly linear with the pigeon erythrocyte system (Pfeuffer and Helmreich, 1975). Other similarities between binding and action include inhibition of both processes by EDTA (Spiegel and Aurbach, 1974; Glossmann, 1975b; Spiegel et al., 1976), temperature-dependence (Spiegel et al., 1976), and the ability of GTP to displace bound nucleotide and decrease the activity of the previously activated enzyme (Pfeuffer and Helmreich, 1975). Thus, the bulk of the binding sites have characteristics that are similar to the sites through which the guanine nucleotides activate adenylate cyclase systems. Nevertheless, the relevance of all of the binding sites remains in doubt, because the concentration of binding sites, usually 50 - 100 pmol/mg membrane protein, is considerably higher than the concentration of hormone receptors, which is generally less than 5 pmol/mg membrane protein. It is possible that each adenylate cyclase unit is associated with multiple guanine nucleotide binding sites. Alternatively, a common guanine nucleotide-linked process may subserve several functions in the membranes, only one of which is to regulate adenylate cyclase activity. Indeed, effects of low concentrations of guanine nucleotides on plasma membrane phenomena apparently not associated with adenylate cyclase have been reported by Sonenberg et al. (1973) and by Glossmann, Baukel and Catt (1974). Therefore serious consideration should be given to a general regulatory role for guanine nucleotides in membrane function.

The mechanism of action of guanine nucleotides remains unknown. Possibilities ruled out from studies with the hepatic adenylate cyclase system include phosphorylation, guanylation and the formation of an intermediate activator, such as cyclic GMP (Salomon et al., 1975). If the binding sites for guanine nucleotides are relevant to the process of activation, then covalent modification, as proposed by Cuatrecasas, Jacobs and Bennett (1975), would be unlikely, since Gpp(NH)p and Gpp(CH$_2$)p can be eluted from the sites as intact molecules (Salomon and Rodbell, 1975; Spiegel and Aurbach, 1974). While the latter evidence argues in favour of the nucleotide activating via allosteric binding to the enzyme system, there is some dispute as to whether the effects of the analogues are reversible, as would be expected if they act as allosteric ligands. Pfeuffer and Helmreich (1975) have reported that the effects of Gpp(CH$_2$)p on the pigeon erythrocyte enzyme system can be reversed with GTP and that, following such reversal, the enzyme can be reactivated with Gpp(CH_2)p. Other investigators have not been able to show reversal by GTP of Gpp(NH)p activation (Glossmann, 1975b; Cuatrecasas et al., 1975; Spiegel et al., 1976). However, if reversal is time- and temperature-dependent, there may be difficulties in distinguishing between reversal and inactivation of labile adenylate cyclase (Lefkowitz and Caron, 1975).

It should be noted that, while both Gpp(NH)p and Gpp(CH_2)p produce strong activation which may be only slowly reversed, another analogue, GTP-γ-S, which contains neither the P–N–P nor the P–C–P group, is a strong activator and its effects are not readily reversed (Pfeuffer and Helmreich, 1975). In this regard, a finding of potential interest is that plasma membranes from liver and fat cells contain GTPases which are highly specific for guanine nucleotides and which are clearly distinct from non-specific nucleotidases in membranes (Salomon and Rodbell, 1975). The GTPases may have a function in the process of activation of adenylate cyclase; it has been proposed that GTPases may be involved in the termination of the GTP-induced activation process (Salomon and Rodbell, 1975; Pfeuffer and Helmreich, 1975), which may account for the differences in the reversibility of the effects of GTP and the analogues, Gpp(NH)p, Gpp(CH_2)p and GTP-γ-S. In fact, another analogue, 3'-deoxy-GTP, which is most probably susceptible to GTPase hydrolysis, activates the hepatic adenylate cyclase system to the same extent as Gpp(NH)p (Salomon et al., 1975), but the effects of 3'-deoxy-GTP are readily reversed upon washing of the membranes (C. Londos, unpublished observations). Thus a possible mechanism consistent with the available data is that guanine nucleotides activate adenylate cyclase systems by binding at an allosteric site, and that binding and action are terminated by hydrolysis of the nucleotide.

Other aspects of guanine nucleotide activation and the possible role of metal ion in this process are discussed below.

EVIDENCE FOR ACTIVATION BY METAL IONS

The conflicting conclusions of investigators who have employed computer fitting procedures to analyse kinetic data (see p. 236) led us to explore other means of investigating the role of metal ion in the activation of adenylate cyclase systems.

Table 13.1 Adenylate cyclase activation by Mn^{2+}

mM Mg^{2+}	Adenylate cyclase activity (pmol cyclic AMP formed/mg protein in 4 min at 30 °C) with	
	no Mn^{2+}	0.2 mM Mn^{2+}
1	8.3	49
5	18	48
10	28	45

Basal activity in liver membranes with 0.007 mM ATP as substrate. Liver membranes were prepared by a modification (Pohl et al., 1971) of the procedure of Neville (1968), and adenylate cyclase was assayed according to Salomon et al. (1974).

From the data discussed below, we conclude that the rat liver adenylate cyclase system is activated directly by divalent cation.

A fortuitous finding was that low concentrations of Mn^{2+}, in the presence of a considerable excess of Mg^{2+}, stimulated activity above that seen with magnesium ion alone. As shown in Table 13.1, as little as 0.2 mM Mn^{2+} in the presence of 5 mM Mg^{2+} nearly tripled basal enzyme activity. One explanation for this phenomenon is that the affinity for MnATP is considerably greater than that for MgATP. However, in several experiments we were unable to detect any differences in K_m for substrate when ATP was combined with Mg or Mn, or with combinations of these cations; under all conditions tested, the K_m values fell within the range of 40 - 70 μM MeATP. Another possibility, consistent with several published models, is that Mn^{2+}, by virtue of its stronger binding of ATP, stimulates by reducing the level of inhibitory, uncomplexed substrate. However, as shown in Table 13.2, activation by Mn^{2+} was independent of ATP concentration. A third, and more plausible, explanation is that Mn^{2+} acts at a site independent of the catalytic site to increase the V_{max}.

Table 13.2 Activation by Mn^{2+} is independent of substrate concentration

mM ATP	Adenylate cyclase activity (pmol cyclic AMP formed/mg protein in 4 min at 30 °C) with	
	5 mM Mg^{2+}	5 mM Mg^{2+} + 1 mM Mn^{2+}
0.01	34 (0.12)	78 (0.07)
0.5	248 (6.6)	556 (4)

Basal activity in liver membranes. The values in parentheses represent the concentration (micromolar) of free, uncomplexed ATP for each of the four conditions tested; these values were calculated assuming the following association constants: MgATP 16 600 and MnATP 60 300 (Tu and Heller, 1974). Note the great differences in uncomplexed ATP concentrations at the two ATP concentrations tested.

Another approach we have employed in establishing the existence of a metal ion-binding site is the use of calcium ion, known to be inhibitory to most adenylate cyclase systems. When the calcium concentration was varied in the presence of different concentrations of Mg^{2+}, the Ca^{2+} concentration required for inhibition increased with increasing Mg^{2+} concentration, suggestive of a competitive relationship (Fig. 13.1). Note that half-maximal inhibition occurred when the concentration of CaATP, which is not a productive substrate, was approximately one-tenth that of MgATP. However, calcium was much less able to inhibit activity when MnATP served as substrate; activity was inhibited by less than 50 per cent even when the concentration of CaATP exceeded that of MnATP (see caption to Fig. 13.1). Since the K_ms for MnATP and MgATP do not differ by more than twofold, the markedly different inhibitory effects of calcium seen in the presence of Mn^{2+} and Mg^{2+} can best be explained by a metal ion site that binds Mn^{2+}, Mg^{2+} and Ca^{2+} with differing affinities, and with calcium exerting inhibitory

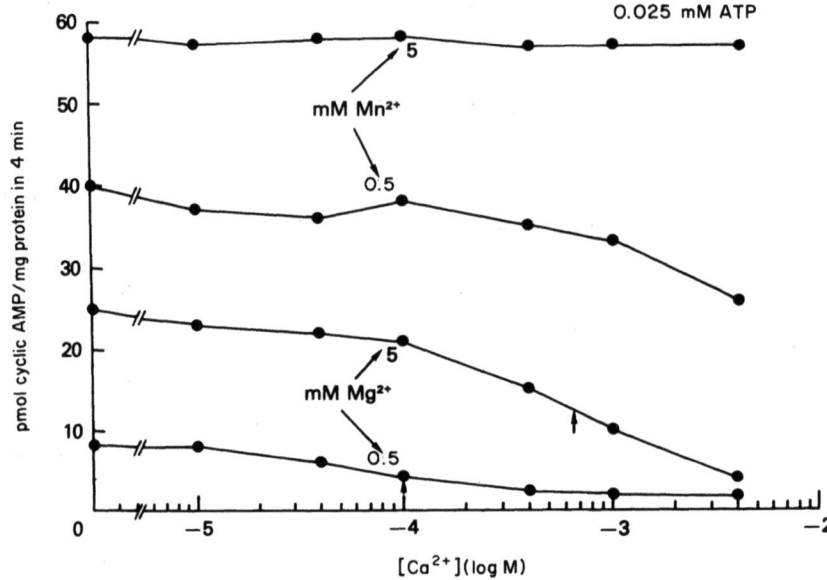

Figure 13.1 Inhibition by Ca^{2+} in the presence of Mg^{2+} and Mn^{2+}. The arrows indicate the $[Ca^{2+}]$ at which activity was inhibited by 50 per cent. Assuming an association constant for CaATP of 9300 (see also footnote to Table 13.2), the CaATP concentration was approximately one-tenth of the MgATP concentration at the point of half maximal inhibition in both curves obtained with Mg^{2+}. At the highest calcium concentration (4 mM) tested in the presence of 0.5 mM Mn^{2+}, the CaATP concentration exceeded the MnATP concentration

Table 13.3 Preactivation of adenylate cyclase by Gpp(NH)p and Me^{2+}

Preincubation conditions	Adenylate cyclase activity (pmol cyclic AMP produced/mg protein in 4 min at 30 °C) with	
	no Gpp(NH)p	10 µM Gpp(NH)p
No additions	47	205
Gpp(NH)p	125	260
Gpp(NH)p + 1 mM Mg^{2+}	243	320
Gpp(NH)p + 1 mM Mn^{2+}	289	370

Preactivation conditions were: 0.1 mM App(NH)p, 1 mM cyclic AMP, 1 mM dithiothreitol, 0.1% bovine serum albumen, 20 mM Tris-HCl, pH 7.6, liver membranes at 0.8 mg membrane protein/ml and, where indicated, 10 µM Gpp(NH)p. After incubation for 10 min at 30 °C, the mixture was centrifuged, and the membranes were washed and resuspended in 20 mM Tris-HCl, pH 7.6, 1 mM dithiothreitol. Adenylate cyclase activity was assayed in the presence of 0.1 mM ATP and 4 mM Mg^{2+}.

Adenylate Cyclase: Actions and Interactions of Regulatory Ligands   241

effects when occupying this site. Indeed, these were the conclusions reached by Drummond and Duncan (1970) and by Birnbaumer et al. (1969). It should be stressed, however, that calcium is inhibitory only to the extent that activation by Mg^{2+} or Mn^{2+} is impeded; under some conditions, calcium activates the hepatic system (see below).

Further evidence for a site which reacts with Me^{2+} comes from experiments in which the enzyme system was activated with Gpp(NH)p and washed prior to testing for adenylate cyclase activity (Table 13.3). The addition of Mg^{2+} or Mn^{2+} to the pretreatment medium considerably enhanced the persistent activation obtained with Gpp(NH)p. Similar, although somewhat weaker, effects are seen with calcium.

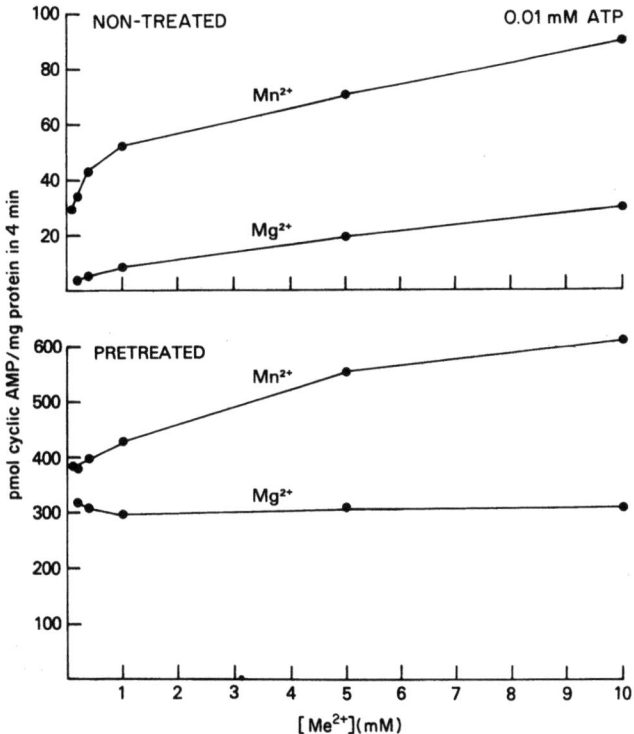

Figure 13.2   Effects of Me^{2+} on adenylate cyclase activity in pretreated and non-treated membranes. (Bottom) Liver plasma membranes at 0.8 mg membrane protein/ml were pretreated with 0.1 mM App(NH)p, 5 mM $MgCl_2$, 1 mM $MnCl_2$, 10 μM Gpp(NH)p, 1 mM dithiothreitol, 1 mM cyclic AMP and 20 mM Tris-HCl, pH 7.6, for 10 min at 30 °C. Membranes were centrifuged, washed and resuspended in 20 mM Tris-HCl, 1 mM dithiothreitol, and tested for adenylate cyclase activity in the presence of varying concentrations of Mg^{2+} and Mn^{2+}. (Top) Non-treated membranes were those pretreated in a medium containing only Tris-HCl and dithiothreitol, but otherwise carried through the procedures described above

Figure 13.2 shows the results of experiments in which the hepatic enzyme system was pretreated with Me^{2+} plus Gpp(NH)p, washed and then tested for the effects of varying Mg^{2+} or Mn^{2+} concentrations in the adenylate cyclase assay medium. The upper diagram shows the effects of Mg^{2+} and Mn^{2+} on the untreated enzyme; the concentrations of Mg^{2+} and Mn^{2+} required for half-maximal activation were 4 mM and 0.3 mM, respectively. However, as shown in the lower diagram, after pretreatment with the metal ion in the presence of Gpp(NH)p there was no further activation by Mg^{2+} and the effects of Mn^{2+} were diminished considerably; such results were found to be independent of the ATP concentration in the assay medium. Therefore it would appear that activation at the Me^{2+}-binding site can be achieved in pretreatment. Similar effects of Me^{2+} on preactivation by fluoride ion have been reported by Perkins and Moore (1971).

As noted above, Spiegel et al. (1976) and Glossmann (1975b) have shown that EDTA completely blocks the activation of adenylate cyclase systems by Gpp(NH)p in pretreatment. We have made a similar observation with liver membranes (Table 13.4). While it is tempting to speculate that activation of Gpp(NH)p is absolutely dependent upon the presence of Me^{2+}, and that EDTA inhibits activation by removal of endogenous membrane-bound Me^{2+}, both Spiegel et al. (1976) and we (Table 13.4) have observed that EGTA was not effective in preventing activation by the nucleotide. On the contrary, EGTA stimulated the hepatic system.

Table 13.4 Effects of chelators on activation by Gpp(NH)p in pretreatment

Pretreatment conditions	Adenylate cyclase activity (pmol cyclic AMP formed/mg protein in 4 min at 30 °C) with	
	no Gpp(NH)p	10 μM Gpp(NH)p
No additions	46	363
EDTA	45	334
EGTA	50	397
Gpp(NH)p	152	320
Gpp(NH)p + EDTA	69	358
Gpp(NH)p + EGTA	314	523

Pretreatment conditions were: 25 mM Tris-HCl, pH 7.6 and 1 mM dithiothreitol at 30 °C for 10 min. Gpp(NH)p concentration was 10 μM, and the chelators were added at 1 mM. The membranes were centrifuged, washed and tested for adenylate cyclase activity with 5 mM Mg^{2+} and 0.1 mM ATP.

Despite its lesser ability to chelate Mg^{2+}, one would have expected 1 mM EGTA to remove most of the endogenous, loosely bound Me^{2+} from the membranes. Therefore it is questionable whether activation by guanine nucleotides is absolutely dependent upon the presence of divalent cations, as would be expected if Me-nucleotide were the active species. In fact, activation by Me^{2+} occurs in the absence of added nucleotide, as is seen in Table 13.1, where activation by Mn^{2+} (and Mg^{2+}) was observed when the only added nucleotide was 0.007 mM ATP, a concentration far too low to expect action at the nucleotide regulatory site. These data suggest that divalent cations and nucleotides act at separate sites on the enzyme system.

In the model of de Haen (1974) and of Rendell et al. (1975) activation by metal ions was attributed to the lowering of the concentration of inhibitory uncomplexed substrate. Our data are more compatible with a model in which the metal ions interact with a metal ion site. In this model, hormones may act by inducing the formation of a state that has a higher affinity for the metal ion, as recently proposed by Hammes and Rodbell (1976). While there are no direct data for this process, Jard et al. (1975) have shown that there is a Mg^{2+}-dependent phenomenon which occurs subsequent to vasopressin binding, and which seems to link hormone – receptor interaction with the process of adenylate cyclase activation in the renal medulla. A similar consideration has been suggested for the role of GTP (or other nucleotides) in coupling glucagon – receptor interaction to the activation of the hepatic enzyme system (Rodbell, Lin and Salomon, 1974) and catecholamine – receptor action on the turkey erythrocyte system (Brown et al., 1976). Thus it would appear that guanine nucleotides and metal ions participate, in an allosteric manner, in the transduction of the hormone message.

EFFECTS OF ADENOSINE

Adenosine, either as an activator or inhibitor, is known to affect several adenylate cyclase systems. The nucleoside promotes cyclic AMP production in brain slices (Sattin and Rall, 1970; Daly et al., 1972), in lymphocytes (Wolberg et al., 1975) and in neuroblastoma cells (Blume and Foster, 1975), and depresses cyclic AMP production in adipocytes (Fain, Pointer and Ward, 1972). Adenosine both inhibits (Fain et al., 1972; Weinryb and Michel, 1974) and activates (Blume and Foster, 1975) adenylate cyclase in broken cell preparations. We were led to investigate the effects of adenosine on the hepatic enzyme system by the observation that membranes incubated with an adenylate cyclase assay mixture produced a dialysable factor which appeared to inhibit selectively the metal ion-activated state of the enzyme. The production of this substance depended on the presence of ATP in the medium, which led us to suspect that a product of ATP metabolism may be responsible. Indeed, adenosine inhibited enzyme activity with a K_i which was dependent on the concentration and species of Me^{2+} in the assay medium. As shown in Table 13.5, the K_i with Mn^{2+} alone was tenfold lower than that seen with Mg^{2+}; note that the concentration of Mn^{2+} in this experiment was near maximal, while Mg^{2+} was submaximal, with respect to the Me^{2+} site (see above). In other experiments we have observed that with increasing Mg^{2+} concentrations the K_i for adenosine is lowered. An Mg^{2+}-dependent lowering of the K_i for adenosine on the lung adenylate cyclase system has been reported by Weinryb and Michel (1974). It is also seen in Table 13.5 that glucagon, but not Gpp(NH)p, produced a dramatic effect on the K_i for adenosine inhibition even with Mg^{2+} as the sole divalent cation.

Table 13.5 Inhibition of adenylate cyclase by adenosine under various assay conditions

Additions to assay medium	Adenylate cyclase assayed with	
	1 mM Mg^{2+}	1 mM Mn^{2+}
	K_i for adenosine (μM)	
None (basal)	800	70
Gpp(NH)p, 50 μM	400	25
Glucagon, 0.1 μM	90	40
Gpp(NH)p plus glucagon	250	25

Adenylate cyclase was assayed in the presence of 0.1 mM ATP.

The inhibitory effects of adenosine were highly selective for this nucleoside, since, among a variety of purine and pyrimidine nucleosides and nucleotides tested, only adenosine and, to a lesser extent, 5'-AMP, were potent enzyme inhibitors; the effects of 5'-AMP may be explained by the presence of 5'-nucleotidase in the membranes. The inhibitory effects of adenosine were reversed completely by low concentrations of calf mucosal adenosine deaminase (Table 13.6). Surprisingly, the deaminase, at higher concentrations than required to reverse the effects of adenosine, stimulated adenylate cyclase activity, and this stimulation was inhibited by 70 per cent by the potent adenosine deaminase inhibitor *erythro*-9-(2-hydroxy-3-nonyl) adenine (Table 13.7). These data indicate that the activation by adenosine deaminase is probably not the result of a contaminating enzyme, and suggest that adenosine or a derivative susceptible to attack by the deaminase may be liganded to the hepatic adenylate cyclase system.

The tentative conclusions from the data on adenosine are that the liver system contains an adenosine binding site and that divalent cations increase the affinity of this site for adenosine. When present in the assay medium, adenosine acts as an inhibitor; however, we found that under certain incubation conditions adenosine acts as an activator. Recall that Gpp(NH)p activates the hepatic system in pre-

Table 13.6 Reversal of adenosine inhibition by adenosine deaminase and activation of adenylate cyclase by adenosine deaminase

	Adenylate cyclase activity (pmol cyclic AMP formed/mg protein in 4 min at 30 °C)			
	units adenosine deaminase per tube			
	0	0.1	0.5	2.3
No adenosine	692	873	1054	1401
1 mM adenosine	70	829	–	–

Adenylate cyclase was assayed with 0.1 mM ATP, 1 mM Mn^{2+}, 10 μM Gpp(NH)p and 0.1 μM glucagon. Calf mucosal adenosine deaminase (E. C. 3.5.4.4) was from Sigma (Type I).

Table 13.7 Reversal of adenylate cyclase activation by adenosine deaminase with the use of the adenosine deaminase inhibitor *erythro*-9-(2-hydroxy-3-nonyl)adenine

Inhibitor	Adenylate cyclase activity (pmol cyclic AMP formed/mg protein in 4 min at 30°C) with	
	no additions	2.3 units adenosine deaminase per tube
0	779	1861
4 µM	778	1628
400 µM	829	1174

Adenylate cyclase was assayed with 0.1 mM ATP, 1 mM Mn^{2+}, 10 µM Gpp(NH)p and 0.1 µM glucagon. The inhibitor, *erythro*-9-(2-hydroxy-3-nonyl)adenine, was a gift of the Burroughs Wellcome Co.

treatment, and that activation was enhanced in the presence of divalent cations (Table 13.3). In those experiments pretreatment was performed in the presence of App(NH)p and cyclic AMP. However, in the absence of adenine nucleotide, metal ions did not enhance the stimulatory effects of Gpp(NH)p, as is shown in Table 13.8. It can be seen that the effects of Me^{2+} were restored in the presence of adenosine. These data suggest that adenosine increases the interactions of divalent cations with the enzyme, just as the cations were shown to increase the inhibitory effects of adenosine (Table 13.5). Provided that Gpp(NH)p is present, the stimulatory effects of metal ions and adenosine persisted, even after extensive washing of the membranes. It remains to be determined whether the activating effects of adenosine, which requires metal ion plus guanine nucleotide, is related to the stimulatory effects of adenosine observed in other cell types (see above).

Table 13.8 Effects of adenosine on preactivation by Gpp(NH)p

	Preincubation conditions		Adenylate cyclase activity (pmol cyclic AMP formed/mg protein in 4 min at 30 °C)
Me^{2+}	10 µM Gpp(NH)p	0.1 mM adenosine	
−	−	−	40
−	−	+	28
−	+	−	282
−	+	+	257
1 mM Mg^{2+}	+	−	270
1 mM Mg^{2+}	+	+	327
1 mM Mn^{2+}	+	−	270
1 mM Mn^{2+}	+	+	442

Pretreatment conditions were as described in the footnote to Table 13.4, the pretreatment medium containing 0.1 mM adenosine, 10 µM Gpp(NH)p, 1 mM Mg^{2+} and 1 mM Mn^{2+}. Adenylate cyclase assay was with 0.1 mM ATP and 5 mM Mg^{2+}.

SUMMARY AND CONCLUSIONS

Our studies suggest that adenosine and metal ions interact at sites which may be structurally linked, since the binding of one of these ligands increases the binding of the other. Glucagon and guanine nucleotides, binding at their respective sites, synergistically promote the activation of the enzyme by a process involving divalent cations. Since glucagon, as well as the divalent cations, increase the affinity of the site for adenosine, it seems logical to conclude that the receptor, nucleotide, regulatory metal ion and adenosine sites are functionally linked in the overall regulatory process. It can be concluded that the adenylate cyclase system is a highly complex regulatory enzyme system, rather than the relatively simple system of receptor and catalytic subunits once considered.

It is little wonder that the kinetic characteristics of the enzyme system have often been conflicting and somewhat confusing, and it would be folly to propose, at this point, a model which would incorporate the actions and interactions of the various ligands discussed above. A particular difficulty in considering kinetic models in the current literature is that none accounts for the effects of adenosine, yet this nucleoside is most likely present, as a contaminant or metabolite, in all adenylate cyclase assay media.

As a final note, we do appreciate the fact that there is as yet no way to distinguish between a direct action of a ligand on the adenylate cyclase system and a non-specific effect on the membrane. However, most of the effects of metal ions, guanine nucleotides and adenosine, as well as the interactions between these ligands discussed in this report, are seen in a detergent-dispersed partially purified adenylate cyclase preparation from liver membranes (A. F. Welton, unpublished observations).

ACKNOWLEDGEMENTS

The authors are indebted to Ms Sue Preston who skillfully conducted the experiments described in this report. For numerous discussions we wish to thank our colleagues, Drs G. G. Hammes, V. H. Hruby, P. M. Lad, M. C. Lin, A. C. Newby, S. Nicosia, A. F. Welton and H. Yamamura, and for assistance in preparing this manuscript we thank Ms Carol King Sartain and Ms Joan K. Shores.

REFERENCES

Birnbaumer, L., Pohl, S. L. and Rodbell, M. (1969). *J. Biol. Chem.*, **244**, 2468
Blume, A. J. and Foster, C. J. (1975). *J. Biol. Chem.*, **250**, 5003
Braun, T. and Dods, R. F. (1975). *Proc. Nat. Acad. Sci. USA*, **72**, 1097
Brown, E. M., Fedak, S. A., Woodard, C. J., Aurbach, G. D. and Rodbard, D. (1976). *J. Biol. Chem.*, **251**, 1239
Burke, G. (1970). *Biochim. Biophys. Acta*, **220**, 30
Cuatrecasas, P., Jacobs, S. and Bennett, V. (1975). *Proc. Nat. Acad. Sci. USA*, **72**, 1739
Daly, J. W., Huang, M. and Shimizu, H. (1972). *Advances in Cyclic Nucleotide Research*, Vol. 1 (ed. P. Greengard, R. Paoletti and G. A. Robison), Raven Press, New York, p. 375
de Haen, C. (1974). *J. Biol. Chem.*, **249**, 2756

Drummond, G. I. and Duncan, L. (1970). *J. Biol. Chem.*, **245**, 976
Drummond, G. I., Severson, D. L. and Duncan, L. (1971). *J. Biol. Chem.*, **246**, 4166
Fain, J. N., Pointer, R. H. and Ward, W. F. (1972). *J. Biol. Chem.*, **247**, 6866
Garbers, D. L. and Johnson, R. A. (1975). *J. Biol. Chem.*, **250**, 8449
Glossmann, H. (1975a). *Naunyn-Schmiedebergs Arch. Pharmacol.*, **289**, 99
Glossmann, H. (1975b). *Naunyn-Schmiedebergs Arch. Pharmacol.*, **291**, 89
Glossmann, H., Baukel, A. and Catt, K. J. (1974). *J. Biol. Chem.*, **249**, 664
Glossmann, H. and Gips, H. (1974). *Naunyn-Schmiedebergs Arch. Pharmacol.*, **286**, 239
Hammes, G. G. and Rodbell, M. (1976). *Proc. Nat. Acad. Sci. USA* (in press)
Harwood, J. P., Low, H. and Rodbell, M. (1973). *J. Biol. Chem.*, **248**, 6239
Jard, S., Roy, C., Barth, T., Rajerison, R. and Bockaert, J. (1975). *Advances in Cyclic Nucleotide Research*, Vol. 5 (ed. G. I. Drummond, P. Greengard and Robison, G. A.), Raven Press, New York, p. 31
Lefkowitz, R. J. (1974). *J. Biol. Chem.*, **249**, 6119
Lefkowitz, R. J. (1975). *J. Biol. Chem.*, **250**, 1006
Lefkowitz, R. J. and Caron, M. G. (1975). *J. Biol. Chem.*, **250**, 4418
Londos, C., Salomon, Y., Lin, M. C., Harwood, J. P., Schramm, M., Wolff, J. and Rodbell, M. (1974). *Proc. Nat. Acad. Sci. USA*, **71**, 3087
Londos, C. and Rodbell, M. (1975). *J. Biol. Chem.*, **250**, 3459
Neville, D. R. (1968). *Biochim. Biophys. Acta*, **154**, 540
Perkins, J. P. and Moore, M. M. (1971). *J. Biol. Chem.*, **246**, 62
Pfeuffer, T. and Helmreich, E. J. M. (1975). *J. Biol. Chem.*, **250**, 867
Pohl, S. L., Birnbaumer, L. and Rodbell, M. (1971). *J. Biol. Chem.*, **246**, 1849
Rendell, M., Salomon, Y., Lin, M. C., Rodbell, M. and Berman, M. (1975). *J. Biol. Chem.*, **250**, 4235
Rodbell, M., Birnbaumer, L., Pohl, S. L. and Krans, H. M. J. (1971a). *J. Biol. Chem.*, **246**, 1877
Rodbell, M., Krans, H. M. J., Pohl, S. L. and Birnbaumer, L. (1971b). *J. Biol. Chem.*, **246**, 1872
Rodbell, M., Lin, M. C. and Salomon, Y. (1974). *J. Biol. Chem.*, **249**, 59
Rodbell, M., Lin, M. C., Salomon, Y., Londos, C., Harwood, J. P., Martin, B. R., Rendell, M. and Berman, M. (1975). *Advances in Cyclic Nucleotide Research*, Vol. 5 (ed. G. I. Drummond, P. Greengard and G. A. Robison), Raven Press, New York, p. 3
Rosen, O. M. and Rosen, S. M. (1969). *Arch. Biochem. Biophys.*, **131**, 449
Salomon, Y., Lin, M. C., Londos, C., Rendell, M. and Rodbell, M. (1975). *J. Biol. Chem.*, **250**, 4239
Salomon, Y., Londos, C. and Rodbell, M. (1974). *Anal. Biochem.*, **58**, 541
Salomon, Y. and Rodbell, M. (1975). *J. Biol. Chem.*, **250**, 7245
Sattin, A. and Rall, T. W. (1970). *Molec. Pharmacol.*, **6**, 13
Schramm, M. and Rodbell, M. (1975). *J. Biol. Chem.*, **250**, 2232
Sonenberg, M., Swislocki, N. I., Bockman, R. S., Aizona, Y., Postal-Vinay, M. C., Rubin, M. and Roberts, J. (1973). *J. Supramol. Struct.*, **1**, 356
Spiegel, A. M. and Aurbach, G. D. (1974). *J. Biol. Chem.*, **249**, 7630
Spiegel, A. M., Brown, E. M., Fedak, S. A., Woodard, C. J. and Aurbach, G. D. (1976). *J. Cyclic Nucleotide Res.*, **2**, 47
Sutherland, E. W. and Rall, T. W. (1960). *Pharmacol. Rev.*, **12**, 265
Tao, M. and Lipmann, F. (1969). *Proc. Nat. Acad. Sci. USA*, **63**, 86
Tu, A. T. and Heller, M. J. (1974). *Metal Ions in Biological Systems*, Vol. 1 (ed. H. Sigel), Marcel Dekker, New York, p. 1
Weinryb, I. and Michel, I. M. (1974). *Biochim. Biophys. Acta*, **334**, 218
Wolberg, G., Zimmerman, T. P., Hiemstra, K., Winston, M. and Chu, L. C. (1975). *Science, N.Y.*, **187**, 957

14
Properties and function of the acetylcholine receptor of vertebrate skeletal muscle

E. A. Barnard (Dept. of Biochemistry, Imperial College, London, UK)

INTRODUCTION

The vertebrate neuromuscular junction — or motor endplate — has been *par excellence* a classical object for the study of impulse transmission controlled by a chemical synapse. An impressive history of electrophysiological and pharmacological investigation has revealed the outline of the events involved in transmission there (Katz, 1966; Hubbard, 1974; Rang, 1974). The quantal release of ACh,* the activation of receptors by the transmitter, the depolarisation of the post-synaptic membrane and the triggering of the muscle membrane action potential are successive stages that have been elucidated, aided by the particular accessibility of this site to electrophysiological and pharmacological analysis. The underlying molecular determinants of the synaptic activity have not, however, yet been defined. The molecular biology of the functioning cholinergic synapse is still at an early stage.

The vertebrate motor endplate probably offers at present the most promising case for approaching such an analysis of an entire synapse. Along with its relative simplicity and its extensive physiological characterisation, there is the recent acquisition, in a number of laboratories throughout the world, of molecular information on the ACh receptor of a closely related synapse, that of the electroplaque of the electric fishes (as reviewed recently, for example, by several authors — Karlin, 1974, Changeux, 1975; Eldefrawi and Eldefrawi, 1975; Landowne *et al*, 1975). The limitation of sparsity of material in the isolation of the neuromuscular ACh receptor can be overcome if we can integrate such biochemical data on the relatively abundant electroplaque receptor with evidence on the receptor at the motor endplate and the functioning of the endplate system.

A necessary first step in this analysis is the isolation of the muscle ACh receptor in pure form, and scrutiny of the tacit assumption that this and the electroplaque

---
*Abbreviations: ACh, acetylcholine; AChE, acetylcholinesterase; BuTX, α-bungarotoxin; deca, decamethonium; DFP, di-isopropylfluorophosphate; TC, D-tubocurarine; EM, electron microscope.

ACh receptor are in essence one and the same molecular component. I shall describe here recent work in our laboratory that has led to this stage. Quantitative molecular information on many components and parameters of the synapse will have to be collected. Again as a first step, I shall consider evidence accumulated now on the numbers, types and spatial distributions of the ACh receptor molecules at the neuromuscular synapse. Functional features of the receptor in its *in situ* state in the membrane will also be discussed. These data are merely a starting-point for the lengthy future task of building a valid functional model of the nicotinic cholinergic synapse.

NUMBERS OF FUNCTIONAL MACROMOLECULES AT THE NERVE – MUSCLE JUNCTION

In counting the number of functional macromolecules of a given type, such as those of AChE, at the synapse, methods of fine spatial resolution are required to avoid overlap or confusion with extrasynaptic molecules of similar properties present in the rest of the muscle, and to recognise functionally distinct zones. Autoradiography of labelled irreversible inhibitors, bound specifically, was applied to achieve this counting (Barnard, 1970), initially for AChE molecules (Rogers *et al.*, 1966, 1969). DFP, labelled with either ^{32}P or ^{3}H, was employed for reaction with the active centres of AChE, the contribution of these being distinguished from other DFP-reactive sites by the use of selective blocking or reactivating agents (Barnard *et al.*, 1973). By confining the counting to the endplate areas microscopically — using light or electron microscope autoradiography — AChE molecules actually at the synapse could thus be counted (Rogers *et al.*, 1966, 1969; Salpeter, 1969; Barnard *et al.*, 1973). By these methods it was found that, for example, the diaphragm muscle red fibre of the adult mouse has 1×10^7 active centres of AChE at each endplate, and these molecules are on or close to the post-synaptic membrane at a mean density of $3000/\mu m^2$.

To measure the endplate receptors in muscles, we (Barnard, Wieckowski and Chiu, 1971a,b) and Miledi and Potter (1971) began about 1970 to prepare and use a radioactive form of the snake venom neutotoxin α-bungarotoxin (BuTX), following the pharmacological characterisation by Lee and co-workers (Chang and Lee, 1966) of the specific antinicotinic, postsynaptic, near-irreversible action of these α-neurotoxins, and parallelling the application of BuTX to give blockade of cholinergic ligand binding in electroplaque membranes (Changeux, Kasai and Lee, 1970). Studies in a variety of laboratories on the electroplaque receptor (reviewed as noted above) have confirmed that, indeed, a specific combination of the receptor and such a toxin occurs, which abolishes the receptor binding of both cholinergic agonists and antagonists.

We employ α-bungarotoxin in [^{3}H]-acetylated forms ([^{3}H]BuTX) which have been separated and characterised chemically and which possess the same specificity for the muscle endplate receptor as the native BuTX molecule (Porter *et al.*, 1973b; Chiu *et al.*, 1974). Either a mono-acetylated species, which has the same affinity

Acetylcholine Receptor of Vertebrate Skeletal Muscle

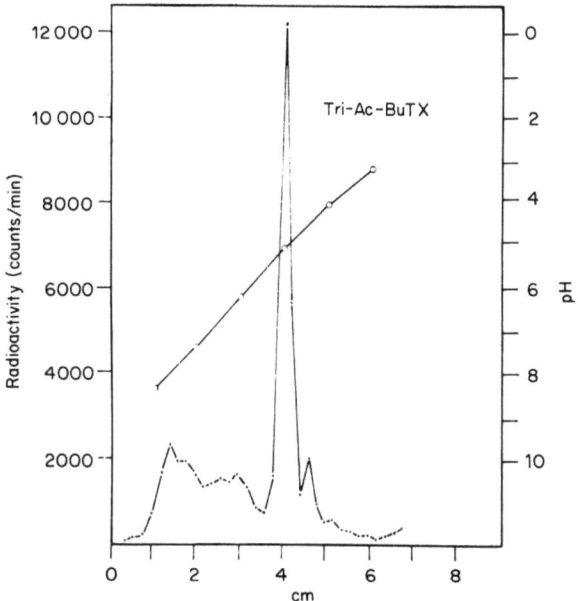

Figure 14.1 Homogeneity of the labelled toxin. To avoid ambiguity in kinetic determinations, it is desirable to use a single species of the modified toxin. Acetylation gives a mixture of mono-, di- and triacetylated derivatives, which are separated by ion exchange chromatography until homogeneous species of a monoacetyl, and one of several suitable triacetyls, are obtained. The most stringent criterion for homogeneity of each of these is isoelectric focusing in a narrow pH range. Here is illustrated a preparation of a triacetyl species, focused in a gradient (○) from pH 3 - 8 on polyacrylamide gel. The radioactivity across the gel was measured on 0.2 mm slices (• — •). From data of R. G. Shorr and E. A. Barnard

and reactivity as native BuTX (Chiu et al., 1974; Barnard et al., 1975), or, to give greater labelling (e.g. for preparative work), a tri-acetylated form (Fig. 14.1) is used; the latter has a threefold lower affinity for the receptor than native BuTX, but is equally specific (Dolly et al., 1977a).

Measurements of the number of ACh receptors at a single junction have been reported from several laboratories based simply upon the uptake of a labelled α-neurotoxin by a muscle or muscle strip and estimates of the number of endplates contained therein. It is easy, however, to incur artefacts in performing such a reaction in intact muscle, due both to the very slow diffusion of the toxin protein through the muscle and to the existence of sites outside the endplates that have a weaker but distinctive affinity for BuTX (Porter et al., 1973b; Chiu, Dolly and Barnard, 1973). There are also questions about the heterogeneity of fibre types, and, hence, of endplate types, within a single muscle, and the assumption of uniformity in all endplates of one type. All of these problems can be avoided by the alternative mentioned above, i.e. by the selective counting in autoradiographs (by light or electron microscopy) of the labelled sites actually associated with each endplate. When a sufficient number are counted, the uniformity for a given muscle fibre type can be tested, and has been found to hold true if the fibre size is constant (Porter and Barnard, 1975c) and the amount of radioactivity bound at a single endplate is determined accurately. Calibration using [^{32}P]DFP applied as an internal standard (Barnard et al., 1971b) yields absolute numbers of toxin-binding sites per endplate. The results have shown that those sites, presumed (see below) to be receptor active centres, number between 2×10^6 and 1×10^8 per endplate in a variety of vertebrate muscles (Barnard et al., 1973, 1975), depending on the muscle type and the fibre diameter (Porter and Barnard, 1975c). Outside the endplate the numbers of these receptor sites are negligibly small, except after denervation or in embryonic muscles.

TYPES OF TOXIN-BINDING SITES AT THE ENDPLATE

It is assumed in the above discussion that each BuTX-binding site is one ACh-binding active centre of the receptor. While reaction with such a toxin does totally abolish the postsynaptic response to ACh (Lester, 1972; Albuquerque et al., 1973b), this does not prove, of course, that the same sites are involved for each agent, or that their numbers are equal. These relationships have been explored by studying the ability of antagonists and of ACh to block the specific uptake of [^{3}H]BuTX.

D-Tubocurarine (TC) prevents the uptake of [^{3}H]BuTX specifically at the endplates in intact muscle specimens (Porter et al, 1973b; Chiu et al., 1974). As shown in Fig. 14.2, when the measurements are made by solubilisation and liquid scintillation counting of the labelled muscle, this protection by TC reaches, at its maximum, a level of about 90 per cent of the total sites. Increase of TC concentration to several orders of magnitude greater than its apparent half-saturation value never abolishes all of the reactivity with [^{3}H]BuTX, there being a fraction, which is observed always to be about 10 per cent of the total toxin-binding sites, which is completely resistant to TC. The other 90 per cent or so of the sites are, however, highly sensitive to TC.

Reaction rates at endplates in intact muscles become complicated, however, by the slow diffusion of a protein such as BuTX into (Porter et al., 1973b) and out of the tissue. This situation earlier gave rise to the impression that a fraction, variously reported as 35-50 per cent, of the endplate BuTX-binding sites is insensitive to TC (Miledi and Potter, 1971; Berg et al.; Porter et al., 1973b; Albuquerque et al., 1973a). Not all of these cases can be attributed, as has been supposed (Colquhoun, Rang and Ritchie, 1974; Colquhoun, 1975), to competition by the reversible inhibitor being (after long reaction times) surmounted by the irreversible reaction, as may not be recognised if a measurement is made only of the final extent of toxin uptake: we had been careful to make (Porter et al., 1973b; Chiu et al., 1974) initial rate measurements and also to demonstrate a

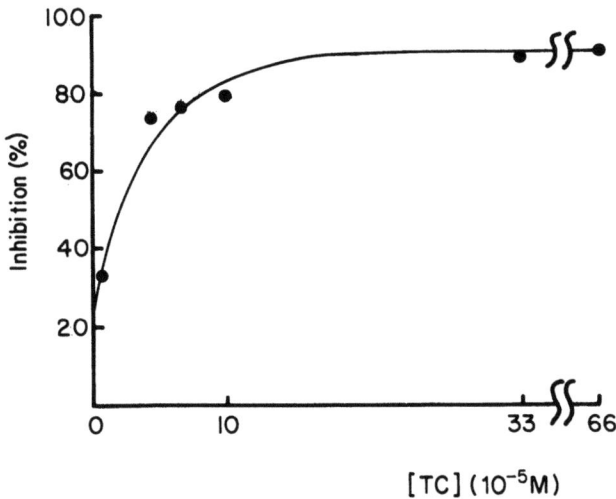

Figure 14.2 The effect of increasing concentrations of TC in suppressing the reaction of endplate receptors in intact mouse diaphragm with [^{3}H]BuTX. The extent of reaction in a 2 h period at 25°C was expressed in each case as a percentage of the control value (TC absent), after correction for non-endplate uptake. In this period 75 per cent of the total receptor present would react with [^{3}H]BuTX in the control case. Each point is the mean for four hemidiaphragms. A suppression to more than 90 per cent of the non-inhibited reaction is never seen at any TC concentration, even up to 10^{-3} M (not shown), in intact muscle or muscle strips (from Barnard et al., 1977)

plateau of reduced toxin uptake in the presence of TC in conditions where no detectable uptake would be predicted (Mildvan and Leigh, 1964) kinetically if all sites had the same high affinity for TC. This phenomenon is due, rather, to the reversible binding at other sites in the muscle of a pool of labelled toxin which can, at later stages in the processing for the measurement (owing to the very slow diffusion out or exchange of this molecule), react at the endplates. When greatly prolonged washes are given with a high concentration of TC always present, this secondary phase of the reaction is prevented and intact muscle specimens then show the suppression of toxin reaction by TC, about 90 per cent at its maximum, as shown in Fig. 14.2 (Barnard et al., 1977). The same true 90 per cent TC-sensitivity was found similarly for the toxin-binding sites in chronically denervated mouse diaphragm muscle (Dolly et al., 1977a).

To confirm this by eliminating diffusion problems, and assess the meaning of the residual 10 per cent of TC-resistant sites observed, it is preferable to conduct the reaction on dispersed membrane fragments from muscle that contain the receptors. This permits reliable kinetic measurements to be made for the reaction of [^{3}H]BuTX with the muscle receptor in its membrane-bound state. Such a preparation of receptor-rich sarcolemmal fragments can be obtained by breakage

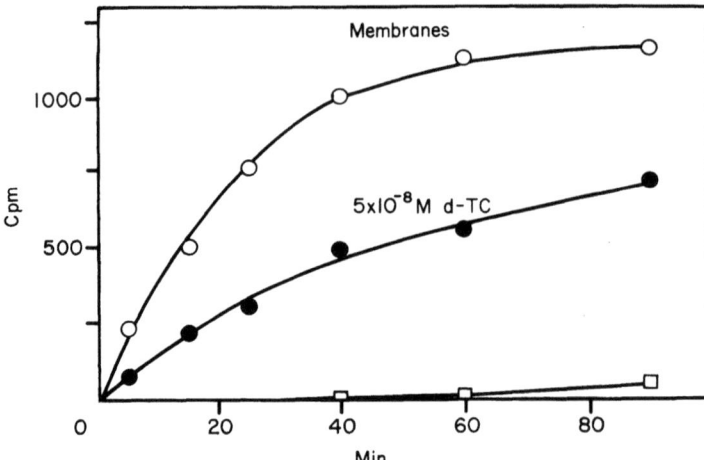

Figure 14.3 Reaction of membrane-bound ACh receptor with [^{3}H]BuTX, and its inhibition by TC. The receptor-rich preparation from denervated muscle is incubated with [^{3}H]BuTX (50 nM, a large excess) at 25°C, pH 7, and the amount of complex found is measured (○) in aliquots by their radioactivity that can be firmly bound to DEAE – cellulose discs when washed with 0.2 per cent Triton X-100 medium; the cationic toxin does not adhere in these conditions. The reaction is first-order with respect to the disappearance of receptor. The maximum suppression of this binding by TC (present at 10^{-3} M in a parallel experiment, □) is illustrated. Another curve shows the retardation of the toxin reaction at a subsaturating TC concentration (here 5×10^{-8} M, ●), one of a set used in estimating the K_D value; these curves proceed to the same final plateau value as in the unprotected case, when the incubation is prolonged sufficiently. From data of E. A. Barnard and B. Mallick

and fractionation of denervated cat leg muscles, or denervated or innervated rat diaphragm muscles, and shows rapid saturation of binding of [^{3}H]BuTX (Fig. 14.3). A monophasic first-order rate characterises the reaction throughout its course, when one employs a homogeneous species of [^{3}H] triacetyl-BuTX (as assessed by isoelectric focusing in a narrow pH range, when a single peak is obtained; Fig. 14.1). With this membrane preparation, TC and cholinergic agonists at about 10^{-4} M concentration give complete or near-complete protection from the toxin-binding (Table 14.1). Non-cholinergic ligands have very little effect. Considering, therefore, the sites in muscle that bind BuTX to saturation in the rapid phase of its reaction at low concentrations, we see that all of those sites have the properties of the ACh receptor active centre, and we henceforth identify them as such.

The 10 per cent of the toxin uptake of intact muscle specimens which is not blocked by reversibly binding cholinergic ligands is attributed to a non-receptor component of muscle also binding the toxin pseudo-irreversibly, but more slowly than the receptor. Such a component was recognised (Chiu *et al.*, 1973) after its

Table 14.1 Maximum inhibition by cholinergic ligands of [^{3}H] BuTX binding to muscle and to receptor preparations

Preparation	Source	Inhibition (%)	
		TC ($3 - 10 \times 10^{-4}$ M)	ACh^a or deca^b ($10^{-3} - 10^{-4}$ M)
1. Intact diaphragm a. Normal b. Denervated	Mouse	 90 90	
2. Muscle membrane fraction (denervated)	Cat leg Rat diaphragm	97 96^c	100
3. Isolated receptor (denervated)	Cat leg	100	100

The binding of [^{3}H] BuTX, at 25°C, pH 7.0 or 7.5, was followed to a final plateau value, in the presence or the absence of the concentration of ligand noted. The percentage of the total uptake that could be suppressed, using the mean value of 2 - 7 separate determinations, in each case is shown. From Barnard et al. (1977).

^{a}The preparations were pretreated with 10^{-5} M DFP.
^{b}The same effect was obtained with both drugs.
^{c}Using a homogenate of rat diaphragm and another assay method, Colquhoun and Rang (1976) observed that about 80 per cent of the observed uptake of [^{125}I] BuTX can be suppressed by maximally effective concentrations of TC in denervated muscle, or 50 per cent in innervated.

separation from the receptor-[^{3}H] BuTX complex on the basis of size: the latter has an apparent molecular weight (by gel filtration in 1.5 per cent Triton X-100 medium) of approximately 500 000, while the non-receptor complex is apparently ~ 200,000, and could be obtained alone when all of the receptor sites were previously blocked by their fast reaction with unlabelled BuTX. When the latter condition obtains, or when the labelling is conducted in 10^{-3} MTC, the degree of muscle labelling still produced is not, we have found by autoradiography of sections of such specimens, associated with any detectable concentration of sites at the synaptic membranes, but appears to be extra-junctional. When the muscle specimens showing about 10 per cent residual labelling after reaction with [^{3}H] BuTX with 10^{-3} M TC present were extracted completely in 1.5 per cent Triton X-100 (at pH 8, 4°C), gel filtration showed (if efficient muscle postlabelling washing procedures had been used) that the residual label is not due to persisting [^{3}H] BuTX in the muscle, but resides in the extra-junctional component of apparent weight 200 000. Since an equal weight of a muscle zone devoid of endplates was always used as a control, and since the TC-resistant label was invariably found in the endplate-containing strips after such subtractive correction, this component must be concentrated near the endplates. It is largely lost when the

Table 14.2 Dissociation constants for TC at the denervated mammalian muscle receptor

Muscles	Preparation	Method	K_D or K_{app} (M)	Ref.
A. Membrane-bound				
Cat leg (mixed)	Membranes	BuTX binding (25°C)	0.4×10^{-7}	Barnard et al. (1977)
Rat diaphragm	Homogenate	BuTX binding (20°C)	4×10^{-7}	Colquhoun et al. (1974)
Rat soleus	Muscle fibre	Electrophysiological[a] (23°C)	8×10^{-7}	Dolly et al. (1977)
Rat diaphragm	Muscle fibre	Electrophysiological[a] (23°C)	6×10^{-7}	Beranek and Vyskocil (1967)
B. Solubilised				
Cat leg (mixed)	Purified	BuTX binding (25°C)	1.0×10^{-7}	Barnard and Dolly (1975)
Rat diaphragm	Crude extract	BuTX binding (RT)[b]	1.2×10^{-8}	Alper, Lowy and Schmidt (1974)
Rat diaphragm	Partly purified	BuTX binding (35°C)	5.5×10^{-7}	Brockes and Hall (1975)

[a]By measurement of the sensitivity to ACh; K_{app}, measured here, is the concentration of TC required for half-maximal inhibition.
[b]RT = Room temperature.

membranes are prepared. Owing to its minor and non-specific nature it has not been investigated further, but we can note that an α-neurotoxin-binding component of similar character has been detected in lobster axons and in mammalian brain (Denburg, Eldefrawi and O'Brien, 1972). Consistent with all of this evidence, a detailed investigation of the blockade by BuTX of the post-synaptic response to neurally released ACh has shown that there is no fraction of that response which is not highly sensitive, also, to TC (Dolly et al., 1977a). Using focal depolarisation of the nerve terminal in the presence of tetrodotoxin and neostigmine (cf. Katz and Miledi, 1967), the endplate potential could be followed over its full range, and no evidence was found for any class of functional receptors having other than a high sensitivity to TC (see values of K_{app} in Table 14.2), or (in protection experiments) not susceptible to complete blockade by BuTX or TC. Hence, functionally a single class of the BuTX-binding sites that are on receptors appears to exist at the endplate.

For the specific toxin-binding receptors in the membrane preparation, nicotinic cholinergic ligands applied at subsaturating concentrations produce measurable retardations of the reaction with [^{3}H]BuTX (Fig. 14.3), and these rates follow expected ligand affinities for this receptor, as will be illustrated below.

LOCATION OF THE RECEPTORS IN THE SYNAPTIC MEMBRANES

The detailed distribution of these receptors at the endplate can be obtained by means of autoradiography at the ultrastructural level. After [^{3}H]BuTX is applied to muscles *in vivo*, this method confirms that the concentrations of label are entirely synaptic (Porter et al., 1973b). The same method can be applied with *in vitro* labelling (to ensure that saturation of the sites has occurred) if precautions are taken to ensure good preservation of ultrastructure and removal of unreacted toxin. Analysis of a large number of EM sections from such a muscle has permitted plots to be made (Porter, Barnard and Chiu, 1973a) of the distribution of the labelled sites, with the synaptic membranes as reference points. We find that the labelling is always associated with the postsynaptic membrane and not with the presynaptic (axonal) membrane. The fidelity with which the grain distribution follows the complex contours of the post-synaptic membrane, as shown by the coincidence of the plot with a theoretical one for a source in the latter membrane (Porter et al., 1973a; Porter and Barnard, 1975a), appears to be sufficient to locate the ACh receptors on that membrane. This analysis has been performed for two different mammals, the mouse and the bat, with identical results (Porter and Barnard, 1975a).

The postsynaptic membrane location has been confirmed by means of the experimental removal of the axonal membrane alone. This can be accomplished (Hall and Kelly, 1971; Betz and Sakmann, 1973) by a limited proteolytic digestion, e.g. by collagenase. Despite such removal of the presynaptic membrane, the EM autoradiographs obtained are as from normal muscle specimens (Barnard et al., 1975). An alternative approach to the same end employs denervation: up to about

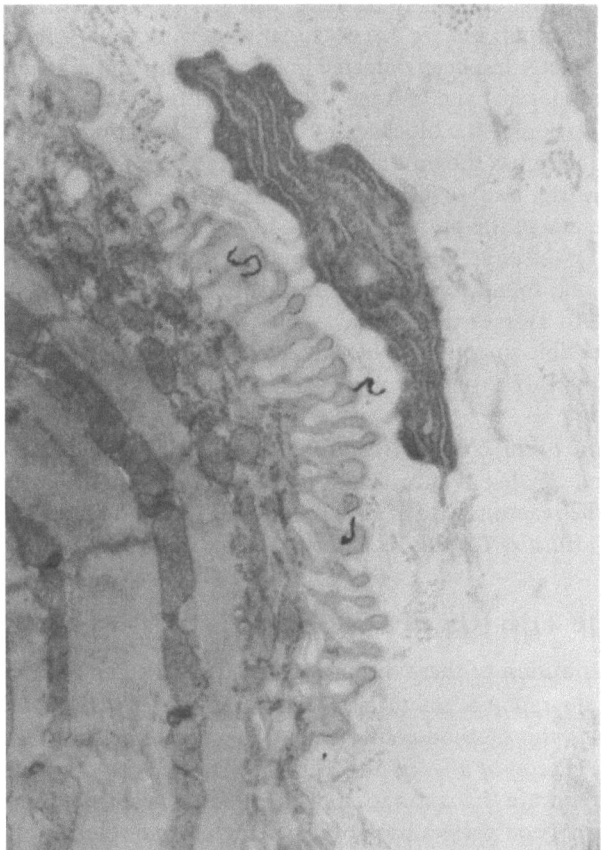

Figure 14.4 The application of denervation to determine the extent of confinement to the postsynaptic membrane of the [^{3}H]BuTX-binding sites. About 5 days after section of the phrenic nerve, the mouse diaphragm endplates have lost their nerve terminals, as seen in this electron micrograph, the postsynaptic zone being covered now by Schwann cells (one seen here) or connective tissue infiltration, but the junctional folds (a row is seen here) are left unaltered at this stage. Comparison of the mean grain density per μm^2 of this postsynaptic membrane shows it to be the same as that at the corresponding innervated endplate, and the same is true for the crest grain density. Hence, any contribution to the latter from scatter due to nearby receptor sites on the presynaptic membrane is less than the experimental error of the method. Note also the 'thickenings' at the fold crests, which are visible here.

one week after nerve section, the postsynaptic morphology is preserved unchanged, but the nerve terminals have disappeared (Fig. 14.4). Using such specimens, the histogram plots are quantitatively unchanged from those derived from endplates of the innervated muscle (Porter and Barnard, 1975b). From all of the evidence just cited, we conclude that the density of receptor sites can be related to the postsynaptic membrane alone (although the inherent limitations of the method mean that up to about 5 per cent of the sites could be on the presynaptic membrane and remain undetected). For any endplate type, therefore, the mean density is measured over the total length of postsynaptic membrane found in the sections. A constant value is obtained for all muscles so far examined (Table 14.3). This includes the endplates in the 5 day denervated mouse hemidiaphragm.

It is important to note that the density of the ACh receptors reported above is the *mean* density, i.e. averaged over the entire postsynaptic membrane. However, we now know that the density of the receptor active centres in that membrane is, in fact, far from uniform. When the distribution of silver grains in EM autoradiographs of [^{3}H]BuTX-labelled mouse diaphragm endplates is analysed, instead, with respect to the distance down the junctional folds (i.e. moving away from the

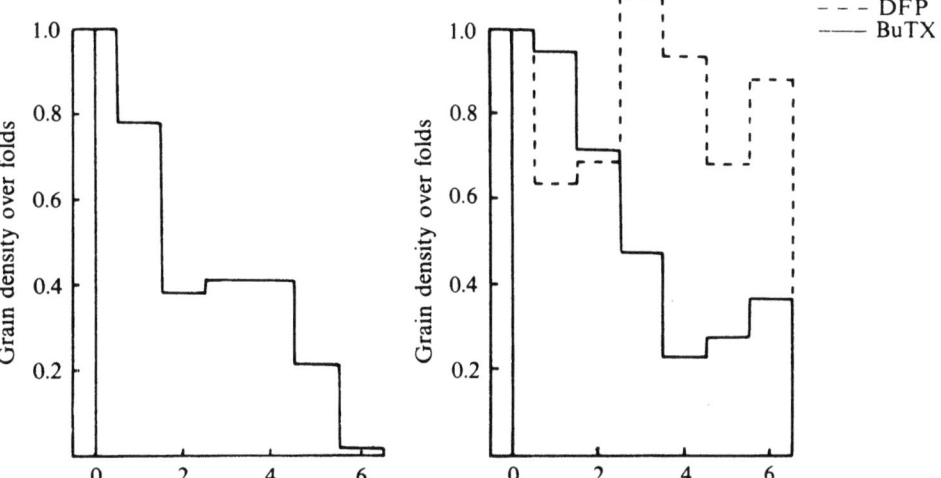

Figure 14.5 Relative silver grain densities in EM autoradiographs of labelled muscle, over the region of the postsynaptic folds. The measured densities (per μm^2, normalised, and corrected for radial dilution) are plotted in relation to the distance down the folds from the axonal membrane as origin. These distances along the abscissa are in arbitrary units, such that the fold crest region occurs mostly within the zone 0 - 1, and entirely in the zones 0 - 2, with the grain densities in zones 3 - 6 being due to radiation scatter from the crest zone plus any isotope along the fold depths. (*Left*) Bat diaphragm endplates, labelled with [^{3}H]BuTX. (*Right*) Mouse diaphragm endplates, labelled with [^{3}H]BuTX (solid line) or with [^{3}H]DFP (broken line). Note that the distribution for [^{3}H]BuTX fits that expected for a concentration of 25 000 sites per μm^2 in the crest zone (upper 30 per cent of the postsynaptic profile, in these particular endplate types) and less than 10 per cent of that level in the fold depths below that zone. In the case of [^{3}H]DFP, the deviations are not significant from an even density throughout all zones. Data from Porter and Barnard (1975a). Note that when 5-day-denervated mouse diaphragm was used, instead, with [^{3}H]BuTX, the same distribution as that shown for normal mouse diaphragm (solid line, right), was obtained (Porter and Barnard, 1975b)

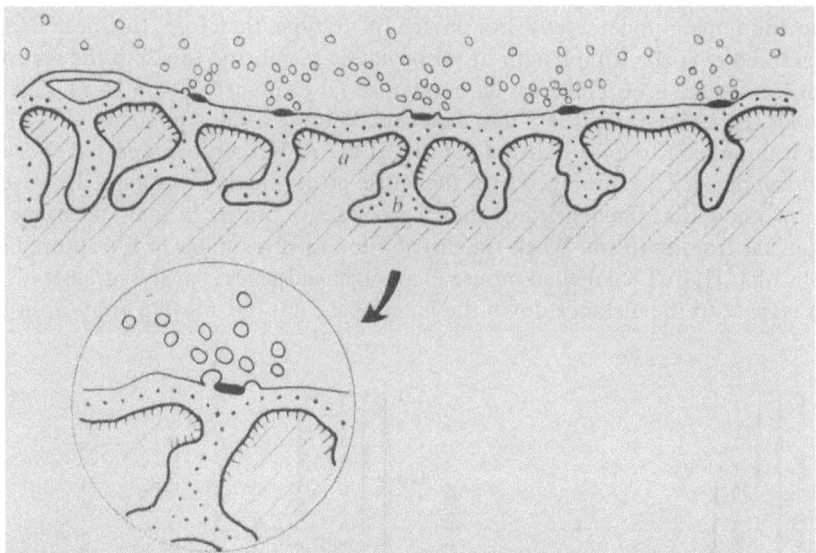

Figure 14.6 Interpretative diagram of frog motor endplate to show the spatial relationships between sites of transmitter release and concentrations of ACh receptors and acetylcholinesterase. The basic morphology was traced from micrographs of frog muscle endplates published by Couteaux and Pecot-Dechavassine (1970). The vesicles characteristically stack opposite the mouths of the postjunctional folds. Dense bars on the presynaptic membrane opposite the fold mouths represent ridges seen in freeze-etch preparations. The striations along the postjunctional membrane at the fold crest correspond to the receptor-rich region (a) of the subneural apparatus. Dotted lines show the extent of visible cleft substance and, it is presumed, of the AChE (see Fig. 14.5).

The inset shows, in detail, the fusion of vesicles with the presynaptic membrane as determined by Heuser et al. (1974) and Peper et al. (1974). The dense presynaptic ridge prevents the vesicles from releasing transmitter directly into the receptor-poor, acetylcholinesterase-rich region of the fold depths (b). Instead, the ACh is released from vesicles at specific sites on either side of the presynaptic ridge (the 'zones actives' of Couteaux) so that it is expelled onto the receptor-rich crests of the folds (a). It is proposed that upon release from receptors on the fold crests part of the ACh escapes, mostly being hydrolysed en route, while the rest must diffuse into the fold depths where likewise it is hydrolysed by the AChE located there. Taken from Porter and Barnard (1975a)

presynaptic membrane along every fold, no matter how it lies) it becomes clear (see Fig. 14.5) that the ACh receptors are located asymmetrically there (Albuquerque et al., 1974; Porter and Barnard, 1975a). A high concentration is present at the crests of the folds, i.e. those regions of the postsynaptic membrane nearest to the presynaptic membrane and mostly lying parallel to the latter (Fig. 14.6). The membrane receptor density near and at the bottom of a fold is low, it being estimated from histograms of the grain counts over the crest zone

Table 14.3 Densities of receptor active centres on the postsynaptic membrane (PSM)

Muscle fibre type	Fold depth	% Thickened[a] zone on PSM	Density (per μm^2) of receptor sites on PSM		Ref.
			Mean	At crests[a]	
Mouse diaphragm (red)	0.50	28	8500	25 000 – 30 000	Porter et al. (1973a); Porter and Barnard (1975a,b)[b]
Mouse diaphragm, 5-day-denervated	0.50	28	9200	25 000 – 30 000	Porter and Barnard (1975b)[b]
Mouse sternomastoid	0.80	31	8800[c]	30 500	Fertuck and Salpeter (1976)
Bat diaphragm (red)	0.35	31	8800	25 000 – 30 000	Porter and Barnard (1975a)[b]
(Adjacent sarcolemma)[d]			(140)		Porter and Barnard (1975a)

[a]See text for definition of these terms.

[b]We had originally estimated 20 000 – 25 000/μm^2 (Porter and Barnard, 1975a), but that was based on reports of intramembranous particles on the lower walls of the folds at a mean of about one-sixth the density in the crests. Since this has been found to be highly variable and there is some question as to whether these are the same particle type as those on the crests, we subsequently (Porter and Barnard, 1975b) employed only the grain density histograms for the folds, which suggest about one-tenth for that relative density in the fold depths, and this is borne out in further counts made of such specimens. With a mean density of 30 per cent of the total post-synaptic membrane lying in the crests here, and with an overall mean density of 9000/μm^2, this gives a value of 25 000/μm^2 for the crest density. The upper limit, given by the possibility that there are no receptors at all below the crests (cf. the 3 per cent of the crest value estimated for the fold depths by Fertuck and Salpeter, 1976), is similarly obtained as 30 000/μm^2. All of the density values in this table are subject to the additional limits of inaccuracy inherent in the EM autoradiographic techniques used.

[c]Value derived for this muscle by an indirect method by Porter and Barnard (1975a). While Fertuck and Salpeter (1976) do not report a mean density for this case, from their data one can calculate the same value for it, within experimental error.

[d]Muscle cell membrane adjacent to (about 3 μm from) endplate zone in mouse diaphragm fibres: value given for comparison, to show the enrichment in receptors at the PSM over the normal muscle membrane, irrespective of the folding at the endplate. At much greater distances, this value becomes much lower still (Porter et al., 1973a; Fertuck and Salpeter, 1976).

alone (this being defined by its electron-dense characteristic — see below) that the crests contain ~ 90 per cent of the total labelled sites (Porter and Barnard, 1975b). From the extent of labelling, measured as before but with respect to the receptor-bearing crest region only, we now find the true local density of receptors to be 25 000 - 30 000/μm^2 (Table 14.3).

Confinement of toxin-binding sites to the fold crests as viewed in EM autoradiographs was independently noted by Fertuck and Salpeter (1974). In [^{125}I] BuTX-labelled mouse sternomastoid endplates the same authors (1976) measured the density there (Table 14.3); their value is derived on the basis that there are no receptors at all below the crests, and if we were to make the same assumption, we would obtain, from our mean density and the value (see below) of 30 per cent for the relative crest area on the postsynaptic membrane, an identical value, 30 000/μm^2, for the receptor density at the fold crests. In a second species examined, a bat, the same polarised distribution and density was found (Porter and Barnard, 1975a; Fig. 14.5).

An important correlation with this distribution comes from two types of independent ultrastructural evidence. Firstly, it is known that the region that we term the crest of the fold is seen as a selectively 'thickened' line (see Fig. 14.4) on the postsynaptic membrane in electron micrographs of endplates, especially after osmication and lead or uranyl staining (Birks, Huxley and Katz, 1960; Zacks, 1973). We have measured the extent of this electron-dense layer in endplates in several twitch muscle types, and find that in these it represents about 30 per cent of their total postsynaptic area (Table 14.3). This fits well the fraction of the surface with high receptor density needed to produce the asymmetric histograms for fold-depth distance seen with the toxin labelling (Fig. 14.5). Since the folds vary considerably in depth (Table 14.3), this indicates that — in the muscle types sampled — the thickened zone expands proportionately as the total postsynaptic membrane area increases. If the thickening is due to the dense layer of receptors, then we can readily understand on that basis the constancy (at about 9000/μm^2) seen above for the receptor density when averaged over the entire postsynaptic membrane. It seems likely that the local crest density of 25 000 - 30 000/μm^2 is the characteristic packing for the ACh receptors of mammalian muscle endplates; the value quoted for the overall (mean) density may well vary, however, if very diverse types of muscle fibres were to be compared, since we have never assumed that the proportion of 30 per cent noted above holds for fibres other than the types cited. It is likely to be greater in certain endplate types known to have very little postsynaptic foldings, such as those on tonic muscle fibres and on some slow twitch fibres. Thus in the mouse soleus muscle, or some frog muscles (Rosenbluth, 1974), the thickened zone in such electron micrographs can be seen to extend along the segments of the postsynaptic membrane running between the infrequent folds and apposed to the presynaptic membrane, suggesting that the receptors are concentrated there over a greater proportion of the total membrane.

The second morphological correlate of the observed location of these sites is the distribution of heavy concentrations of intramembranous characteristic particles of about 120 Å mean diameter, seen in recent freeze-etch studies of mammalian and frog muscle endplates (Peper et al., 1974; Heuser, Reese and Landis, 1974; Rash and Ellisman, 1974). These particles are almost entirely confined to the same crest region, and have been seen in patches of $6000/\mu m^2$ (Heuser et al., 1974) or $7500/\mu m^2$ (Peper et al., 1974) local density. While it seems inescapable that these particles contain the receptors that we label, the number of receptor active centres per particle cannot be deduced with assurance until we know the significance of the patchy distribution of these particles in the crest zones. Possible redistribution from an original pattern there, or loss of particles between the islands seen, must first be firmly ruled out. In electroplaque postsynaptic membranes continuous arrays of rather similar particles are seen, at densities of $6000 - 12\,000/\mu m^2$ (Cartaud et al., 1972; Nickel and Potter, 1973; Landowne, Potter and Terrar, 1975). Labelled α-neurotoxin binding sites have also been measured there by EM autoradiography, and a value of about $50\,000/\mu m^2$ has been found (Bourgeois et al., 1972, Cohen and Changeux, 1975). It seems possible that the arrangement of the ACh receptors in the electroplaque membrane differs from that at muscle endplates. If, at the endplate postsynaptic membrane, we simply compare the mean density over the crest zone only, of its particles in both the rat and the frog, $2000 - 3000/\mu m^2$ (Heuser et al., 1974; Ellisman et al., 1976), with that of the [^{3}H] BuTX-binding sites there, this is compatible with six subunits, or with the eight per particle discerned by Rash et al. (1975) at the highest resolution, if the subunits considered carry two or one toxin sites each, i.e. the uncertainties in these various parameters do not as yet permit us to be more precise than that.

While, as noted earlier, the total number of ACh receptor active centres at a single endplate can vary over a 50-fold or greater range among different vertebrate muscle fibres, their surface density in the receptor-bearing zone appears to be, as far as present evidence goes, at a constant level. Consistent with this, it has been shown that the response to applied saturating doses of ACh, measured by intracellular recording, is — within experimental error — constant (3.5 mV per 10^6 molecules of ACh) for twitch fibre endplates, for a range of muscle types and vertebrate species tested, of widely differing total contents of receptors per endplate (Albuquerque et al., 1974; Barnard et al., 1975; Kuffler and Yoshikami, 1975). When a fixed quantity of ACh is released at the endplate, the response evoked is determined by the local surface density of receptors and not by their total number. That density is so high that the ACh content of one synaptic vesicle, or quantum, cannot saturate the receptors in the postsynaptic area on which it impinges (Barnard et al., 1975). The arrangement there permits the highest efficiency of activating encounters to be realised during the brief lifetime (~ 0.5 ms) of ACh in the synaptic cleft, and maintains a high margin of safety in transmission.

A direct determination of this margin of safety has been made by measuring progressive receptor occupancy by BuTX and the resultant degrees of suppression of the endplate potential (Albuquerque et al., 1973b), and shows, indeed, a high degree of efficiency of the postsynaptic activation, consistent with this model.

FUNCTIONAL ARRANGEMENT OF POSTSYNAPTIC MACRO-MOLECULES AT THE ENDPLATE

We have seen that the receptor active centres are present essentially only in the crest regions of the postsynaptic membrane, at a density of about $25\,000/\mu m^2$. The distribution of AChE molecules down the postsynaptic folds is also of interest. We use [^{3}H] DFP labelling: the distribution of the AChE active centres labelled by DFP follows quite closely that of the total of DFP-labelled sites at the endplate (Salpeter, 1969; Salpeter, Plattner and Rogers, 1972). With this method we find that AChE molecules are essentially uniformly spread over the entire fold surface (Fig. 14.5). Hence, there is a clear distinction between the arrangement of the receptors and the arrangement of the AChE molecules over the postsynaptic membrane.

There is evidence to show that the AChE molecules are in a more external situation than the receptor molecules. The AChE can be detached from the endplate in intact muscles by limited proteolysis, and the receptor properties of the synapse are then left intact (Hall and Kelly, 1971; Betz and Sakmann, 1973). When this removal is accomplished, there is a loss of the inter-synaptic matrix or 'cleft substance' layer which is to be seen in the electron micrographs of endplates as a fuzzy line above the postsynaptic membrane. This line always, in untreated muscle, extends to the bottom of every fold. It seems likely that this intersynaptic matrix contains the AChE (Barnard, 1974). The evidence now available on the structure of the synaptic AChE from the electroplaque as source (Dudai, Herzberg and Silman, 1973; Rieger, Bon and Massoulié, 1973) shows that it contains, when undamaged, a long protein tail attached to the globular enzyme. In frog muscle endplates projections are seen from the postsynaptic membrane into the cleft substance layer which suggests a comparable structure (Rosenbluth, 1974). In a plausible model a tail attaches the active enzyme to, or is in a layer above, the membrane (Rieger et al., 1973; Barnard, 1974), accounting for the selective dissociability of the AChE.

We have a situation, therefore, in which certain postsynaptic membrane regions lining or close to the primary synaptic cleft carry about 25 000 receptor active centres per μm^2 and about 3000 AChE active centres per μm^2, while lower in the folds there is very largely only the AChE, at its same density. What is the functional significance of this arrangement?

At first sight the actual arrangement of receptors discovered thus would seem to be inefficient for their combination with ACh as liberated in the synaptic cleft. The presynaptic ACh-laden vesicles tend to concentrate in stacks exactly over the *mouths* of the subneuronal folds (Birks et al., 1960; Zacks, 1973). Characteristic 'vesicle release sites' have been discerned in transmission EM and freeze-etch studies of the presynaptic membranes of endplates (Peper et al., 1974; Heuser et al., 1974; Rash and Ellisman, 1974), from which the vesicles release the transmitter. It would seem, then, that AChE is expelled down into every fold, into lower regions of the folds where, paradoxically, the receptors are sparse. The freeze-etch studies provide further information that can resolve this contradiction. A definite ridge on the presynaptic membrane defines, in fact, the edge of each vesicle release site, as illustrated in Fig. 14.6. This geometry leads one to suppose that the vesicle contents are expelled onto the crest of each folded postsynaptic unit, and do not find a direct path into the mouth of the fold. This means that the patches of high receptor density are, in fact, well situated for primary interception of the ACh.

The local coexistence in the crest region of high surface concentrations of receptors and AChE is well understandable in the light of the known important role of enzymic destruction of ACh (Barnard, 1974) in restricting the period of endplate excitation. They must be arranged in some manner that minimises interception by AChE of ACh on its primary outward path to the receptors (Barnard, 1974). The reason for having AChE but little receptor in the depths of the folds is less obvious. Why are the folds often so deep? Clearly, not so as to accommodate more receptors, as was previously usually supposed. To act as an enzyme sink for residual ACh would seem less efficient than the simple absence of folding to avoid ACh entrapment.

Postsynaptic folding is greater in frequency and in depth in thicker muscle fibres and as the speed of muscle contraction becomes more important, as the data of Padykula and Gauthier (1970), and our own observations on various muscles, indicate. It could be, therefore, that these folds are needed to provide a more rapid conductance channel for the wave of postsynaptic membrane depolarisation to the sarcolemma and sarcoplasmic reticulum in such thick fibres. Direct connections thereto from the base of the folds have been claimed (Zacks and Saito, 1970). Such a channel might be passive or active. It has to be examined in detail whether there is any electrogenic component in the membrane lining these fold depths. Recent evidence by Thesleff, Vyskocil and Ward (1974) indicates that the endplate contains local, distinctive sites of action potential generation. An alternative possibility is that these receptor-free regions are needed as sites of ion-pumps in the membrane, to recover ions exchanged into the synaptic cleft. Only such hypothetical explanations can be offered at present. Certainly, where there is a functional demand that leads to the development of these receptor-free postsynaptic membrane extensions, it must be necessary (at synapses relaying impulses at high speeds) to cover them with AChE throughout, as is observed, to prevent local trapping of ACh therein.

When the nerve terminal is removed, the well-known appearance of ACh sensitivity all over the muscle membrane has been shown to be due to the actual appearance of BuTX-binding sites there (Miledi and Potter, 1971; Berg et al., 1972; Hartzell and Fambrough, 1972; Chiu et al., 1973; Libelius, 1974). It is clear that these molecules did not simply migrate from the endplates. Firstly, the overall number of receptor sites in a denervated muscle is many times that of its original endplate, e.g. in the 15-day-denervated rat diaphragm, eighteenfold (Chiu et al., 1973). Secondly, EM autoradiographic analysis of the endplates of a denervated muscle — mouse diaphragm — after an interval in which several-fold multiplication of the receptors has occurred in each fibre shows that the original number, density and crest localisation are maintained unchanged at those endplates (Porter and Barnard, 1975b). We do not know if these extrajunctional muscle receptor molecules are chemically identical with those at the endplate — although they are very similar in most properties — but the former must be synthesised or unmasked from another source.

ISOLATION OF THE ACh RECEPTOR PROTEIN FROM DENERVATED MUSCLES

As has been found with the electroplaque ACh receptor, the muscle receptor can be extracted efficiently into solution by detergents, both ionic and non-ionic (Chiu et al., 1973). The overall concentration of ACh receptor in normal muscle is so low, however, compared with that in the *Torpedo* electric organ, that purification is much more difficult than in the latter case. An improvement is obtained by making use of the elevated receptor content of chronically denervated muscles.

In measuring the free receptor concentration in such extracts, an assay is used based upon reaction with [^{3}H]BuTX and retention of the receptor-toxin complex on a DEAE-cellulose filter disc (Dolly and Barnard, 1974). We employ homogenisation of denervated muscles, followed by an aqueous wash of the particulate fraction, and its extraction in 1.5 per cent Triton X-100 or Emulphogene at 4°C for 3 h, all in the presence of protease inhibitors and with de-aeration. This gives 80-90 per cent solubilisation of the total content of the BuTX-binding component of the muscle. The extract can be initially fractionated by gel filtration

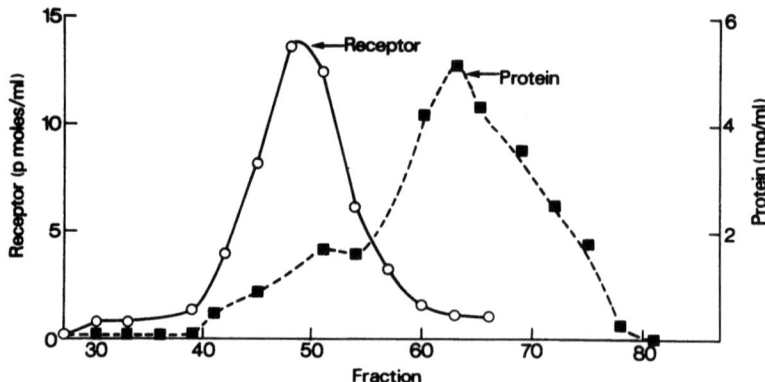

Figure 14.7 Gel filtration of ACh receptor from denervated cat leg muscles. The extract in 1.5 per cent Triton X-100 medium was passed through a column of Ultrogel AcA 22, at 4°C. The receptor, as measured in picomoles per ml by the [^{3}H]BuTX-binding assay, is present only in the single peak shown, which is centred at a value corresponding, if the column is calibrated with globular proteins, to a Stokes radius of 70 Å, as found with *Torpedo* receptor (Raftery et al., 1972). The protein was measured by the Folin-Lowry method. AChE in the extract is separated as a single peak centred at fraction 56

on Sepharose 6B or Ultragel AcA 22 (Fig. 14.7). A single broad peak of receptor activity is obtained, separated from most of the protein present. AChE is also separated from the muscle receptor at this stage (Barnard and Dolly, 1975).

Further purification of the muscle receptors has been made by affinity chromatography. We have employed a column of Agarose to which has been covalently bound either (a) cobratoxin or (b) a cholinergic ligand of structure

$$-HN-\!\!\left\langle\!\!\bigcirc\!\!\right\rangle\!\!-\overset{+}{N}(CH_3)_3$$

attached by a long side-arm; the latter type of column was previously used (Berman and Young, 1971) for electroplaque AChE purification. After removal of other proteins by appropriate washes, a biospecific elution is accomplished using either Flaxedil (2 mM) in (b) (Fig. 14.8) or carbamylcholine (1 M) in (a). As can be seen, a highly efficient purification occurs, with almost all of the extraneous protein still present completely separated from the receptor. An alternative affinity chromatography, (c), can be obtained with a resin carrying a TC group bound through an azo linkage (provided by Dr B. Belleau, Montreal), which we have found can also give in suitable conditions (again with Flaxedil as eluent) a profile similar to that of Fig. 14.8. Dr J. O. Dolly has studied the system using bound cobratoxin and carbamylcholine, which gives equally satisfactory purification, with details to be described elsewhere (Dolly et al., 1977b).

The final stage of purification employs a DEAE-Sephadex column and a salt gradient (Dolly and Barnard, 1975). This yields a single peak of receptor, and removes the remaining extraneous protein, as shown by gel electrophoresis (Fig. 14.9). The final product has a specific activity of up to 6000 nmol receptor/g protein (in terms of BuTX-binding sites). A purification of about 4000-fold overall, from the crude extract, is achieved.

Criteria of purity of the final product are (1) its homogeneity in rechromatography, or in isoelectric focussing; (2) its homogeneity in polyacrylamics gel electrophoresis (Fig. 14.9); and (3) its high specific activity, which is of the same order as that of the pure preparations reported of the electroplaque ACh receptor (listed by Changeux, 1975). The specific activity noted is based upon protein estimation by a micro adaptation of the Folin-Lowry protein method, using serum albumin arbitrarily as a standard. Since for the electroplaque receptor it has been found (Eldefrawi and Eldefrawi, 1973) that this gives values 30 per cent lower than those determined by amino acid analysis, this correction, assuming it holds here, too, would give a final specific activity of about 8000 nmol/g for the purest preparations obtained. The activity, in toxin-binding assays, is completely stable upon storage. Isoelectric focusing in a narrow (pH 4-6) range of the complex of this receptor with homogeneous [^{3}H] monoacetyl-BuTX, a stringent test, has provided further evidence that a single active protein is isolated, if precautions to prevent proteolysis or ageing have been applied. The isolectric point of the free receptor is close to 5.0 (in 0.05 per cent Triton X-100).

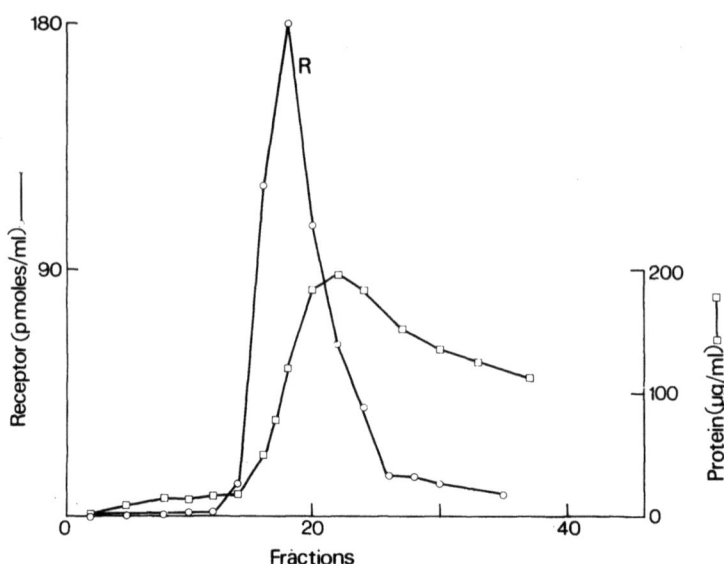

Figure 14.8 Affinity chromatography of the gel-filtered (see Fig. 14.7) ACh receptor at 4 °C. The column contained a bound cholinergic ligand (type (b); see text). Prior to the stage shown, the receptor solution was applied to the column in 0.05 M potassium phosphate/0.2 per cent Triton X-100 and washed in that medium until protein was entirely absent in the effluent; a breakthrough peak of protein was obtained which was 50 times the height of the protein peak shown here, but contained 0.5 per cent of the receptor activity shown here. At fraction 0 here, 2.1 mM Flaxedil (gallamine triethiodide) was applied in the same medium. The protein here was measured by a micro adaptation of the Folin – Lowry method. The Flaxedil was removed from the effluent by continuous-flow dialysis through hollow fibre assemblies in series, against 0.1 per cent Triton X-100 solution, prior to assay. No AChE activity is detectable in the receptor peak. A pool of the first two-thirds of the receptor peak was passed onto a column of DEAE – Sephadex in 0.1 per cent Triton X-100/0.025 M potassium phosphate, pH 8.0 (when all the receptor became bound); this was washed with 0.1 M NaCl in that medium until no more protein was eluted, and a gradient from 0.1 M to 1.2 M NaCl in that medium applied, with continuous-flow dialysis as before. This eluted a peak of the receptor, separated from all other protein initially present. For further details, see Dolly and Barnard (1975)

PROPERTIES OF THE ACh RECEPTOR IN SOLUTION

When the receptor - toxin reaction is performed with the purified soluble material in the presence of a nicotinic cholinergic ligand, the reaction is retarded (Fig. 14. 10), with behaviour that conforms kinetically to that expected for a reversible ligand protecting from an irreversible inhibitor. Thus the apparent dissociation constant (or protection constant), K_D, for each ligand used could be estimated

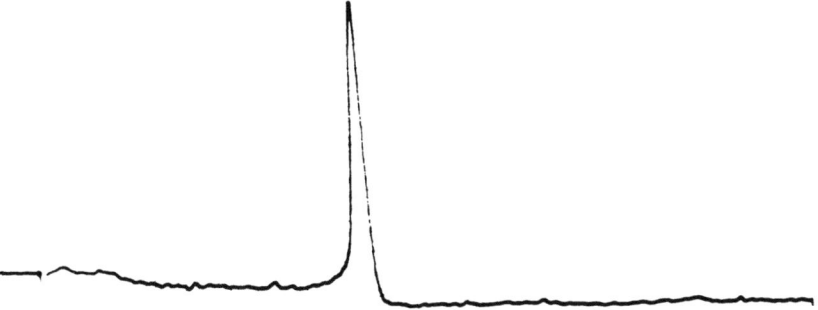

Figure 14.9 Electrophoresis on polyacrylamide gel of the final product of the ACh receptor purification, stained for protein with Amido-Schwartz. Migration is from the right, a scan of the gel, in a laser densitometer at 570 nm, is shown. For other details see Dolly and Barnard (1975)

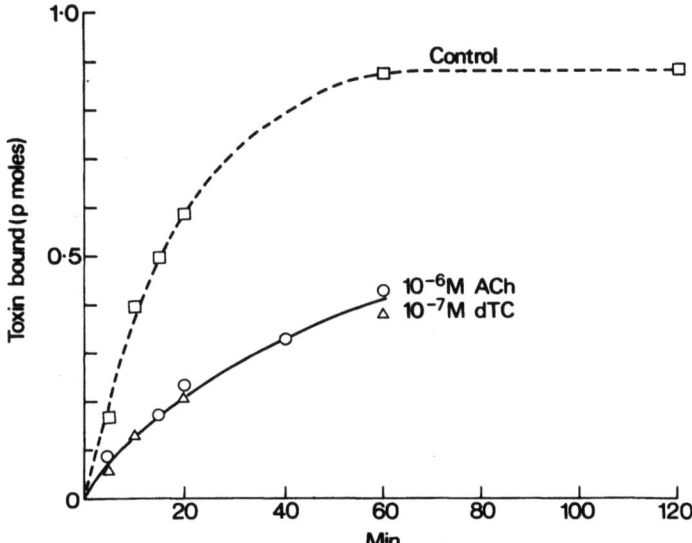

Figure 14.10 Reaction of pure ACh receptor with [^{3}H]BuTX, and the protections exerted by specific ligands. [^{3}H]BuTX (6 nM) was reacted with a fixed amount of receptor solution, and the amount bound per ml of solution (□) as a function of time was determined in a 100 μl aliquot by the DEAE-cellulose filter disc assay. The medium was 25 mM phosphate buffer, pH 8, in 0.2 per cent Triton X-100, at 25 °C. The broken curve is theoretical for second-order behaviour. Parallel reactions conducted in the presence of 1.0×10^{-7} M TC (△) or 1.0×10^{-6} M ACh (○) are shown as examples of those used, in second-order plots, to determine the initial retardation in the series for K_D estimation. A 20 min preincubation with each ligand was given at 25 °C: in the case of ACh, 3×10^{-6} M DFP was added at the outset

from the equation (Mildvan and Leigh, 1964)

$$\frac{v_i}{v} = \frac{K_D}{K_D + [L]} \tag{14.1}$$

where v_i and v are the initial velocities in the presence of the ligand, concentration [L], and in its absence, respectively. With higher concentrations of ACh or TC, all of the BuTX-reactive sites become protected (Table 14.1). The dissociation constants (K_D) for a series of such ligands at these sites were determined (Fig. 14.10) on the basis of Eq. 14.1.

The dissociation constants for five ligands, derived thus from protection experiments (Table 14.4), are in agreement with their known pharmacological relative effectiveness on skeletal muscle. Hexamethonium, which is only a weak antagonist at endplates, has the largest K_D value. The muscarinic ligands atropine and pilocarpine, used at concentrations (1×10^{-5} M and 5×10^{-6} M, respectively) where they completely block muscarinic receptors, produced no protection at all in this system. Likewise, choline (used at 2×10^{-5} M) had no effect.

The same treatment was applied to the binding of nicotinic ligands at the receptor in denervated muscle membrane fragments, following experiments of

Table 14.4 Dissociation constants (K_D) for ligands on ACh receptors

Ligand	K_D (muscle) (μM)		K_D (*Electrophorus*) (μM)
	Purified	Membranes	Membranes[a]
Agonists			
ACh[b]	0.01, 1.0[c]	0.2	1.5
Carbachol[b]	1.0	3.0	22
Decamethonium	0.5	0.3	0.8
Antagonists			
TC	0.1	0.04	0.17
Flaxedil		0.5	0.4
Hexamethonium	340		61
Atropine			
Pilocarpine	> 100	> 100	
Choline			

All were determined from the protection afforded from labelled toxin binding by a suitable range of concentrations of the ligand, at 25°C. For soluble receptor, the medium contained 0.2 per cent Triton X-100.
[a] Meunier et al., 1974; 22°C, Ringer medium.
[b] DFP (10^{-5} M) pretreatment given, and 3×10^{-6} M phospholine present in the reaction mixture, to inhibit traces of AChE, for the muscle case. For *Electrophorus*, 10^{-4} M Tetram was used.
[c] Two apparent classes of site were detected.

the type illustrated in Fig. 14.3. Similar behaviour was observed, and Eq. 14.1 was followed. In all cases the K_D values quoted (Table 14.4) are for receptors that had been pre-equilibrated with the ligand. If an effect occurs here of time-dependent affinity increase upon contact with an agonist, as found by Weber et al. (1975) for membrane-bound (but not soluble) Torpedo receptor, then this must be much faster in the muscle membrane than that found (half-time 5 - 10 min) with Torpedo membranes, since no time-dependence occurs on the scale of measurement used here. The final affinity, in those terms, is always reported here.

The constants obtained for the soluble and membrane-bound muscle ACh receptors for various ligands are quite similar to those obtained by Changeux and colleagues for the electroplaque receptor of *Electrophorus electricus*, in the membrane fragment preparation (Table 14.4). However, solubilisation of that receptor causes the affinities for agonists to become 10 - 40-fold stronger (Meunier et al., 1974). Identity of the affinity values for a ligand of the soluble receptor from the two sources is not to be expected, however, since even in the case of electroplaques there is a considerable difference between types: the ACh receptor from *Torpedo* sp. shows different affinities for particular ligands, and different behaviour upon solubilisation, than the receptor from *Electrophorus electricus* (Meunier et al., 1974; Changeux, 1975), and there are considerable differences reported even between *Torpedo* receptor preparations from different laboratories (Eldefrawi and Eldefrawi, 1975).

The affinity of TC for the muscle receptor in determining its physiological response has also been estimated pharmacologically (Dolly et al., 1977a). Those values are in agreement with that found here for the binding of TC, as measured by protection from [^{3}H]BuTX uptake (Table 14.2). This is further evidence that the binding of BuTX occurs at a functionally active receptor molecule.

In summary, the ACh receptor has been purified from mammalian skeletal muscle. It is a single protein, with an apparent molecular weight, as assessed by gel filtration in 0.2 per cent Triton X-100, similar to that found for the electroplaque ACh receptor in similar media (assuming the same partial specific volume), and since the latter has been found to have a true molecular weight of about 250 000 when corrected for bound detergent (Changeux, 1975; Landowne et al., 1975), this is presumably the size of the muscle ACh receptor, too. It has the receptor properties of a rapid reaction with BuTX and the binding of cholinergic ligands, with affinities in line with their pharmacological effects on this receptor.

An impure preparation of this muscle receptor has been shown to possess some ionic translocation modulator (ITM) properties of the intact system, since it could be reconstituted into a synthetic bilayer which responds to applied ACh at physiological concentrations (Kemp et al., 1973). This effect has been confirmed in another laboratory (Romine et al., 1974). The same effect has recently been obtained by Dr G. Kemp at Buffalo on this receptor purified on the cobratoxin affinity column. An equivalent effect has been reported for vesicles of *Torpedo* lipids containing the purified electroplaque ACh receptor (Michealson et al., 1974). It will be of importance to see if, in the pure receptor, the ITM property resides in the same protein as the receptor active centre. There is a great deal that we must yet learn, for the muscle ACh receptor, of the structural basis of its synaptic activity.

ACKNOWLEDGEMENTS

The results presented are based upon the work performed in our laboratories at State University of New York, Buffalo, USA — where my co-workers were Vivian Coates, M. H. Hudeck, V. Kumar, B. Mallick, C. W. Porter and R. G. Shorr (without mention of earlier contributors to this work there) — and also upon the work with J. O. Dolly firstly when I was on leave (1975) at Molecular Pharmacology Division, National Institute for Medical Research, Mill Hill, London, and more recently in our new location at Imperial College. The former work was aided by grant GM-11754 from the National Institutes of Health (USA) and a Fellowship to Dr Dolly from the Muscular Dystrophy Association of America, and the latter by a programme grant from the Medical Research Council (UK). For making electrophysiological correlations, we acknowledge the collaboration of E. X. Albuquerque and colleagues, formerly at Buffalo and now at Department of Pharmacology and Experimental Therapeutics, University of Maryland, Baltimore, USA.

REFERENCES

Albuquerque, E. X., Barnard, E. A., Chiu, T. H., Lapa, A. J., Dolly, J. O., Jansson, S. E., Daly, J. and Witkop, B. (1973a). *Proc. Nat. Acad. Sci. USA*, 70, 949
Albuquerque, E. X., Barnard, E. A., Jansson, S. E. and Wieckowski, J. (1973b). *Life Sci.*, 12, 545
Albuquerque, E. X., Barnard, E. A., Porter, C. W. and Warnick, J. E., (1974). *Proc. Nat. Acad. Sci. USA*, 71, 2818
Alper, R., Lowy, J. and Schmidt, J. (1974). *FEBS Lett*, 48, 130
Barnard, E. A. (1970). *Int. Rev. Cytol.*, 29, 213
Barnard, E. A. (1974). *The Peripheral Nervous System* (ed. J. I. Hubbard), Plenum Press, New York, 201-224
Barnard, E. A., Chiu, T. H., Jedrzejczyk, J., Porter, C. W. and Wieckowski, J. (1973). *Drug Receptors* (ed. by H. P. Rang), Macmillan, London, p. 225
Barnard, E. A., Coates, V., Dolly, J. O. and Mallick, B. (1977). *Cell Biol. Int. Rep.*, 1, 99
Barnard, E. A. and Dolly, J. O. (1975). *Proc. 6th Internat. Cong. Pharmacol., Helsinki*, Vol. 1 (ed. J. Tuomisto and M. K. Paasonen), p. 77
Barnard, E. A., Dolly, J. O., Porter, C. W. and Albuquerque, E. X. (1975). *Exp. Neurol.*, 48
Barnard, E. A., Wieckowski, J. and Chiu, T. H. (1971a). *Proc. First Eur. Biophysics Congress*, Vol. XII (ed. E. Broda, A. Locker and H. Springer Lederer), Med. Acad. Vienna Press, Vienna, p. 371
Barnard, E. A., Wieckowski, J. and Chiu, T. H. (1971b). *Nature*, 234, 207
Beranek, R. and Vyskocil, F. (1967). *J. Physiol.*, 188, 53
Berg, D. K., Kelly, R. B., Sargent, P. B., Williamson, P. and Hall, Z. W. (1972). *Proc. Nat. Acad. Sci. USA*, 69, 147
Berman, J. B. and Young, M. (1971). *Proc. Nat. Acad. Sci. USA*, 68, 395
Betz, W. and Sakmann, B. (1973). *J. Physiol.*, 230, 673

Birks, R., Huxley, H. E. and Katz, B. (1960). *J. Physiol.*, 150, 134
Bourgeois, J. P., Ryter, A., Menez, A., Fromageot, P., Boquet, P. and Changeux, J. P. (1972). *FEBS Lett.*, 25, 127
Brockes, J. P. and Hall, Z. W. (1975). *Biochemistry*, 14, 2092
Cartaud, J., Beneditti, E. L., Cohen, J. B., Meunier, J. C. and Changeux, J. P. (1972). *FEBS Lett.*, 33, 109
Chang, C. C. and Lee, C. Y. (1966). *Br. J. Pharmacol. Chemother.*, 28, 172
Changeux, J. P. (1975). *Handbook of Psychopharmacology*, Vol. 6 (ed. L. L. Iverson, S. D. Iverson and S. H. Snyder), Plenum Press, New York, p. 235
Changeux, J. P., Kasai, M. and Lee, C. Y. (1970). *Proc. Nat. Acad. Sci. USA*, 67, 1241
Chiu, T. H., Dolly, J. O. and Barnard, E. A. (1973). *Biochem. Biophys. Res. Commun.*, 51, 205
Chiu, T. H., Lapa, A. J., Barnard, E. A. and Albuquerque, E. X. (1974). *Exp. Neurol.*, 43, 399
Cohen, J. B. and Changeux, J. P. (1975). *Ann. Rev. Pharmacol.*, 15, 83
Colquhoun, D. (1975). *Ann. Rev. Pharmacol.*, 15, 307
Colquhoun, D. and Rang, H. P. (1976). *Molec. Pharmacol.*, 12, 519
Colquhoun, D., Rang, H. P. and Ritchie, J. M. (1974). *J. Physiol.*, 240, 199
Couteaux, R. and Pecot-Dechavassine, M. (1970). *C. R. Acad. Sci., Paris, Ser. D.*, 271, 2346
Denburg, J. L., Eldefrawi, M. E. and O'Brien, R. D. (1972). *Proc. Nat. Acad. Sci. USA*, 69, 177
Dolly, J. O. and Barnard, E. A. (1974). *FEBS Lett.*, 46, 145
Dolly, J. O. and Barnard, E. A. (1975). *FEBS Lett.*, 57, 267
Dolly, J. O., Barnard, E. A. and Shorr, R. G. (1977b). Trans. Biochem. Soc., 168
Dolly, J. O., Albuquerque, E. X., Sarvey, J. M., Mallick, B. and Barnard, E. A. (1977a). *Molec. Pharmacol.*, 11, 1
Dudai, Y., Herzberg, M. and Silman, I. (1973). *Proc. Nat. Acad. Sci. USA*, 66, 651
Eldefrawi, M. E. and Eldefrawi, A. T. (1973). *Biochem. Biophys. Acta*, 159, 362
Eldefrawi, M. E. and Eldefrawi, A. T. (1975). *Ann. N. Y. Acad. Sci.*, 264, 183
Ellisman, M. H., Rash, J. E., Staehelin, L. A. and Porter, M. R. (1976). *J. Cell Biol.*, 68, 752
Fertuck, H. C. and Salpeter, M. M. (1974). *Proc. Nat. Acad. Sci. USA*, 71, 1376
Fertuck, H. C. and Salpeter, M. M. (1976). *J. Cell Biol.*, 69, 144
Hall, Z. W. and Kelly, R. B. (1971). *Nature New Biol.*, 232, 62
Hartzell, H. C. and Fambrough, D. M. (1972). *J. Gen. Physiol.*, 60, 248
Heuser, J. E., Reese, T. S. and Landis, D. M. D. (1974). *J. Neurocytol.*, 3, 109
Hubbard, J. I. (1974). *The Peripheral Nervous System* (ed. J. I. Hubbard), Plenum Press, New York, p. 151
Karlin, A. (1974). *Life Sci.*, 14, 1385
Katz, B. (1966). *Nerve, Muscle and Synapse*, McGraw-Hill, New York
Katz, B. and Miledi, R. (1967). *Proc. Roy. Soc. B*, 167, 8
Kemp, G., Dolly, J. O., Barnard, E. A. and Wenner, C. E. (1973). *Biochem. Biophys. Res. Commun.*, 54, 607-613
Kuffler, S. W. and Yoshikami, D. (1975). *J. Physiol.*, 224, 703
Landowne, D., Potter, L. T. and Terrar, D. A. (1975). *Ann. Rev. Physiol.*, 37, 485
Lester, H. (1972). *Molec. Pharmacol.*, 6, 623
Libelius, R. (1974). *J. Neurol. Trans.*, 35, 137
Meunier, J. C., Sealock, R., Olsen, R. and Changeux, J. P. (1974). *Eur. J. Biochem.*, 45, 371
Michealson, D., Vandlen, R., Bode, J., Moody, T., Schmidt, J. and Raftery, M. A. (1974). *Arch. Biochem. Biophys.*, 165, 796
Mildvan, A. S. and Leigh, R. A. (1964). *Biochim. Biophys. Acta*, 89, 393
Miledi, R. and Potter, L. T. (1971). *Nature*, 233, 599
Nickel, E. and Potter, L. T. (1973). *Brain Res.*, 57, 508

Padykula, H. A. and Gauthier, G. F. (1970). *J. Cell Biol.*, **46**, 27
Peper, K., Dreyer, F., Sandri, C., Akert, K. and Moor, H. (1974). *Cell Tissue Res.*, **149**, 437
Porter, C. W. and Barnard, E. A. (1975a). *J. Memb. Biol.*, **20**, 31
Porter, C. W. and Barnard, E. A. (1975b). *Exp. Neurol.*, **48**, 542
Porter, C. W. and Barnard, E. A. (1975c). *Ann. N. Y. Acad. Sci.*, **264**
Porter, C. W., Barnard, E. A. and Chiu, T. H. (1973a). *J. Memb. Biol.*, **14**, 383
Porter, C. W., Chiu, T. H., Wieckowski, J. and Barnard, E. A. (1973b). *Nature New Biol.*, **241**, 3
Rang, H. P. (1974). *Quart. Rev. Biophys.*, **7**, 283
Rash, J. E. and Ellisman, M. H. (1974). *J. Cell Biol.*, **63**, 457
Rash, J. E., Warnick, J. E., Ellisman, M. H. and Albuquerque, E. X. (1975). *J. Cell Biol.*, **67**, 354
Rieger, F., Bon, A. and Massoulié, J. (1973). *Eur. J. Biochem.*, **34**, 534
Romine, W. O., Goodall, M. T., Peterson, J. and Bradley, R. J. (1974). *Biochim. Biophys. Acta*, **316**, 316
Rogers, A. W., Darzynkiewicz, Z., Barnard, E. A. and Salpeter, M. M. (1966). *Nature*, **210**, 1003
Rogers, A. W., Darzynkiewicz, Z., Salpeter, M. M., Ostrowski, K. and Barnard, E. A. (1969). *J. Cell Biol.*, **41**, 665
Rosenbluth, J. (1974). *J. Cell Biol.*, **62**, 755
Salpeter, M. M. (1969). *J. Cell Biol.*, **42**, 122
Salpeter, M. M., Plattner, H. and Rogers, A. W. (1972). *J. Histochem. Cytochem.*, **20**, 1059
Thesleff, S., Vyskocil, F. and Ward, M. P. (1974). *Acta Physiol. Scand.*, **91**, 196
Weber, M., David-Pfeuty, T. and Changeux, J. P. (1975). *Proc. Nat. Acad. Sci. USA*, **72**, 3443
Zacks, S. I. (1973). *The Motor Endplate*, Krieger, Huntington, N. Y.
Zacks, S. I. and Saito, A. (1970). *J. Histochem. Cytochem.*, **18**, 302

Author index*†

Adair, G. S., 114, *125*
Adler, L., *see* Kannan, K. K., 73, 74, *90*
Ahlquist, R. P., 13, *36*
Aizona, Y., *see* Sonenberg, M., 237, *247*
Akera, T., 221, 222, 223, 225, 230, 231, 232, *233*. *See also* Ku, D., 223, *233*; Tobin, T., 215, 216, 217, 218, 219, 225, 226, 227, 228, 229, 230, 231, 232, *233*
Akert, K., *see* Peper, K., 260, 263, 264, *274*
Albert, A., 1, 8, 11, 12, 13, 20, *36*
Alberty, R. A., 94, *107*
Albuquerque, E. X., 252, 260, 263, *272*. *See also* Barnard, E. A., 251, 252, 257, 263, *272*; Chiu, T. H., 250, 251, 252, *273*; Dolly, J. O., 251, 253, 256, 257, 271, *273*; Rash, J. E., 263, *274*
Allen, D. W., 112, 121, *125*
Allen, R. C., *see* Cammarata, A., ' 8, *36*
Allison, J. L., *see* O'Brien, R. L., 177, *189*
Almaula, P. I., *see* Baker, B. R., 134, *149*
Alper, R., 256, *272*
Alvares, A. P., 203, *211*
Amadori, E., *see* Ullrich, V., 210, *212*
Andersson, B., 73, *90*
Antikainen, P. J., 13, *36*
Aoki, M., *see* Kakeya, N., 89, 90, 104, *107*
Armstrong, J. McD., 74, *90*
Armstrong, M. D., *see* Kappe, T., 13, *37*
Arnone, A., 116, 125, *125*
Asahi, Y., *see* Watanabe, A., 11, *39*
Aschman, D. G., *see* Richards, W. G., 46, 47, *54*
Ash, A. S. F., 23, *36*
Aurbach, G. D., *see* Brown, E. M., 243, *246*; Spiegel, A. M., 236, 237, 242, *247*
Aust, S. D., *see* Wetton, A. F., 204, *212*

Baczynskyj, L., *see* Martin, D. G., 170, 179, *189*
Bag, S. P., *see* Rigler, N. E., 35, *38*
Baker, B. R., 130, 131, 132, 134, *149*
Bald, R., 191, 195, *199*. *See also* Pongs, O. 191, 193, 195, *199*

Bambas, L. L., *see* Rebstock, M. C., 191, *200*
Banerjee, S. P., *see* Tobin, T., 226, *233*
Barber, J., *see* Le Pecq, J. B., 169, 188, *189*
Barcroft, J., 112, 113, 114, 115, *125*. *See also* Adair, G. S., 114, *125*
Barlin, G. B., *see* Albert, A., 20, *36*
Barlow, R. B., 1, *36*
Barnard, E. A., 250, 251, 252, 253, 255, 256, 257, 263, 264, 265, 267, *272*. *See also* Albuquerque, E. X., 252, 260, 263, *272*; Chiu, T. H., 250, 251, 254, 265, 266, *273;* Dolly, J. O., 251, 253, 256, 257, 266, 267, 268, 269, *273*; Kemp, G., 271, *273*; Porter, C. W., 250, 251, 252, 257, 258, 259, 260, 261, 262, 266, *274*; Rogers, A. W., 250, *274*
Barnoux, C., *see* Gefter, M., 153, *165*
Baron, J., *see* Estabrook, R. W., 209, *211*
Barry, C. D., 66, 67, *71*
Barth, T., *see* Jard, S., 243, *247*
Baskin, S. I., *see* Akera, T., 221, 222, 223, 231, 232, *233*; Tobin, T., 231, *233*
Bass, G. E., *see* Purcell, W. P., 5, *38*
Bauer, W., 169, *188*
Baugh, C. M., 142, *149*
Baukel, A., *see* Glossmann, H., 237, *247*
Bazill, G., 153, *165*
Beddell, C. R., 121, 122, *125*. *See also* Paterson, R. A., 121, *126*
Bedford, G. R., *see* Feeney, J., 69, *71*
Bell, P. H., 8, *36*
Benedetti, E. L., *see* Cartaud, J., 263, *273*
Benesch, R., 112, *125*. *See also* Benesch, R. E., 18, *36*
Benesch, R. E., 18, *36*. *See also* Benesch, R., 112, *125*
Bengtsson, U., *see* Bergstén, P. C., 77, 84, 88, *90*; Kannan, K. K., 73, *90*
Benkovik, S., *see* Bruice, T. C., 12, *36*
Bennett, C. D., *see* Poe, M., 130, *150*
Bennett, V., *see* Cuatrecasas, P., 237, 238, *246*
Beranek, R., 256, *272*
Berg, D. K., 252, 265, *272*

---

*Numbers in *italics* indicate the page on which the full reference is to be found.
†Multiple-author papers are indexed as follows: a paper by Jones and Brown will appear under 'Jones' and under 'Brown, *see* (or *see also*) Jones', with the page numbers given under each entry.

Bergstén, P. C., 77, 84, 88, *90*. *See also* Kannan, K. K., 73, 74, *90*; Liljas, A., 73, 83, 84, *90*; Vaara, I., 85, 88, *91*
Berkoff, C. E., *see* Blank, B., 18, *36*; Di Tullio, N. W., 18, *37*
Berman, J. B., 267, *272*
Berman, M., *see* Rendell, M., 236, 243, *247*; Rodbell, M., 236, *247*
Bertino, J. R., 128, *149*. *See also* Johns, D. G., 131, *150*; Perkins, J. R., 136, *150*
Beveridge, D. L., 42, *54*
Betz, W., 257, 264, *272*
Biles, C., *see* Martin, D. G., 170, 179, *189*
Birdsall, B., 67, *71*, 133, 134, 138, 140, 141, 142, 148, *149*. *See also* Feeney, J., 133, 143, 144, 146, *150*; Way, J. L., 133, 136, *150*
Birdsall, N. J. M., *see* Birdsall, B., 67, *71*
Birks, R., 262, 264, *273*
Birnbaumer, L., 235, 241, *246*. *See also* Pohl, S. L., 238, *247;* Rodbell, M., 236, *247*
Bjur, R. A., *see* Dann, J. G., 133, 134, 140, *150*; Roberts, G. C. K., 133, 134, 136, 138, 142, 144, *150*
Black, J. W., 21, 23, 28, 30, 31, 32, 33, *36*. *See also* Durant, G. J., 33, *37*
Blair, L. K., *see* Brauman, J. I., 50, *54*
Blakemore, R. C., *see* Parsons, M. E., 33, *38*
Blakley, R. L., 127, 128, 129, 132, *149*
Blank, B., 18, *36*. *See also* Di Tullio, N. W., 18, *37*
Bleich, H. E., 69, *71*
Blow, D. M., 74, *90*
Blumberg, W. E., *see* Peisach, J., 206, *212*
Blume, A. J., 243, *246*
Bock, A. V., *see* Adair, G. S., 114, *125*
Bockhart, J., *see* Jard, S., 243, *247*
Bockman, R. S., *see* Sonenberg, M., 237, *247*
Bode, J., *see* Michealson, D., 266, 271, *273*
Bohr, C., 114, *125*
Boicelli, C. A., 63, 64, *71*
Bon, A., *see* Rieger, F., 264, *274*
Bonetti, G., *see* Visconti, M., 11, *38*
Bonting, S. L., 224, *233*
Boquet, P., *see* Bourgeois, J. P., 263, *273*
Boson, S. F., *see* Olander, J., 102, *107*
Bourgeois, J. B., 263, *273*
Bourns, A. N., *see* Sheppard, W. A., 121, *126*
Bovey, F. A., *see* Dorman, D. E., 64, *71*; Tonelli, A. E., 62, *72*
Boyce, P., 152, *165*

Bradbury, A. F., 56, 57, *71*. *See also* Boicelli, C. A., 63, 64, *71*
Bradley, R. J., *see* Romine, W. O., 271, *274*
Bragg, W. L., 109, *125*
Bram, S., 177, *188*
Brauman, J. I., 50, *54*
Braun, T., 236, *246*
Braunitzer, G., *see* Matsuda, G., 112, *126*
Braverman, E., *see* Baugh, C. M., 142, *149*
Breslow, R., 11, 12, *36*
Brewster, A. I., 56, 57, *71*
Brimblecombe, R. W., 33, 34, 35, *36*
Brittain, R. T., 13, *36*
Brockes, J. P., 256, *273*
Brodie, B. B., 202, *211*
Brody, T. M. *see* Akera, T., 221, 222, 223, 230, 231, 232, *233*; Ku, D., 223, *233*; Tobin, T., 215, 216, 217, 219, 220, 225, 226, 227, 228, 229, 230, 231, 232, *233*
Brown, D. J., 11, *36*
Brown, E. M., 243, *246*. *See also* Spiegel, A. M., 237, 242, *247*
Brown, J. P., 142, *149*
Brown, J. P., *see* Feeney, J., 69, *71*
Brown, N. C., 151, 152, 154, *165*. *See also* Clements, J., 153, 154, 156, 157, 158, 161, 163, *165*; Mackenzie, J., 153, 154, 155, 159, 160, *166*; Neville, M., 153, 154, *166*; Wright, G. E., 160, 161, *166*
Brugnoni, G. P., *see* Hopmann, R. F. W., 11, 12, *36*
Bruice, T. C., 12, *36*
Bryan, R. F., *see* Kretzinger, R. H., 88, *90*
Buckingham, A. D., 1, *36*
Buehring, K. U., 142, *149*
Bünemann, H., *see* Müller, W., 170, *189*
Burchall, J. J., 131, 132, *149*. *See also* Ferone, R., 132, *150*; Hitchings, G. H., 132, 133, *150*
Burgen, A. S. V., 69, 70, *71*, 95, *107*. *See also* Birdsall, B., 133, 134, 138, 140, 141, 142, 148, *149*; Bradbury, A. F., 56, 57, *71*; Dann, J. G., 133, 134, *150*; Feeney, J., 56, 61, 62, 63, 69, *71*, 133, 143, 144, 146, *150*; King, R. W., 96, 98, 100, 102, 105, *107*; Roberts, G. C. K., 133, 134, 136, 138, 142, 144, *150*; Taylor, P. W., 88, 89, *91*, 94, 95, 98, 102, 104, *107*; Way, J. L., 133, 136, *150*
Burger, A., 1, *36*. *See also* Leffler, E. B., 13, *38*
Burgess, R. W., 69, *71*
Burke, G., 235, *246*
Bystrov, V. F., 60, 61, 63, *71*

Cammarata, A., 8, *36*

Campbell, I. D., 86, *90*
Canady, M. R., *see* Bonting, S. L., 224, *233*
Canellakis, E. S., 185, *188*
Cantor, C., *see* Oen, H., 196, *199*
Carey, P. R., *see* Kumar, K., 96, 106, *107*
Carlbom, U., *see* Kannan, K. K., 73, *90*; Liljas, A., 73, 83, 84, *90*
Caron, M. G., *see* Lefkowitz, R. J., 238, *247*
Cartaud, J., 263, *273*
Casy, A. F., *see* Ham, N. S., 23, *37*
Catt, K. J., *see* Glossmann, H., 237, *247*
Celma, M. L., 191, *199*
Chand, N., 23, *36*
Chang, C. C., 250, *273*
Changeux, J. P., 249, 250, 267, 271, *273*. *See also* Bourgeois, J. P., 263, *273*; Cartaud, J., 263, *273*; Cohen, J. B., 263, *273*; Meunier, J. C., 270, 271, *273*; Weber, M., 271, *274*
Chanutin, A., 114, *125*. *See also* Sugita, Y., 114, *126*
Charton, M., 25, 33, *36*
Chaykovsky, M., 134, *150*
Chen, K. K. N., *see* Chaykovsky, M., 134, *150*
Chisholm, J. W., *see* Waring, M. J., 169, *189*
Chiu, T. H., 250, 251, 252, 254, 256, 266, *273*. *See also* Albuquerque, E. X., 252, *272*; Barnard, E. A., 250, 252, *272*; Porter, C. W., 250, 251, 252, 257, 261, *274*
Chou, D., *see* Kang, S., 23, *37*
Chu, L. C., *see* Wolberg, G., 243, *247*
Church, C., *see* Leo, A., 5, *38*
Clayton, J. M., *see* Purcell, W. P., 5, *38*
Clement, G. E., 18, *36*
Clements, J., 153, 154, 156, 157, 158, 161, 163, *165*
Coates, V., *see* Barnard, E. A., 253, 255, 256, *272*
Cohen, G., 169, 171, *188*
Cohen, J. B., 263, *273*. *See also* Cartaud, J., 263, *273*
Colburn, R. W., *see* Rajan, K. S., 13, *38*
Cole, S. J., *see* Harding, M. M., 88, *90*
Coleman, J. E., 73, *90*, 100, *107*
Collatz, E. E., *see* Czernilofsky, A. P., 196, *199*
Collin, R., 130, *150*
Colquhoun, D., 252, 255, 256, *273*
Conney, A. H., 203, 210, *211*. *See also* Alvares, A. P., 203, *211*
Connolly, T. N., *see* Good, N. E., 121, *126*
Controulis, M., 190, *199*
Coon, M. J., *see* Haugen, D. A., 204, *212*;
Lu, A. Y. H., 203, *212*; Strobel, H. W., *212*
Cooper, D. Y., *see* Conney, A. H., 203, 210, *211*; Estabrook, R. W., 203, *211*; Remmer, H., 206, *212*
Corcoran, J. W., 167, *188*
Costello, R. J., *see* Topliss, J. G., 4, *38*
Cotton, F. A., *see* Kretzinger, R. H., 88, *90*
Coulter, C., 159, *165*
Couteaux, R., 260, *273*
Cox, J. M., *see* Perutz, M. F., 112, *126*
Cozzarelli, N., 153, 163, *165*. *See also* Coulter, C., 159, *165*: Gass, K., 153, 154, 155, *165*; Low, R., 153, 156, 157, 158, *166*
Craig, L. C., *see* Gibbons, W. A., 61, 63, *71*
Craig, P. N., 5, *36*
Cranfield, R., *see* Wooton, R., 5, *39*
Crawford, E. J., *see* Plante, L. T., 134, *150*
Crawford, L. V., 169, *188*
Crick, F. H. C., *see* Blow, D. M., 74, *90*; Watson, J. D., 167, *189*
Crooks, H. M., *see* Controulis, M., 190, *199*
Crothers, D. M., 185, *188*. *See also* Müller, W., 170, *189*
Cuatrecasas, P., 237, 238, *246*
Curnish, R. R., *see* Chanutin, A., 114, *125*
Czernilofsky, A. P., 196, *199*

Daly, J. W., 243, *246*. *See also* Albuquerque, E. X., 252, *272*; Jerina, D., 210, *212*
D'Ambrosio, J., *see* Clements, J., 153, 154, 156, 157, 158, 161, 163, *165*
Dann, J. G., 133, 134, 140, *150*. *See also* Roberts, G. C. K., 133, 134, 136, 138, 142, 144, *150*
Darzynkiewicz, Z., *see* Rogers, A. W., 250, *274*
Das, H. K., 193, *199*
Datta, S. P., 30, *36*
Dattagupta, N., *see* Müller, W., 170, *189*
David-Pfeuty, T., *see* Weber, M., 271, *274*
Davidson, G. E., *see* Brown, J. P., 142, *149*
Davie, E. W., *see* So, A. G., 191, *200*
Davis, J. M., *see* Rajan, K. S., 13, *38*
Davis, S. S., *see* Higuchi, T., 5, 6, *37*
Dean, S. M., 49, *54*
De Haen, C., 235, 236, 243, *246*
Delarge, J., *see* Blank, B., 18, *36*
Dell, A., 170, 179, 182, *188*
De Moss, J. A., *see* Weber, M. J., 192, *200*
Denburg, J. L., 256, *273*

Deniserich, P., see Hansch, C., 191, *199*
De Santis, P., 182, *188*
Deslauriers, R., 56, 64, 65, 67, 68, 69, *71*. See also Smith, I. C. P., 56, 64, *72*; Walter, R., 56, *72*
Dessert, A. M., see Miller, W. H., 104, *107*
Deutsch, E. W., see Hansch, C., 5, *37*
Deutsch, H. F., see Kuang-Tzu, D. L., 73, *90*
Diamond, L. K., see Farber, S., 128, *150*
Dickerson, R. E., 74, *90*. See also Kendrew, J. C., 112, *126*
Diehl, H., 206, 207, *211*
Di Tullio, N. W., 18, *37*
Dobbs, F., see Brown, J. P., 142, *149*
Dodds, R. F., see Braun, T., 236, *246*
Dolly, J. O., 251, 253, 256, 257, 266, 267, 268, 269, 271, *273*. See also Albuquerque, E. X., 252, *272*; Barnard, E. A., 251, 252, 253, 255, 256, 257, 263, 267, *272*; Chiu, T. H., 251, 254, 265, 266, *273*; Kemp, G., 271, *273*
Donoghue, D., see Poe, M., 130, *150*
Dorman, D. E., 64, *71*
Douglas, C. G., 114, 115, *126*
Drabkin, D.L., 112, *126*
Dreyer, F., see Peper, K., 260, 263, 264, *274*
Drummond, G. I., 235, 241, *247*
Dudai, Y., 264, *273*
Duncan, L., see Drummond, G. I., 235, 241, *247*
Duncan, W. A. M., see Black, J. W., 23, 28, 33, *36*; Brimblecombe, R. W., 33, 34, 35, *36*
Durant, G. J., 24, 25, 28, 33, *37*. See also Black, J. W., 23, 28, 30, 31, *36*; Brimblecombe, R. W., 34, 35, *36*; Parsons, M. E., 33, *38*
du Vigneaud, V., see Von Dreele, P. H., 56, *72*
Dyckes, D. F., see Von Dreele, P. H. 56, *72*

Eagles, P. A. M., see Paterson, R. A., 121, *126*
Ebnöther, C., see Visconti, M., 11, *38*
Edelfrawi, A. T., see Edelfrawi, M. E., 249, 267, 271, *273*
Edelfrawi, M. E., 249, 267, 271, *273*. See also Denburg, J. L., 251, *273*
Edsall, J. T., see Armstrong, J. McD., 74, *90*; Martin, R. B., 35, *38*
Eilat, D., see Oen, H., 196, *199*
Eisenberg, H., see Cohen, G., 169, 171, *188*

Elion, G. A., see Hitchings, G. H., 132, *150*
Ellisman, M. H., 263, *273*. See also Rash, J. E., 263, 264, *274*
Emmett, J. C., see Black, J. W., 30, 31, 33, *36*; Brimblecombe, R. W., 34, 35, *36*
Erdmann, V. A., see Bald, R., 191, 195, *199*; Pongs, O., 191, 193, 195, 196, 197, *199*
Erickson, J. S., 130, *150*
Ernster, L., see Hrycay, E., 209, *212*
Estabrook, R. W., 203, 209, *211*. See also Remmer, H., 206, *212*; Schenkman, J.B., 206, *212*; Waterman, M. R., 206, *212*
Eyre, P., see Chand, N., 23, *36*

Fain, J. N., 243, *247*
Falco, E. A., see Hitchings, G. H., 132, *150*
Falkbring, S. O., see Kannan, K. K., 73, 74, *90*
Famborough, D. M., see Hartzell, H. C., 265, *273*
Farber, S., 128, *150*
Farnell, L., 46, *54*
Fedak, S. A., see Brown, E. M., 243, *246*; Spiegel, A. M., 237, 242, *247*
Feeney, J., 56, 60, 61, 62, 63, 64, 66, 69, *71*, 133, 143, 144, 146, *150*. See also Birdsall, B., 67, *71*, 133, 134, 138, 140, 141, 142, 148, *149*; Boicelli, C. A., 63, 64, *71*; Bradbury, A. F., 56, 57, *71*; Burgen, A. S. V., 69, 70, 71, *71*; Dell, A., 170, 179, 182, *188*; Hansen, P. E., 61, 66, *71*; Roberts, G. C. K., 133, 134, 136, 138, 142, 144, *150*; Way, J. L., 133, 136, *150*; Wessels, P. L., 69, *72*
Ferger, M. F., see Von Dreele, P. H., 56, *72*
Fernandez-Munoz, R., 191, 192, 193, *199*
Ferone, R., 131, 132, *150*
Fertuck, H. C., 261, 262, *273*
Fohlen, G. M., see Kumler, W. D., 34, *37*
Forsythe, A. B., see Hansch, C., 5, *37*
Fosbinder, R. J., see Walter, L. A. 25, *38*; Hunt, W. H., 25, *37*
Foster, C. J., see Blume, A. J., 243, *246*
Foveau, D., see Marriq, C., 73, *90*
Frankel, R. B., see Koch, S., 206, *212*
Franklin, K., see Richardson, M. F., 12, *38*
Freeman, M., see Osborn, M. J., 128, *150*
Fridborg, K., see Kannan, K. K., 73, 74, 77, 83, *90*; Liljas, A., 73, 83, 84, *90*; Strandberg, B., 73, 74, *91*
Frieden, E., 2, *37*
Friedkin, M., see Plante, L. T., 134, *150*

Friedman, P. A., see Goldberg, I. H., 167, 188
Friedman, S., see Haselkorn, D., 97, *107*
Fromageot, P., see Bourgeois, J. B., 263, *273*
Frommer, U., 203, 204, 210, *211*, *212*
Fujita, T., 104, *107*
Fuller, W., 168, 169, *188*
Furness, M. E., see Harrap, K. R., 131, *150*
Futterman, S., 128, *150*

Gabers, D. L., 236, *247*
Galardy, R. E., see Bleich, H. E., 69, *71*
Ganellin, C. R., 23, 24, 25, 26, 28, *37*, 46, 47, *54*. See also Black, J. W., 21, 23, 28, 30, 31, 33, *36*; Brimblecombe, R. W., 34, 35, *36*; Durant, G. J., 24, 25, 28, *37*; Farnell, L., 46, *54*; Parsons, M. E., 33, *38*
Garrett, E. R., see Hansch, C., 191, *199*
Gass, K., 153, 154, 155, *165*
Gaumont, Y., see Chaykovsky, M., 134, *150*
Gauthier, G. F., see Padykula, H. A., 265, *274*
Gautier, F., see Müller, W., 171, *189*
Gefter, M., 153, *165*
Gehring-Müller, R., see Matsuda, G., 112, *126*
Gibbons, W. A., 61, 63, *71*. See also Sogn, J. A., 63, *71*
Gigon, P. L., 206, *212*
Gill, E. W., 2, *37*
Gillette, J. R., see Brodie, B. B. 202, *211*; Gigon, P. L., 206, *212*; Remmer, H., 206, *212*
Gips, H., see Glossmann, H., 236, *247*
Giraud, N., see Mariq, C., 73, *90*
Girol, D., see Haselkorn, D., 97, *107*
Glasel, J. A., 68, *71*. See also Barry, C. D., 66, 67, *71*; Brewster, A. I., 56, *71*
Gleason, J. G., see Blank, B., 18, *36*
Glickson, J. D., see Walter, R., 56, *72*
Glossman, H., 236, 237, 238, 242, *247*
Go, A., see Kopple, K. D., 64, *71*
Goaman, L. C. G., see Perutz, M. F., 112, *126*
Goldacre, R., see Albert, A., 11, 12, *36*
Goldberg, I. H., 167, *188*
Goldman, I. D., 131, *150*
Goldstein, A., see Das, H. K., 193, *199*
Good, N. E., 121, *126*
Goodall, M. T., see Romine, W. O., 271, *274*
Goodford, P. J., 6, *37*, 119, *125*. See also Beddell, C. R., 121, 122, *125*; Wooton, R., 5, *39*

Gore, W. E., see Risinger, G. E., 11, *38*
Gorin, M., see Hansch, C., 191, *199*
Gormley, J. J., see Wessels, P. L., 69, *72*
Göthe, P. O., 85, *90*. See also Kannan, K. K., 73, 74, *90*
Grafuis, M. A., 18, *37*
Gram, T. E., see Gigon, P. L., 206, *212*
Green, J. P., 13, *37*. See also Margolis, S., 23, *38*
Green, R. W., 20, *37*
Greenberg, D. M., 134, *150*
Greenfield, N. J., 136, *150*. See also Poe, M., 130, 136, *150*
Greenwald, I., 114, *126*
Gregory, H., see Feeney, J., 69, *71*; Wessels, P. L., 69, *72*
Griffin, B. W., 206, *212*
Griffiths, D. V., see Birdsall, B., 134, 138, 140, 142, *149*; Feeney, J., 143, 144, 146, *150*
Gross, J., see Brazill, G., 153, 165
Grzybowski, A. K., see Datta, S. P., 30, *36*
Guest, G. M., see Rapoport, S., 114, *126*
Guiliani, A. M., see Birdsall, B., 67, *71*
Guldberg, C. M., 109, *126*
Gund, P., see Hahn, F. E., 190, 193, 194, *199*
Gunsalus, I. C., 209, *212*. See also Wilson, G. S., 207, *212*
Gurevich, A. I., see Kolosov, M. N., 191, *199*
Gustafsson, J. A., see Hrycay, E., 209, *212*
Gustari, K., see Schill, G., 35, *38*
Guthe, K. F., see Allen, D. W., 112, 121, *125*

Hahn, F. E., 190, 191, 193, 194, *199*. See also Corcoran, J. W., 167, *188*; O'Brien, R. L., 177, *189*
Hakala, M. T., 131, *150*
Haldane, J. B. S., see Douglas, C. G., 114, 115, *126*
Haldane, J. S., see Barcroft, J., 112, *125*; Douglas, C. G., 114, 115, *126*
Hall, Z. W., 257, 264, *273*. See also Berg, D. K., 252, 265, *272*; Brockes, J. P., 256, *273*
Ham, N. S., 23, *37*
Hammes, G. G., 243, *247*. See also Alberty, R. A., 94, *107*
Hammond, J., see Richards, W. G., 46, 47, *54*
Handschumacher, R. E., see Brown, N. C., 152, *165*
Hanners, W. E., see Canellakis, E. S., 185, *188*

Hansch, C., 5, 6, 7, *37*, 191, *199*. See also Fujita, T., 104, *107*; Leo, A., 5, *38*; Silipo, C., 5, *38*
Hansen, P. E., 61, 66, *71*
Harding, M. M., 88, *90*
Harding, N. G. L., *see* Dann, J. G., 133, 134, 140, *150*
Harrap, K. R., 131, *150*
Hart, L. I., *see* Harrap, K. R., 131, *150*
Hartz, T. P., *see* Clement, G. E., 18, *36*
Hartzell, H. C., 265, *273*
Harwood, J. P., 236, *247*. See also Londos, C., 236, *247*; Rodbell, M., 236, *247*
Haselkorn, D., 97, *107*
Haugen, D. A., 204, *212*
Hawkins, N. M., *see* Bonting, S. L., 224, *233*
Hayes, J. E., *see* Hahn, F. E., 191, *199*
Hehri, W. J., 50, *54*
Heidema, J., *see* Strobel, H. W., 203, *212*
Heller, M. J., *see* Tu, A. T., 239, *247*
Helmreich, E. J. M., *see* Pfeufter, T., 236, 237, 238, *247*
Henderson, L. E., 73, *90*. See also Lindskog, S., 73, 89, *90*
Henderson, R., *see* Tobin, T., 220, 230, *233*
Henley, S. M., *see* Waring, M. J., 169, *189*
Henriksson, O., 73, *90*. See also Henderson, L. E. 73, *90*
Herlem, M., 34, *37*
Hershberger, W. K., *see* Pedersen, M. G., 202, *212*
Herzberg, M., *see* Dudai, Y., 264, *273*
Hesselbo, T., *see* Black, J. W., 33, *36*; Wyllie, J. H., 32, *39*
Heuser, J. E., 260, 263, 264, *273*
Hiemstra, K., *see* Wolberg, G., 243, *247*
Higashijima, T., 60, *71*
Higuchi, T., 5, 6, *37*
Hildebrandt, A. G., *see* Estabrook, R. W. 209, *211*
Hill, B. T., *see* Harrap, K. R., 131, *150*
Hine, J., 6, *37*
Hirota, Y., *see* Gefter, M., 153, *165*
Hirshfield, J. M., *see* Poe, M., 130, 136, *150*
Hirt, R. C., 34, *37*
Hitchings, G. H., 132, 133, *150*. See also Burchall, J. J., 131, 132, *149*; Ferone, R., 132, *150*
Ho, B. T., *see* Baker, B. R., 134, *149*
Hoerger, E., *see* Brown, D. J., 11, *36*
van der Hoeven, T. A., *see* Haugen, D. A., 204, *212*
Hollingworth, B. R., *see* Martin, R. B., 35, *38*
Holm, R. H., *see* Koch, S., 206, *212*

Holmes, F., 24, *37*
Homann, H. E., 194, *199*
Hoogsteen, K., *see* Poe, M., 130, 136, *150*
Hopmann, R. F. W., 11, 12, *37*
Hopps, H. E., *see* Hahn, F. E., 191, *199*
Horsley, J., *see* Richards, W. G., 42, *54*
Howard-Flanders, P., *see* Boyce, R. P., 152, *165*
Hruby, V. J., *see* Brewster, A. I., 56, 57, *71*; Glasel, J. A., 68, *71*
Hrycay, E., 209, *212*
Huang, M., *see* Daly, J. W., 243, *246*
Hubbard, J. I., 249, *273*
Huennekens, F. M., *see* Osborn, M. J., 128, *150*
Hughes, E. W., 34, *37*
Hultquist, M. E., *see* Seeger, D. R., 128, *150*
Hunt, W. H., 25, *37*. See also Walter, L. A., 25, *38*
Hutchison, D. J., 131, *150*
Huxley, H. E., *see* Birks, R., 262, 264, *273*

Ianotti, A. T., *see* Johns, D. G., 131, *150*
Ibers, J. A., *see* Koch, S., 206, *212*
Ing, H. R., 4, *37*
Ingelmann-Sundberg, M., *see* Hrycay, E., 209, *212*
Ishimura, Y., 209, *212*
Ison, R. R., *see* Ham, N. S., 23, *37*
Iyanagi, T., 203, *212*
Izawa, S., *see* Good, N. E., 121, *126*

Jack, D., *see* Brittain, R. T., 13, *36*
Jacobs, S., *see* Cuatrecasas, P., 237, 238, *246*
Jacobson, M., *see* Conney, A. H., 203, 210, *211*
Jaffé, H. H., 11, *37*
Jain, S. C., *see* Sobell, H. M., 168, 170, *189*; Tsai, C., 168, *189*
Jamison, R. F., 13, *37*
Janssen, M. J., 34, *37*
Jannsson, S. E., *see* Albuquerque, E. X., 252, 263, *272*
Jarup, L., 74, *90*. See also Kannan, K. K., 73, *90*; Liljas, A., 73, 83, 84, *90*
Jard, S., 243, *247*
Jarke, F. H., *see* Rajan, K. S., 13, *38*
Jedrzejczyk, J., *see* Barnard, E. A., 250, 252, *272*
Jeffrey, G. A., 120, *126*
Jencks, W. P., 135, *150*
Jenkins, D. J. A., *see* Milton-Thompson, G. J., 32, *38*
Jenny, E., *see* Greenberg, D. M., 134, *150*

Author Index

Jerina, D., 210, *212*
Johns, D. G., 131, *150*
Johnson, C. K., 75, *90*
Johnson, C. L., *see* Green, J. P., 13, *37*
Johnson, G. L., *see* Kahn, J. B., 224, *233*
Johnson, L. F., 56, *71*
Johnson, R. A., *see* Gabers, D. L., 236, *247*
Jones, F., *see* Holmes, F., 24, *37*
Jones, H. L., *see* Jaffé, H. H., 11, *37*
Jones, R. G., *see* Lee, H. M., 25, *38*
Juchan, M. R., *see* Pedersen, M. G., 202, *212*
Junk, K. W., *see* Lu, A. Y. H., 203, *212*

Kahn, J. B., 224, *233*
Kaiser, E. T., *see* Olander, J., 102, *107*
Kakeya, N., 89, *90*, 104, *107*
Kamada, A., *see* Kakeya, N., 89, *90*, 104, *107*
Kameyama, N., 34, *37*
Kang, S., 23, *37. See also* Green, J. P., 13, *37*; Margolis, S., 23, *38*
Kannan, K. K., 73, 74, 77, 83, *90. See also* Bergstén, P. C., 77, 84, 88, *90*; Jarüp, L., 74, *90*; Liljas, A., 73, 83, 84, *90*; Lindskog, S., 73, 89, *90*; Notstrand, B., 73, 75, *90*; Vaara, I., 85, 88, *90*
Kanner, L. C., *see* Das, H. K., 193, *199*
Kappas, A., *see* Alvares, A. P., 203, *211*
Kappe, T., 13, *37*
Karlin, A., 249, *273*
Karrer, P., *see* Visconti, M., 11, *38*
Kasai, M., *see* Changeux, J. P., 250, *273*
Katagiri, K., 179, *188*
Katritzky, A. R., 11, 29, *37*
Katz, B., 249, 257, *273. See also* Birks, R., 262, 264, *273*
Keilin, D., *see* Mann, T., 73, 90, 98, *107*
Keller-Schierlein, W., 179, *188*
Kellie, G. M., 7, *37*
Kelly, M. M., *see* Beveridge, D. L., 42, *54*
Kelly, R. B., *see* Berg, D. K., 252, 265, *272*; Hall, Z. W., 257, 264, *273*
Kemp, G., 271, *273*
Kernohan, J. C., 98, *107*
Kendrew, J. C., 112, *126. See also* Dickerson, R. E., 74, *90*
Khokhlov, A. S., *see* Kolosov, M. N., 191, *199*
Kier, L. B., 23, *37*, 53, *54*
Kim, K. H., *see* Hansch, C., 5, 7, *37*
King, R. W., 96, 98, 100, 102, 105, *107*. *See also* Dann, J. G., 133, 134, 140, *150*; Feeney, J., 143, 144, 146, *150*; Kumar, K., 96, 106, *107*; Taylor, P. W., 88, 89, *91*, 94, 95, 98, 102, 104, *107*

Kisliuk, R. L., *see* Chaykovsky, M., 134, *150*
Koch, S., 206, *212*
Kolosov, M. N., 191, *199*
Kopple, K. D., 64, *71*
Koren, J. G., *see* Hirt, R. C., 34, *37*
Kornberg, T., *see* Gefter, M., 153, *165*
Korolkovas, A., 4, *37*
Korte, F., 12, *37*
Kostos, V., *see* Di Tullio, N. W., 18, *37*
Kotelchuck, D., 56, 63, *71*
Krampitz, L. O., 11, *37*
Krans, H. M. J., *see* Rodbell, M., 236, *247*
Kraut, J., 12, *37*
Kretzinger, R. H., 88, *90*
Krugh, T. R., 170, *188*
Ku, D., 223, *233. See also* Tobin, T., 218, 231, *233*
Kuang-Tzu, D. L., 73, *90*
Küchler, E., *see* Czernilofsky, A. P., 196, *199*
Kuffler, S. W., 263, *273*
Kumar, K., 96, 106, *107*
Kume, S., *see* Post, R. L., 213, 223, 228, *233*
Kumler, W. D., 34, *37*
Kuntzman, R., 203, *212. See also* Conney, A. H., 203, 210, *211*
Kuwahara, S., *see* Mannering, G. J., 208, *212*

Lackner, H., 179, *188*
LaDu, B. N., *see* Brodie, B. B., 202, *211*
Lagowski, J. M., *see* Katritzky, A. R., 11, 29, *37*
Landis, D. M. D., *see* Heuser, J. E., 260, 263, 264, *273*
Landis, W., *see* Jerina, D., 210, *212*
Landowne, D., 249, 263, 271, *273*
Langley, J. N., 109, *126*
Lanir, A., 98, 100, *107*
Lapa, A. J., *see* Albuquerque, E. X., 252, *272*; Chiu, T. H., 250, 251, 252, *273*
Lapiere, C. L., *see* Blank, B., 18, *36*
Larsen, F. S., *see* Akera, T., 230, *233*
Larson, J. E., *see* Wartell, R. M., 169, *189*; Wells, R. D., 170, 176, *189*
Laurent Tabusse, G., *see* Marriq, C., 73, *90*
Le Bret, M., *see* Le Pecq, J. B., 169, 188, *189*
Lee, C. Y., *see* Chang, C. C., 250, *273*; Changeux, J. P., 250, *273*; Tobin, T., 217, 219, 226, *233*
Lee, H. M., 25, *38*
Lee, J. S., *see* Waring, M. J., 173, *189*
Leffler, E. B., 13, *38*
Lefkowitz, R. J., 236, 237, 238, *247*

Lehrmann, C., 202, *212*
Leibman, K., *see* Estabrook, R. W., 209, *211*
Leigh, R. A., *see* Mildvan, A. S., 253, 270, *273*
Leigh, S., *see* Alvares, A. P., 203, *211*
Leo, A., 5, *38*. *See also* Hansch, C., 6, *37*
Leong, J. L., *see* Wattenberg, L. W., 202, 203, *212*
Le Pecq, J. B., 169, 188, *189*
Lerman, L. S., 168, 169, *189*
Lester, H., 252, *273*
Levin, W., *see* Alvares, A. P., 203, *211*; Conney, A. H., 203, 210, *211*
Levine, B. A., 66, *72*
Levy, G. C., *see* Deslauriers, R., 69, *71*
Lewis, G. P., 13, *38*
Leyden, D. E., *see* Walters, D. B., 18, *38*; Rigler, N. E., 35, *38*
Libelius, R., 265, *273*
Lichtenberger, F., 210, *212*. *See also* Staudt, H., 208, *212*
Lien, E. J., 5, *38*. *See also* Hansch, C., 5, 7, *37*
Liler, M., 11, *38*
Liljas, A., 73, 83, 84, *90*. *See also* Bergstén, P. C., 77, 84, 88, *90*; Jarüp, L., 74, *90*; Kannan, K. K., 73, 74, *90*; Lindskog, S., 73, 89, *90*; Vaari, I., 85, 88, *90*
Lin, M. C., *see* Londos, C., 236, *247*; Rendell, M., 236, 243, *247*; Rodbell, M., 236, 243, *247*; Salomon, Y., 236, 237, 238, *247*
Lindskog, S., 73, 89, *90*, 96, 98, *107*. *See also* Campbell, I. D., 86, *90*; Strandberg, B., 73, 74, *91*
Lipmann, F., *see* Tao, M., 236, *247*
Logan, R. H., *see* Kopple, K. D., 64, *71*
Londos, C., 236, *247*. *See also* Rodbell, M., 236, *247*; Salomon, Y., 236, 237, 238, *247*
Lövgren, S., *see* Bergstén, P. C., 77, 84, 88, *90*; Kannan, K. K., 73, 74, 77, 83, *90*; Liljas, A., 73, 83, 84, *90*; Vaara, I., 85, 88, *90*
Low, H., *see* Harwood, J. P., 236, *247*
Low, R., 153, 156, 157, 158, *166*. *See also* Cozzarelli, N., 153, 163, *165*; Gass, K., 153, 154, 155, *165*
Lowy, J., *see* Alper, R., 256, *272*
Lu, A. Y. H., 203, *212*. *See also* Strobel, H. W., 203, *212*
Lu, M. C., *see* Tobin, T., 218, 231, *233*
Luck, G., 169, *189*

McGandy, E. L., *see* Perutz, M. F., 112, *126*

McGhee, J. D., 174, 175, 185, *189*
McGregor, W. H., *see* Deslauriers, R., 69, *71*
McKelvy, J. F., *see* Glasel, J. A., 68, *71*
Mackenzie, J., 153, 154, 155, 159, 160, *166*
Mallick, B., *see* Barnard, E. A., 253, 255, 256, *272*; Dolly, J. O. 251, 253, 256, 257, 271, *273*
Mann, T., 73, 90, 98, *107*
Mannering, G. J., 208, *212*
Maren, T. H., 73, 89, *90*. *See also* King, R. W., 98, *107*
Margolis, S., 23, *38*
Marriq, C., 73, *90*
Martin, B. R., *see* Rodbell, M., 236, *247*
Martin, D. G., 170, 179, *189*
Martin, R. B., 35, *38*
Mason, H. S., 201, *212*. *See also* Iyanagi, T., 203, *212*
Mason, M. S., *see* Waterman, M. R., 207, *212*
Mason, S. F., *see* Brown, D. J., 11, *36*
Massoulie, J., *see* Rieger, F., 264, *274*
Mathews, C. K., *see* Erickson, J. S., 130, *150*
Mathews, F. S., *see* Perutz, M. F., 112, *126*
Matsuda, G., 112, *126*
Matsumoto, K., 34, *38*
Matsushita, T., 152, *166*. *See also* Brown, N. C., 152, *165*
Matsuura, S., *see* Morimoto, T., 207, *212*
Maxwell, R. E., 191, *199*
Mayer, J. R., *see* Tuckerman, M. M., 13, *38*
Meldrum, N. V., 73, *90*
Menez, A., *see* Bourgeois, J. B., 263, *273*
Mercer, R. D., *see* Farber, S., 128, *150*
Messer, W., *see* Pongs, O., 193, 195, 198, *199*
Metzler, D. E., 35, *38*
Meulman, P. A., *see* Martin, D. G., 170, 179, *189*
Meunier, J. C., 270, 271, *273*. *See also* Cartaud, J., 263, *273*
Miao, C. K., *see* Blank, B., 18, *36*
Michealson, D., 266, 271, *273*
Michel, I. M., *see* Weinryb, I., 243, *247*
Mihailovic, M. L., *see* Keller-Schierlein, W., 179, *188*
Mihich, E., 131, 132, *150*
Mildvan, A. S., 253, 270, *273*
Miledi, R., 250, 252, 265, *273*. *See also* Katz, B., 257, *273*
Miller, W. H., 104, *107*
Milton-Thompson, G. J., 32, *38*

Misiewicz, J. J., see Milton-Thompson, G. J., 32, *38*
Miyazawa, T., see Higashijima, T., 60, *71*
Mizsak, S. A., see Martin, D. G., 170, 179, *189*
Modest, E. J., see Chaykovsky, M., 134, *150*
Momany, F. A., see Burgess, R. W., 69, *71*
Monro, R. E., see Celma, M. L., 191, *199*; Fernandez-Manoz, R., 191, 192, 193, , *199*
Moody, T., see Michealson, D., 266, 271, *273*
Mookerjee, P. K., see Hine, J., 6, *37*
Moor, H., see Peper, K., 260, 263, 264, *274*
Moore, M. M., see Perkins, J. P., 242, *247*
Morimoto, T., 207, *212*
Morris, H. R., see Dell A., 170, 179, 182, *188*
Moses, R. E., 152, *166*
Muirhead, H., see Perutz, M. F., 112, *126*
Müller, W., 170, 171, *189*
Mulliken, R. S., 49, *54*
Myers, D. V., see Armstrong, J. McD., 74, *90*

Nachod, F. C., see Tuckerman, M. M., 13, *38*
Nair, M. G., see Baugh, C. M., 142, *149*
Nakamoto, K., see Hansch, C., 191, *199*
Narasimhulu, S., see Remmer, H., 206, *212*
Nastainszyk, W., see Lichtenberger, F., 210, *212*
Nathans, D., 191, *199*
Navon, G., see Lanir, A., 98, 100, *107*
Neilands, J. B., see Grafius, M. A., 18, *37*; Williams, V. R., 35, *39*
Neill, J. M., see van Slyke, D. D., 112, *126*
Neillie, W. F. S., see Jameson, R. F., 13, *37*
Nemethy, G., 2, 38, 62, *72*. See also Gibbons, W. A., 61, 63, *71*
Netter, K. J., see Estabrook, R. W., 209, *211*
Neville, D. R., 238, *247*
Neville, M., 153, 154, *166*. See also Mackenzie, J., 153, 154, 155, 159, 160, *166*
Newton, B. A., 167, *189*
Nichol, C. A., 128, *150*. See also Hakala, M. T., 131, *150*; Zakrzewski, S. F., 128, *150*
Nickel, E., 263, *273*
Nickel, V. S., see Maxwell, R. E., 191, *199*

Nierhans, D., 194, *199*
Nierhans, K. H., see Homann, H. E., 194, *199*; Nierhans, D., 194, *199*; Pongs, O., 196, 197, *199*
Nikaitani, D., see Hansch, C., 5, 6, 7, *37*
Nordman, C. E., see Sobell, M. M., 168, 170, *189*
Norrington, F. E., 112, *126*. See also Beddell, C. R., 121, 122, *125*
North, A. C. T., see Barry, C. D., 66, 67, *71*
Notstrand, B., 73, 75, *91*. See also Kannan, K. K., 73, 77, 83, *90*
Novotny, J., see Baker, B. R., 134, *149*
Nyman, P. O., 73, *91*. See also Anderson, B., 73, *90*; Gothe, P. O. 85, *90*; Henderson, L. E., 73, *90*; Kannan, K. K., 73, 74, *90*; Lindskog, S., 73, 89, *90*, 96, *107*; Strandberg, B., 73, 74, *91*
Nys, G. G., 6, *38*

O'Brien, P. J., see Rahimtula, A. D., 209, *212*
O'Brien, R. D., see Denburg, J. L., 256, *293*
O'Brien, R. L., 177, *189*
Oen, H., 196, *199*
Ohlsson, A., see Kannan, K. K., 73, 77, 83, *90*
Ohnishi, M., see Urry, D. W., 56, 57, 58, 59, 63, *72* .
Olander, J., 102, *107*
Olsen, R., see Neunier, J. C., 270, 271, *273*
Omura, T., 203, *212*. See also Mannering, G. J., 208, *212*; Morimoto, T., 207, *212*
Orcutt, B., see Post, R. L., 213, 216, 223, 228, *233*
Orrenius, S., see Frommer, U., 203, *212*
Osborn, A. R., 11, *38*
Osborn, M. J., 128, *150*
O'Shea, M., see Ferone, R., 131, *150*
Ostler, G., see Dann, J. G., 133, 134, 140, *150*
Ostrowski, K., see Rogers, A. W., 250, *274*
Ostwald, W., 114, *126*
Otsuka, H., 179, 180, *189*
Owings, F. F., see Blank, B., 18, *36*

Pachler, K. G. R., 64, *71*
Padykula, H. A., 265, *274*
Paiva, A., see Paiva, T. B., 21, 30, *38*
Paiva, T. B., 21, 30, *38*
Papathanasopoulos, N., see Chaykovsky, M., 134, *150*
Parsons, M. E., 33, *38*. See also Black, J. W., 23, 28, 33, *36*; Brimblecombe, R. W., 34, 35, *36*; Durant, G. J., 24, 25, 28, 33, *37*
Paterson, R. A., 121, *126*
Payes, B., see Greenberg, D. M., 134, *150*

Pecht, I., see Haselkorn, D., 97, *107*
Pecot–Dechavassine, M., see Couteaux, R., 260, *273*
Pedersen, M. G., 202, *212*
Peisach, J., 206, *212*
Pellegrini, M., 196, *199*. See also Oen, H., 196, *199*
Peper, K., 260, 263, 264, *274*
Pepper, E. S., see Ganellin, C. R., 23, 37, 46, *54*
Perault, A. M., 130, *150*
Perkins, J. P., 242, *247*
Perkins, J. R., 136, *150*
Perrin, D. D., 13, *38*
Perutz, M. F., 112, *126*
Pestka, S., 190, 191, 193, *199*
Petef, M., see Kannan, K. K., 73, 74, 77, 84, *90*; Liljas, A., 73, 83, 84, *90*
Peters, T., 224, 232, *233*
Peterson, J., see Romine, W. O., 271, *274*
Peterson, J. A., see Griffin, B. W., 206, *212*; Ishimura, Y., 209, *212*
Pew, C. L., see Ku, D., 223, *233*
Pfeuffer, T., 236, 237, 238, *247*
Phillips, D. C., see Kendrew, J. C., 112, *126*
Phillips, J., see Albert, 11, 12, *36*
Plante, L. T., 134, *150*
Plattner, H., see Rogers, A. W., 250, *274*; Salpeter, M. M., 264, *274*
Pletcher, J., 12, *38*
Poe, M. 130, 136, *150*
Pohl, S. L., 235, 238, *247*. See also Birnbaumer, L., 241, *246*; Rodbell, M., 236, *247*
Pointer, R. H., see Fain, J. N., 243, *247*
Pongs, O., 191, 193, 195, 196, 197, 198, *199*. See also Bald, R., 191, 195, *199*
Pople, J. A., see Hehre, W. J., 50, *54*
Port, G. N. J., see Pullman, B., 23, *38*; Ganellin, C. R., 23, 24, *37*, 46, *54*
Porter, C. W., 251, 252, 257, 259, 261, 262, 263, 266, *274*. See also Albuquerque, E. X., 260, *272*; Barnard, E. A., 251, 252, 257, 258, 260, 263, *272*
Porter, M. R., see Ellisman, M. H., 263, *273*
Post, R. L., 213, 214, 215, 216, 223, 228, *233*. See also Sen, A. K., 227, 228, *233*
Postal-Vinay, M. C., see Sonenberg, M., 239, *247*
Potter, L. T., see Landowne, D., 249, 263, 271, *273*; Miledi, R., 250, 252, 265, *273*; Nickel, E., 263, *273*
Prasad, K. U., see Walter, R., 56, *72*
Prelog, V., see Keller-Schierlein, W., 179, , *188*
Printz, M. P., see Bleich, H. E., 69, *71*

Pullman, A., 42, *54*
Pullman, B., 23, *38*. See also Collin, R., 130, *150*; Perault, A. M., 130, *150*; Pullman, A., 42, *54*
Pulver, K., see Risinger, G. E., 11, *38*
Purcell, W. P., 5, 6, *38*

Rabin, R. H., see Peters, T., 224, 232, *233*
Radna, R. J., see Beveridge, D. L., 42, *54*
Raftery, M. A., see Michealson, D., 266, 271, *273*
Rahimtula, A. D., 209, *212*
Rajan, K. S., 13, *38*
Rajerison, R., see Jard, S., 243, *247*
Rall, T. W., see Sattin, A., 243, *247*; Sutherland, E. W., 235, *247*
Randall, E. W., see Sogn, J. A., 63, *72*
Rang, H. P., 249, *274*. See also Colquhoun, D., 252, 255, 256, *273*
Rapoport, H., see Matsumoto, K., 34, *38*
Rapoport, S., 114, *126*
Rash, J. E., 263, 264, *274*. See also Ellisman, M. H., 263, *273*
Rashbaum, S., see Low, R., 153, 156, 157, 158, *166*
Rasmussen, A. C., see Parsons, M. E., 33, *38*
Rebstock, 191, *200*. See also Contoulis, M., 190, *199*
Reed, H. J., see Kraut, J., 12, *37*
Reese, T. S., see Heuser, J. E., 260, 263, 264, *273*
Reilley, C. N., see Rigler, N. E., 35, *38*
Reinert, K. E., 169, 171, *189*
Reinhardt, C. G., see Krugh, T. R., 170, *188*
Reinwald, E., see Pongs, O., 193, 195, *199*
Rekker, R. F., see Nys, G. G., 6, *38*
Remmer, H., 206, *212*. See also Schenkman, J. B., 206, *212*
Rendell, M., 236, 243, *247*
Richards, F. M., 75, *91*
Richards, W. G., 43, 46, *47*. See also Dean, S. M., 49, *54*; Farnell, L., 46, *54*; Ganellin, C. R., 23, 24, 46, *54*
Richardson, C. C., see Moses, R. E., 152, *166*
Richardson, M. F., 12, *38*
Riddell, F. G., see Kellie, G. M., 7, *37*
Rieger, F., 264, *274*
Rigler, N. E., 35, *38*
Risinger, G. E., 11, *38*
Ritchie, A. C., see Brittain, R. T., 13, *36*
Ritchie, J. M., see Colquhoun, D., 252, 256, *273*
Riveros, J. M., see Brauman, J. I., 50, *54*

Rizzo, R., *see* De Santis, P., 182, *188*
Roberts, F., *see* Barcroft, J., 113, 114, 115, *125*
Roberts, G. C. K., 13, *38*, 133, 134, 136, 138, 142, 144, *150*. *See also* Birdsall, B., 133, 134, 138, 140, 141, 142, 148, *149*; Bradbury, A. F., 56, 57, *71*; Burgen, A. S. V., 69, 70, 71, *71*; Dann, J. G., 133, 134, 140, *150*; Dell, A., 170, 179, 182, *188*; Feeney, J., 56, 61, 62, 63, 69, 71, *71*, 133, 143, 144, 146, *150*; Hansen, P. E., 61, 66, *71*; Way, J. L., 133, 136, *150*
Roberts, J., *see* Sonenberg, M., 237, *247*
Robertson, J. M., 120, *126*
Robin, R. O., *see* Bell, P. H., 8, *36*. *See also* Miller, W. H., 104, *107*
Rockey, J. H., *see* Feeney, J., 56, 61, 62, 63, *71*
Rodbard, D., *see* Brown, E. M., *246*
Rodbell, M., 236, 243, *247*. *See also* Birnbaumer, L., 235, 241, *246*; Hammes, G. G., 243, *247*; Harwood, J. P., 236, *247*; Londos, C., 236, *247*; Pohl, S. L., 238, *247*; Rendell, M., 236, 243, *247*; Salomon, Y., 236, 237, 238, *247*; Schramm, M., 236, *247*
Rogers, A. W., 250, *274*. *See also* Salpeter, M. M., 264, *274*
Rogers, S. J., 18, *38*
Romine, W. O., 271, *274*
Roques, B., *see* Le Pecq, J. B., 169, 188, *189*
Rosen, O. M., 235, *247*
Rosen, S. M., *see* Rosen, O. M., 235, *247*
Rosenbluth, J., 262, 264, *274*
Rosenthal, A. S., *see* Post, R. L., 214, *233*
Rosenthal, O., *see* Conney, A. H., 203, 210, *211*; Estabrook, R. W., 203, *211*; Remmer, H., 206, *212*
Rosowsky, A., *see* Chaykovsky, M., 134, *150*
Ross, S. T., *see* Blank, B., 18, *36*
Roughton, F. J. W., 114, *126*. *See also* Meldrum, N. U., 73, *90*
Rouvray, D. H., 11, *38*
Roy, C., *see* Jard, S., 243, *247*
Rubin, M., *see* Sonenberg, M., 237, *247*
Ruehle, A. E., *see* Williams, R. R., 11, *39*
Rummel, W., *see* Lehrmann, C., 202, *212*
Russell, P. B., *see* Hitchings, G. H., 132, *150*
Ryter, A., *see* Bourgeois, J. B., 263, *273*

Saito, A., *see* Zacks, S. I., 265, *274*
Saito, H., *see* Smith, I. C. P., 56, 64, *72*
Sakmann, B., *see* Betz, W., 257, 264, *272*

Sakore, T. D., *see* Sobell, H. M., 168, 170, *189*
Salomon, Y., 236, 237, 238, *247*. *See also* Londos, C., 236, *247*; Rendell, M., 236, 243, *247*; Rodbell, M., 236, 243, *247*
Salpeter, M. M., 250, 264, *274*. *See also* Fertuck, H. C., 261, 262, *273*; Rogers, A. W., 250, *274*
Samorjai, R. L., *see* Deslauriers, R., 69, *71*
Sandri, C., *see* Peper, K., 260, 263, 264, *274*
Santi, D. V., *see* Baker, B. R., 134, *149*
Sarantakis, K., *see* Deslauriers, R., 69, *71*
Sargent, P. B., *see* Berg, D. K., 252, 265, *272*
Sartorelli, A. C., *see* Johns, D. G., 131, *150*
Sarvey, J. M., *see* Dolly, J. O., 251, 253, 256, 257, 271, *273*
Sasaki, S., *see* Morimoto, T., 207, *212*
Sasame, H. A., *see* Remmer, H., 206, *212*
Sato, K., *see* Katagiri, K., 179, *188*
Sato, R., *see* Omura, T., 203, *212*
Sattin, A., 243, *247*
Saunders, H. L., *see* Blank, B., 18, *36*; Di Tullio, N. W., 18, *37*
Savoda, J., *see* Kopple, K. W., 64, *71*
Sax, M., *see* Pletcher, J., 12, *38*
Scatchard, G., 175, *189*
Schädelin, J., *see* Diehl, H., 206, 207, *211*
Schenkman, J. B., 206, *212*. *See also* Remmer, H., 206, *212*
Scheraga, H. A., *see* Burgess, R. W., 69, *71*; Kotelchuck, D., 56, 63, *71*; Scott, R. A., 62, *72*; Von Dreele, P. H., 56, *72*
Schild, H. O., *see* Ash, A. S. F., 23, *36*
Schill, G., 35, *38*
Schmidt, J., *see* Michealson, D., 266, 271, *273*
Schmidt, M., *see* Alper, R., 256, *272*
Schmitt, R. G., *see* Hirt, R. C., 34, *37*
Schneider, W. C., 34, *38*
Schofield, K., *see* Osborn, A. R., 11, *38*
Schramm, M., 236, *247*. *See also* Londos, C., 236, *247*
Schwan, T. J., *see* Baker, B. R., 134, *149*
Schwartz, I. L., *see* Johnson, L. F., 56, *71*
Schwartz, R. A., *see* Canellakis, E. S., 185, *188*
Schwyzer, R., *see* Wurthrich, K., 64, *72*
Sciaky, M., *see* Marriq, C., 73, *90*
Scott, J. M., *see* Brown, J. P., 142, *149*
Scott, R. A., 62, *72*
Scudder, P. N., *see* Dann, J. G., 133, 134, 140, *150*; Feeney, J., 143, 144, 146, *150*
Sealock, R., *see* Neunier, J. L., 270, 271, *273*

Seeger, D. R., 128, *150*
Sen, A. K., 227, 228, *233*. See also Post, R. L., 213, 214, 223, 228, *233*; Tobin, T., 218, 219, 220, 226, 230, *233*
Serjeant, E. P., see Albert, A., 11, *36*
Severson, D. L., see Drummond, G. I., 235, *247*
Sexton, W. A., 1, *38*
Seydel, J. K., 8, *38*
Shaw, Y. H., see Canellakis, E. S., 185, *188*
Shemiakin, M. M., see Kolosov, M. N., 191, *199*
Sheppard, W. A., 121, *126*
Sheppey, G. C., see Wooton, R., 5, *39*
Shimizu, H., see Daly, J. W., 243, *246*
Shoji, J., see Otsuka, H., 179, 180, *189*
Shore, V. C., see Kendrew, J. C., 112, *126*
Short, L. N., see Osborn, A. R., 11, *38*
Silipo, C., 5, *38*
Silman, I., see Dudai, Y., 264, *273*
Sims, P., see Waterfall, J. F., 211, *212*
Singh, R. M. M., see Good, N. E., 121, *126*
Sinistri, C., 13, 15, 16, 18, *38*
Smadel, J. E., see Hahn, F. E., 191, *199*
Smith, G. A., see Dell, A., 170, 179, 182, *188*
Smith, I. C. P., 56, 64, *72*. See also Deslauriers, R., 56, 64, 65, 67, 68, 69, *71*; Walter, R., 56, *72*
Smith, J. M. Jr., see Seeger, D. R., 128, *150*
Smith, R. N., see Hansch, C., 5, *37*
Smyth, D. G., see Bradbury, A. F., 56, 57, *71*
Snell, E. E., see Metzler, D. E., 35, *38*
So, A. G., 191, *200*
Sobell, H. M., 168, 170, *189*. See also Tsai, C., 168, *189*
Sogn, J. A., 63, *72*
Sonenberg, M., 237, *247*
Sonenberg, N., 195, 196, *200*
Spatola, A. F., see Glasel, J. A., 68, *71*
Spencer, H. M., see Leffler, E. B., 13, *38*
Spiegel, A. M., 236, 237, 242, *247*
Stack, E. J., see Di Tullio, N. W., 18, *37*
Staehelin, L. A., see Ellisman, M. H., 263, *273*
Stamatoyannopoulos, G., 112, *126*
Staudinger, Hj., see Frommer, U., 203, 204, 211, *212*; Ullrich, V., 209, 210, *212*
Staudt, H., 208, *212*
Stern, A., see Gibbons, W. A., 61, 63, *71*
Stewart, J. C., see Martin, D. G., 170, 179, *189*

Stewart, R. F., see Hehre, W. J., 50, *54*
Stokstad, E. L. R., see Buehring, K. U., 142, *149*
Stöffler, G., 200. See also Czernilofsky, A. P., 196, *199*
Strand, P. J., see Wattenberg, L. W., *212*
Strandberg, B. E., 73, 74, *91*. See also Dickerson, R. E., 74, *90*; Järup, L., 74, *90*; Kannan, K. K., 73, 74, *90*; Kendrew, J. C., 112, *126*; Liljas, A., 73, 83, 84, *90*; Lindskog, S., 73, 89, *90*
Strauss, H. L., see Hirt, R. C., 34, *37*
Strid, L., see Andersson, B., 73, *90*
Strobel, H. W., 203, *212*
Sudmeier, J. L., see Rigler, N. E., 35, *38*
Sueoka, N., see Matsushita, T., 152, *166*
Sugita, Y., 114, *126*
Sutherland, E. W., 235, *247*
Sutton, L. E., 45, *54*
Swislocki, N. I., see Sonenberg, M., 237, *247*
Sylvester, R. J. Jr., see Farber, S., 128, *150*

Tam, B. D., see Greenberg, D. M., 134, *150*
Tamura, T., see Buehring, K. U., 142, *149*
Tang, S. C., see Koch, S., 206, *212*
Tao, M., 236, *247*
Tashian, R. E., 76, *91*
Tashiro, Y., see Morimoto, T., 207, *212*
Tasumi, M., see Higashijima, T., 60, *71*
Taylor, P. W., 88, 89, *91*, 94, 95, 98, 102, 104, *107*
Terrar, D. A., see Landowne, D., 249, 263, 271, *273*
Thesleff, S., 265, *274*
Thomas, W. A., 64, *71*
Thompson, D. M., see Richardson, M. F., 12, *38*
Thornton, J., see Birdsall, B., 67, *71*
Thorslund, A., see Lindskog, S., 98, *107*
Tilander, B., see Strandberg, B., 73, 74, *91*
Tischendorf, G. W., see Stöffler, G., 197, *200*
Tobin, T., 215, 216, 217, 218, 219, 220, 225, 226, 227, 228, 229, 230, 231, 232, *233*. See also Akera, T., 221, 222, 223, 231, *233*; Ku, D., 223, *233*; Post, R. L., 213, 223, 228, *233*; Sen, A. K., 227, *233*
Tolstoouhov, A. V., 8, *38*
Tominana, M., see Paiva, T. B., 21, *38*
Topliss, J. G., 4, *38*
Tong, H. K., see Green, R. W., 20, *37*
Tonelli, A. E., 62, *72*. See also Brewster, A. I., 56, *71*
Torres-Pinedo, R., see Fernandez-Munoz, R., 191, 192, 193, *199*
Tougard, P., see Bram, S., 177, *188*

Tratton, C. D., *see* Rebstock, M. C., 191, 200
Triebel, H., *see* Luck, G., 169, *189*
Truitt, E. B., *see* Kier, L. B., 53, *54*
Truter, M., 34, *38*
Tsai, C., 168, *189*
Tsay, K. Y., *see* Williams, R. C. Jr., 112, *126*
Tsibris, J. C. M., *see* Wilson, G. S., 207, *212*
Tu, A. T., 239, *247*
Tuckerman, M. M., 13, *38*
Tun-kyi, A., *see* Wüthrich, K., 64, *72*
Turner, P. C., *see* Dann, J. G., 133, 134, 140, *150*
Tute, M. S., 5, *38*

Udenfriend, S., *see* Jerina, D., 210, *212*
Ughetto, G., *see* De Santis, P., 182, *188*
Ullrich, V., 201, 202, 203, 204, 209, 210, *212*. *See also* Diehl, H., 206, 207, *211*; Frommer, U., 204, 210, *211*; Ishimura, Y., 209, *212*; Lehrmann, C., 202, *212*; Lichtenberger, F., 210, *212*; Staudt, H., 208, *212*; Waterman, M. R., 206, *212*
Unger, S. H., *see* Hansch, C., 5, 7, *37*
Urry, D. W., 56, 57, 58, 59, 63, *72*

Vaara, L., 85, 88, *91*. *See also* Bergstén, P. C., 77, 84, 88, *90*; Kannan, K. K., 73, 74, *90*; Liljas, A., 73, 83, 84, *90*; Notstrand, B., 73, 75, *90*
Valerino, D. M., *see* Johns, D. G., 131, *150*
Van Atta, R. A., *see* Kahn, J. B., 224, *233*
Vanderwerff, H., *see* Hitchings, G. H., 132, *150*
Vandlen, R., *see* Michealson, D., 266, 271, *273*
van Slyke, D. D., 112, *126*
Vazquez, D., 191, 192, 193, *200*. *See also* Celma, M. L., 191, *199*; Fernandez-Munoz, R., 191, 192, 193, *199*
Verpoorte, J. A., *see* Armstrong, J. McD., 74, *90*
Villa, L., *see* Sinistri, C., 13, 15, 16, 18, *38*
Vinograd, J., *see* Bauer, W., 169, *188*
Visconti, M., 11, *38*
Von Dreele, P. H., 56, *72*
Von Hippel, P. H., *see* McGhee, J. D., 174, 175, 185, *189*
Vyskocil, F., *see* Beranek, R., 256, *272*; Thesleff, S., 265, *272*

Waage, P., *see* Guldberg, C. M., 109, *126*
Wakelin, L. P. G., 173, 174, 175, 176, 177, 178, 185, 186, *189*. *See also* Waring, M. J., 169, 171, 172, 173, 176, *189*
Walker, T. F., *see* Brimblecombe, R. W., 33, *36*
Walter, L. A., 25, *38*
Walter, R., 56, *72*. *See also* Deslauriers, R., 56, 64, 65, 67, 68, *71*; Johnson, L. F., 56, *71*; Kotelchuck, D., 56, 63, *71*; Smith, I. C. P., 56, *72*; Urry, D. W., 56, 57, 58, 63, *72*
Walters, D. B., 18, *38*
Ward, M. P., *see* Thesleff, S., 265, *274*
Ward, W. F., *see* Fain, J. N., 243, *247*
Waring, M. J., 167, 168, 169, 170, 171, 172, 173, 176, 178, 185, *189*. *See also* Cranford, L. V., 169, *188*; Fuller, W., 168, 169, *188*; Luck, G., 169, *189*; Wakelin, L. P. G., 173, 174, 175, 176, 177, 178, 185, 186, *189*
Warnick, J. E., *see* Albuquerque, E. X., 260, 263, *272*; Rash, J. E., 263, *274*
Wartell, R. M., 169, *181*
Wasserman, O., *see* Peters, T., 224, 232, *233*
Watanabe, A., 11, *39*
Waterfall, J. F., 211, *212*
Waterman, M. R., 206, 207, *212*
Watson, H. C., *see* Kendrew, J. C., 112, *126*
Watson, J. D., 167, *189*
Wattenberg, L. W., 202, 203, *212*
Way, J. L., 133, 136, *150*
Webb, L. E., *see* Perutz, M. F., 112, *126*
Weber, G., 136, *150*
Weber, H. J., 198, *200*
Weber, M., 271, *274*
Weber, M. J., 192, *200*
Weber, P., *see* Ullrich, V., 202, 203, 204, *212*
Wechsler, J., *see* Gefter, M., 153, *165*
Weinryb, I., 243, *247*
Weitkamp, H., *see* Korte, F., 12, *37*
Welch, A. D., *see* Nichol, C. A., 128, *150*
Wells, R. D., 170, 176, *189*. *See also* Wartell, R. M., 169, *189*
Wenner, C. E., *see* Kemp, G., 271, *273*
Werkheiser, W. C., *see* Baker, B. R., 134, *149*
Wessels, P. L., 69, *72*. *See also* Feeney, J., 69, *71*
Wetlaufer, D. B., *see* Martin, R. B., 35, *38*
Wetton, A. F., 204, *212*
White, A. I., *see* Campbell, I. D., 86, *90*
White, K. P., *see* Matsushita, T., 152, *166*
Wieckowski, J., *see* Albuquerque, E. X., 252, 263, *272*; Barnard, E. A., 250, 252,

Wieckowski, *cont.*
272; Porter, C. W., 250, 252, 257, *274*
Wilchek, M., *see* Sonenberg, N., 195, 196, *200*
Wilkinson, S., *see* Beddell, C. R., 121, 122, *125*
Williams, D. H., *see* Dell, A., 170, 179, 182, *188*
Williams, J. G., *see* Milton-Thompson, G. J.,, 32, *38*
Williams, M. K., *see* Thomas, W. A., 64, *72*
Williams, M. N., *see* Poe, M., 130, *150*
Williams, R. C. Jr., 112, *126*
Williams, R. J. P., *see* Barry, C. D., 66, 67, 71; Levine, B. A., 66, *72*
Williams, R. R., 11, *39*
Williams, V. R., 35, *39*
Williamson, P., *see* Berg, D. K., 252, 265, *272*
Wilson, G. S., 207, *212*
Winget, G. D., *see* Good, N. E., 121, *126*
Winston, M., *see* Wolberg, G., 243, *247*
Winter, W., *see* Good, N. E., 121, *126*
Wisseman, C. L., *see* Hahn, F. E., 191, *199*
Wissemann, C., *see* Brown, N. C., 152, *165*
Witikainen, U., *see* Antikainen, P. J., 13, *36*
Witkop, B., *see* Albuquerque, E. X., 252, *272*; Jerina, D., 210, *212*
Wittmann, H. G., 195, *200*. *See also* Pongs, O., 196, 197, *199*
Wolberg, G., 243, *247*
Wolf, J., *see* Ullrich, V., 210, *212*
Wolff, J., *see* Londos, C., 236, *247*
Wolff, J. A., *see* Farber, S., 128, *150*
Wollenberg, P., *see* Ullrich, V., 204, *212*
Won, C. H., *see* Hansch, C., 191, *199*

Woodard, C. J., *see* Brown, E. M., 243, *246*; Spiegel, A. M., 237, 242, *247*
Woolley, P., 88, *91*
Wooton, R., 5, *39*. *See also* Beddell, C. R., 121, 122, *125*
Wright, G. E., 160, 161, *166*. *See also* Mackenzie, J., 153, 154, 155, 159, 160, *165*
Wüthrich, K., 64, *72*
Wylie, J. H., 32, *39*. *See also* Black, J. W. 33, *36*
Wyman, J. Jr., *see* Allen, D. W., 112, 121, *125*

Xavier, A. V., *see* Barry, C. D., 66, 67, *71*

Yoeli, M., *see* Ferone, R., 131, *150*
Yoshida, T., *see* Katagiri, K., 179, *188*
Yoshikami, D., *see* Kuffler, S. W., 263, *273*
Young, D. A. B., *see* Paterson, R. A., 121, *126*
Young, M., *see* Berman, J. B., 267, *272*
Yu, C. I., *see* Benesch, R., 112, *125*
Yuferov, V., *see* Roberts, G. C. K., 133, 134, 136, 138, 142, 144, *150*

Zacks, S. I., 262, 264, 265, *274*
Zakrzewski, S. F., 128, 130, *150*. *See also* Hakala, M. T., 131, *150*
Zamir, A., *see* Sonenberg, N., 195, 196, *200*
Zimmer, C., *see* Luck, G., 169, *189*
Zimmerman, T. P., *see* Wolberg, G., 243, *247*

Subject index

Ab initio molecular orbital calculations 42-3, 49-52
Absorption spectra 96, 130-1, 206, 209
Acetazolamide 77-82, 93, 100
Acetylcholine receptor 249-72
Acetylcholinesterase 250, 259, 264-5
Acridines, 9-amino, 168, 185-8
Adenosine, 243-6
Adenosine deaminase, 244-5
Adenylate cyclase, 235-46
Adrenaline, 13-18
Affinity chromatography, 267-8
Affinity labelling, 191-9
p-Aminobenzoyl-L-glutamate, 133-49
Aminopterin, 128-9, 140
Anions, binding to carbonic anhydrase, 85-6, 88
Apocarbonic anhydrase, 100-1
ATPase, $Na^+ + K^+$, 213-32
Autoradiography, 250, 257-66

Barrier to rotation, 47
Basicity, 11-12, 130
Bisulphite, aldehyde addition complex, 120, 122
Bungarotoxin, 250-72
Burimamide, 28-35

Calcium, 239-41
Calculations, molecular orbital, 41-54
Carbachol, 267, 270
Carbonic anhydrase, 73-89, 93-107
  structure of, 75-7
  sulphonamide binding to, 77-89, 93-107
  kinetics of, 93-107
Cassaine, 224-32
Catecholamines, 13-18
Chloramphenicol, 190-9
Chlorguanide, 128-9
Cimetidine, 28-35
Cobalt in carbonic anhydrase, 96, 98
Conformation
  of drugs, 43-9, 53, 182-5
  of peptides, 55-71, 182-5
Co-operativity in ligand binding, 133-6
Correlation analysis, 4-7
Correlation time, 68
Crystallography, X-ray, 73-89, 109-10, 124

Cyclic AMP, 235-46
Cysteine in carbonic anhydrase, 85
Cytochrome b_5, 208
Cytochrome P450, 201-11
  inhibition of, 204-5
  induction of, 203-4
  mechanism of, 205-11

Decamethonium, 255-70
Denervation, 257, 265, 266-8
Dihydrofolate, 127-8, 140
Dihydrofolate reductase, 127-49
  inhibition of, 128-49
Di-isopropylfluorophosphate, 250, 252, 259, 264
Dimethylsulphoxide, 59
Diphosphoglycerate, 112, 114-5, 115-8, 121-3, 125
DNA
  drug binding to, 167-88
  polymerase, 151-65
  synthesis, 151-65
Drug
  conformation, 43-9, 53
    relation to activity, 47-9, 69-71
  design, 1-8, 118-22
  metabolism, 201-11

Echinomycin, 170-85
  conformation of, 182-5
Electron distribution, calculation of, 49-50
Electrostatic interactions, 95, 116-7, 120-3, 130, 141
Endoplasmic reticulum, 203
Europium, 66-7

Flaxedil, 267-8, 270
Flexibility
  of drugs, 41, 43-9, 69-71
  of peptides, 55-71
Folate, 128-49
Folinic acid, 127-8, 140, 144-6

Gastrin, 69
Glucagon, 236, 243-4, 246
GTP and analogues, 236-43, 244-6

Subject Index

Haemoglobin, 112–25
  diphosphoglycerate, 114–5, 121–3
  oxygen binding 112–4, 121–3
  structure, 115–7
Hexamethonium, 270
Histamine
  analogues, 23–5, 47–9
  antagonists, 28–35
  conformation of, 45–9
  electron distribution, 50–3
  ionisation, 21–3
  tautomerism, 23, 25–8
Histidine
  in carbonic anhydrase, 73–89
  in dihydrofolate reductase, 137–43, 148–9
  in haemoglobin, 116
Hormonal peptides, 55–71
Hydrogen bonds, 57–60, 69, 73–89, 120–3, 154–5, 159–161

Immunoglobulin, hapten binding to, 97
Intercalation, 168–88
Ionisation state, 88, 96, 98, 102–4, 130–1
Iron, in cytochrome P450, 205–11
Isocytosine, 6-(p-hydroxyphenylazo), 151–65
Isoprenaline, 13–18
Isotopic labelling, 57, 143–8

Kinetics
  of drug-receptor interactions, 69–71, 93–107, 219–23, 231–2, 268–70
  stopped flow, 93–107, 148

Lanthanide probes, 66–7
Luteinising hormone releasing hormone, 69

Magnesium, 213–32, 235–46
Manganese, 235–46
3-Mercaptopicolinic acid, 18–20
Mercury, in carbonic anhydrase, 84–7
Methasquin, 128–9
Methotrexate, 128–49
Metiamide, 28–35
Molecular orbital calculations, 41–54
Monoiodoamphenicol, 191–9
Mono-oxygenases, 201–11
Motor endplate, 249–66

NAD (H), 207–8
NADP (H), 136, 146–8, 203, 207–8
Neuromuscular junction, 249–66
p-Nitrobenzoyl-L-glutamate, 144–7
Noradrenaline, 13–18
Nuclear magnetic resonance, 46, 55–68, 98, 121, 124, 136–49, 154–5,

Ouabain, 213–32
Oxygen
  binding to haemoglobin 112–4, 115–7, 121–3
  and cytochrome P450, 209–10
Oxytocin, 56–68
Oxytocinoic acid, 64–7

Partition coefficient, 100–1
Peptide bond
  cis and trans, 63–4
  synthesis, 191–4
Peptides
  conformation of, 55–71, 182–5
  hormonal, 55–71
pH dependence of binding, 98–9, 102
Phosphorylation of ATPase, 214–7, 227–31
Physico-chemical activity relationships, 6, 119
Potassium and sodium ATPase, 213–32
Potential energy calculations, 43–9, 53, 63, 182–4
Protein synthesis, 152, 190–3
Protonation equilibria, 8–35, 137–43
  (see also Ionisation state)
Purification of acetylcholine receptor, 266–8
Purine deoxyribonucleotide triphosphates, 152–8, 160–1
Pyrimethamine, 128–9
Pyrimidines
  amino, 12
  6-(arylhydrazano), 151–65
  2, 4-diamino, 128–49
  2-amino-4-keto, 130

Quinoxaline antibiotics, 167–88

Rate constants, association and dissociation, 94–107
Receptor, acetylcholine, 249–72
Receptors, 109–11, 249–72
Relaxation times, ^{13}C, 67–8
Resonance Raman spectroscopy, 96
Ribosomal proteins, 194–9
Ribosomes, 191–9

Schiff's base, 118–23
Sedimentation coefficient, 169, 172, 177–9, 187
Skeletal muscle, 249–72
Sodium and potassium ATPase, 213–32
Solubilisation, acetylcholine receptor, 266–72
Species differences, 219–23, 229–32

Spin–spin coupling, 46, 57–8, 60–6
  relation to conformation, 60–6
Steric effects, 88–9, 95, 99, 104–6
Structure–activity relationships, 1–35,
  89, 93–107, 128–32, 159–65, 177–82,
  190–1
Sulphanilamide, 82–7, 100
Sulphonamides and carbonic anhydrase,
  73–89, 93–107
Sulphonamides, N-acetyl, 98–100

Tautomerism, 15, 17, 23, 130
Tetrahydrofolate, 127–8
Thiamine, 11–12
Thimidylate synthetase, 127
Thyrotropin releasing factor, 69
Tocinoic acid, 64–7
Transfer RNA, 191–4, 196

Triamterine, 128–9
Triazines, 128–9
Trimethoprim, 128–9, 131, 134–49
Triostin, 179–82
Tubocurarine, 252–7, 269–71
Tyrosine, in dihydrofolate reductase,
  143–9

Ultraviolet spectroscopy, 96, 130–1
Uracil, 6-(p-hydroxyphenylazo), 151–65

Vasopressin, 56–68
Viscosity, 169, 171, 173, 180, 187

Zinc, in carbonic anhydrase, 76, 79, 80–1,
  84, 88–9, 106

If you have any concerns about our products,
you can contact us on
ProductSafety@springernature.com

In case Publisher is established outside the EU,
the EU authorized representative is:
**Springer Nature Customer Service Center GmbH
Europaplatz 3, 69115 Heidelberg, Germany**

Printed by Libri Plureos GmbH
in Hamburg, Germany